Directory of Medical and Health Care Libraries in the United Kingdom and Republic of Ireland

Also available
Libraries in the United Kingdom and the Republic of Ireland
An annual listing of over 600 public, academic, special and government
libraries.

Directory of Medical and Health Care Libraries in the United Kingdom and Republic of Ireland

Seventh Edition

Compiled by Derek J. Wright
for the Medical, Health and Welfare Libraries
Group of the Library Association

LA

The Library Association
London

© The Library Association 1990

Published by
Library Association Publishing Ltd
7 Ridgmount Street
London WC1E 7AE

First published 1957
Second edition 1963
Third edition 1969
Fourth edition 1976
Fifth edition 1982
Sixth edition 1986
Seventh edition 1990

Editions 1 to 4 entitled
*Directory of Medical Libraries
in the British Isles*

British Library Cataloguing in Publication Data

Directory of medical and health care libraries in the United
  Kingdom and Republic of Ireland. – 7th ed.
  1. Great Britain. Medical libraries —— Directories
  I. Wright, Derek J. (Derek James), *1937 –*   II. Library
  Association, *Medical, Health and Welfare Libraries Group*
  026.61

  ISBN 0-85365-779-3

Printed and made in Great Britain by Dotesios Printers Ltd,
Trowbridge, Wiltshire.

CONTENTS

PREFACE

This edition follows the format of earlier editions, and I have included details, where they were available, of fax numbers and electronic mail addresses. Computer data retrieval is now more widely available, especially CD-ROM facilities. Probably , by the time for the next edition, CD-ROM terminals will have overtaken those using online services

There have been many changes since the previous edition. Many hospitals have closed or amalgamated with others, many new libraries have been formed and, regretfully, many have been dispersed. It is particularly sad that the present economic climate has seen the closure of the last two commercial medical lending libraries - Ferriers in Edinburgh and HK Lewis in London. It is sad, too, that with the amalgamations, many familiar names have disappeared - notably amongst the London medical schools.

However, on a brighter note, recent years have seen the rise of the specialist information services, such as BACUP, MIDIRS and, probably one of the first, Help for Health.

It is inevitable that some of the information will be out of date before this edition is printed, but I have tried to ensure that all entries were as complete as I could make them. As in the previous edition, some librarians were unable to send in returns (for one reason or another), so the entries are truncated

As in any work of this nature, it is essentially a team effort - although any errors. or omissions are my fault alone. First I must thank David Stewart and his colleagues at the Royal Society of Medicine for their practical assistance. Desmond Linton gave me much good advice, and supplied a copy of the last edition on disc. As Desmond mentioned in the preface to the 6th edition, most of the information had to be amended, but it made the compilation of this edition much easier. Thanks are also due to Barbara Jover and Kathryn Beecroft of LAPL for their advice, tolerance and seeing this work safely through to publication.

Thanks to all those who replied to the questionnaires, and I hope that I have interpreted their answers correctly. I am grateful, too, to the Regional Librarians who supplied details of changes in their Regions, and to the many librarians who sent information on other libraries to be included. Particular thanks are due to Graeme Barber, Janet Claridge, and Philippa Lane.

Finally, sets of self-adhesive address labels can be obtained from the compiler and copies of the full database can be made available: quotations and specifications will be supplied on request.

Derek Wright

NHS REGIONAL LIBRARIANS GROUP
MEMBERS

East Anglia

Mr PB Morgan MA ALA
Librarian
Cambridge University Medical Library
Addenbrooke's Hospital
Hills Road
Cambridge CB2 2QQ

Tel: 0223 336750
Fax: 0223 336709
Telex: 81240
E-mail: PBM2 @ UK.AC.CAM.PHX

Mersey

Mr DM Crook BA ALA
Librarian
Liverpool Medical Institution
114 Mount Pleasant
Liverpool L3 5SR

Tel: 051 709 9125

North East Thames

Mr JF Hewlett MSc ALA
Regional Librarian
David Ferriman Library
North Middlesex Hospital
Sterling Way
London N18 1QX

Tel: 081 884 3391
Fax: 081 884 2773

North West Thames

Miss FM Picken ALA
Regional Librarian
Charing Cross & Westminster Medical School
17 Horseferry Road
London SW1P 2AR

Tel: 071 630 1574

North West Thames Nurse Education Coordinating Centre

Mrs E Chakrabarty BA DipLib ALA
Principal Librarian, NWT Nurse Education
Riverside College of Nursing (Wolfson)
30 Vincent Square
London SW1P 2NW

Tel: 071 746 8923

North Western

Mrs VA Ferguson BA DipLib FLA
Medical Librarian
John Rylands University Library of Manchester
Oxford Road
Manchester M13 9PP

Tel: 061 275 3729
Fax: 061 273 7488
E-mail: YMULB @ UK.AC.UMIST

Northern

Mrs K O'Donovan BA ALA MIInfSc
Medical Librarian
University of Newcastle upon Tyne Medical
   and Dental Library
The Medical School
Framlingham Place
Newcastle upon Tyne NE2 4HH

Tel: 091 222 6000
E-mail: O'DONOVAN @ UK.AC.
                    NEWCASTLE

Northern Ireland

Mr WD Linton BSc BLS MIBiol ALA ALAI
Librarian
Northern Ireland Health & Social Services
            Library
Queen's University Medical Library
Institute of Clinical Science
Grosvenor Road
Belfast
Northern Ireland BT12 6BJ

Tel: 0232 322043
Telex: 747578 QUBMED G
E-mail: EIIG 4886 @ UK.AC.QUB.
                    V1

Oxford

Dr P Leggate MA DPhil FIInfSc
Regional Librarian
Oxford Region Library and Information Service
Cairns Library
John Radcliffe Hospital
Headington
Oxford OX3 9DU

Tel: 0865 817531
Fax: 0865 742070

Scotland

Mrs JM Payne BA ALA
Librarian
Scottish Health Service Centre
Crewe Road South
Edinburgh EH4 2LF

Tel: 031 332 2335
Fax: 031 315 2369

South East Thames

Mr JA Mills ALA   Tel: 0424 730073 x2271
Regional Librarian   Fax: 0424 730249
Health Care Planning Library
SE Thames RHA
Thrift House
Bexhill on Sea
East Sussex TN39 3NQ

South West Thames

Mr MJ Carmel BA FLA   Tel: 0483 37270
Regional Librarian   Fax: 0483 303691
SW Thames Regional Library Service   E-mail: DATAMAIL (SAWERS)
Royal Surrey County Hospital
Guildford
Surrey GU2 5XX

South Western (SWEHSLinC)

Mrs PK Prior BSc Cert Ed ALA   Tel: 0803 614567 x4704
Librarian   Fax: 0803 616395
Torbay Hospital   E-mail: DATAMAIL (Pamela K
Lawes Bridge   Prior)
Torquay
South Devon TQ2 7AA

Trent

Mr GL Matthews ALA   Tel: 0709 824525
Principal Librarian   Fax: 0709 820007
Libraries Suite   (Specify FAO Library)
District General Hospital
Rotherham S60 2UD

Wales

Vacancy

Wessex

Mr RB Tabor MIInfSc   Tel: 0703 777222 x3750
Regional Librarian   Fax: 0703 785648
Wessex Regional Library Information Service
South Academic Block
Southampton General Hospital
Southampton SO9 4XY

West Midlands

Mrs JM Claridge BA FLA   Tel: 021 414 5862
Sub-Librarian   Fax: 021 414 4036
Barnes Library   E-Mail:
University of Birmingham Medical School   LANET: LLA 2069
Vincent Drive   JANET: CLARIDJM @ UK.AC.
Birmingham B15 2TJ   BHAM.IBM 3090

Yorkshire

Mr IPG King BA ALA   Tel: 0274 542200 x4130
Regional Librarian   Fax: 0274 547509
Bradford Royal Infirmary   (specify FAO IPG KING)
Bradford   E-mail: DATAMAIL
West Yorkshire BD9 6RJ

LIST OF ABBREVIATIONS AND ACRONYMS

AFRS	Agricultural and Food Research Service
ANSLICS	Aberdeen and North of Scotland Library and Information Cooperative Service
ASHSL	Association of Scottish Health Sciences Librarians
AWHILES	All Wales Health Information and Library Extension Service
BCLIP	Black Country Library and Information Providers
CADIG	Coventry and District Information Group
CHIPS	Croydon Health Information Providers
CICRIS	West London Commercial and Technical Library Service
CLIC	Cancer Libraries in Cooperation
CURL	Consortium of University Libraries
EMRLS	East Midlands Regional Library Service
EULOS	Essex University List of Serials
FIRST	Forum for Information Resources in Staffordshire
HATRICS	Hampshire Technical Research Industrial Commercial Service
HCLEA	Health Care Libraries of East Anglia
HERTIS	Hertfordshire Technical Library and Information Consultant
HULTIS	Humberside Libraries Technical Interloan Scheme
LADSIRLAC	Liverpool and District Scientific Industrial and Research Library Advisory Council
LASER	London and South Eastern Region
LINNET	Leicestershire Information Network
LOTS	Librarians in Occupational Therapy Schools
NANTIS	Nottingham and Nottinghamshire Technical Information Service

NISG	Nursing Interest Sub Group [of LA MHWLG]
NORWHSLA	North West Health Services Librarians Association
NRAHSL	Northern Region Association of Health Service Libraries
PLCS	Psychiatric Libraries Cooperative Scheme
S3RBK	Southampton, Surrey, Sussex, Reading, Brunel and Kent University Libraries in Cooperation
SALG	Scottish Agricultural Librarians Group
SASLIC	Surrey and Sussex Libraries in Cooperation
SHIRL	Serial holdings in Irish Libraries
SINTO	Sheffield Interchange Organisation
SULIS	Suffolk Union List of Serials
SWEHSLinC	South West England Health Service Libraries in Cooperation
TRAHCLIS	Trent Regional Association of Health Care Libraries and Information Specialists
WILCO	Wiltshire Libraries in cooperation
WRLIS	Wessex Regional Library Information Service
YRAHCLIS	Yorkshire Regional Association of Health Care Libraries and Information Services

Aberdeen

1
FORESTERHILL COLLEGE
Westburn Road, Aberdeen AB9 2XS
Tel: 0224 681818 x2544
STAFF: Ms M Jaffray MA DipLib ALA, Ms A Clapham MA DipLib
FOUNDED: 1967
TYPE: Nursing, midwifery
HOURS : Mon-Fri 8.45-5.00
READERS: Staff and other users
STOCK POLICY: Books and journals discarded after a period
LENDING: Books and journals. Photocopies provided
COMPUTER DATA RETRIEVAL: Terminal at another library/dept
HOLDINGS: 95 current titles
CLASSIFICATION: RCN
PUBLICATIONS: Accessions list; current awareness journals
BRANCHES: Dr Gray's Hospital, Glen; Ladybridge Hospital,
Banff; Chalmers Hospital, Banff; Gilbert Bain Hospital,
Shetland; Balfour Hospital, Orkney; School of Midwifery,
Aberdeen
NETWORKS: ASHSL, ANSLICS

2
GRAMPIAN SCHOOL OF OCCUPATIONAL THERAPY
Woolmanhill, Aberdeen, AB9 1GS
Tel: 0224 681818 x55494
STAFF: Mrs M Mellis, MA ALA (part-time)
FOUNDED: 1977
TYPE: Nursing, Occupational therapy
HOURS: Mon-Fri 9.00-5.00
READERS: Staff and other users
STOCK POLICY: No stock discarded
LENDING: Books only. Photocopies provided
HOLDINGS: c.4000 books, c.30 journals, 16 current
CLASSIFICATION: Own scheme
NETWORKS: ASHSL, ANSLICS, LOTS, Grampian health Board

3

UNIVERSITY OF ABERDEEN MEDICAL SCHOOL
Foresterhill, Aberdeen AB9 2ZD
Tel: 0224 681818   Telex 73458
Fax: 0224 685157
STAFF: Dr PD Lawrence BSc PhD, Mrs W Pirie MA ALA, Mr M McFarlane
       MA ALA
FOUNDED: 1972
TYPE: Multidisciplinary
HOURS: Mon-Thurs 9-10, Fri, Sat 9-5, Sun 2-5 (vacation Mon-Fri
       9-5, Sat 9-1)
READERS: All users
STOCK POLICY: Some books discarded. All journals kept
LENDING: Books ; journals overnight; av material
COMPUTER DATA RETRIEVAL: DIMDI online - cost recovered.
       CD-ROM: Compact Cambridge from 1987.
HOLDINGS: 20,000 books, 35,000 bound journals; 350 current
       journals. 5 microfilms, 170 tape/slides, 3500 35mm slides,
       200 videotapes (VHS)
CLASSIFICATION: DDC
NETWORK: Local cooperative network

Aberystwyth

4
BRONGLAIS GENERAL HOSPITAL POSTGRADUATE CENTRE
Aberystwyth, Dyfed SY23 2EF
Tel: 0970 623131 x112 Fax: 0970 624930
STAFF: Ms V Baker MA DipLib ALA, Ms S Peacock BA DipLib ALA (job
       share)
FOUNDED: 1973
TYPE: Multidisciplinary
HOURS: Key available at all times. Staffed Mon-Fri 9-5
READERS: Staff and other users
STOCK POLICY: Books and journals discarded as space/demand
 determines
LENDING: Books and journals, small av collection on patient
         information
COMPUTER DATA RETRIEVAL: DATASTAR, DIALOG online - free.
HOLDINGS: 180 journals; 170 current. 200 Tape/slides,
          30 videotapes (VHS),
CLASSIFICATION: NLM
NETWORK: AWHL

Airdrie

5
MONKLANDS DISTRICT GENERAL HOSPITAL MEDICAL LIBRARY
Monkscourt Avenue, Airdrie ML6 0JS
Tel:02364 69344
STAFF: Mrs EM MacDonald ALA (part-time)
FOUNDED: 1977

TYPE: Multidisciplinary
HOURS: Always open. Staffed 28 hours per week
READERS: Staff.
STOCK POLICY: Books and journals discarded after 10 years.
LENDING: Books and journals, videos, tapes, slides;photocopies
provided.
COMPUTER DATA RETRIEVAL: Access to terminal in another dept.
HOLDINGS: 2,500 books, 920 journals; 102 current journals.
Tape/slides, 35 mm slides, videotapes (VHS)
CLASSIFICATION: UDC
PUBLICATIONS: Newsletter, periodicals list

Alton

6
WESSEX REGIONAL ORTHOPAEDIC LIBRARY
Lord Mayor Treloar Hospital,Chawton Park Rd, Alton, Hants GU34 1RJ
Tel:0420 82811
STAFF: Mrs JY Mayhew ALA
TYPE: Multidisciplinary
HOURS: Staffed Mon-Fri 9-5.30. Key available at night.
READERS: Staff, other users at discretion of librarian
STOCK POLICY: Books and journals discarded at variable intervals.
LENDING: Books and journals,videotapes, tape/slides; photocopies
provided.
COMPUTER DATA RETRIEVAL: DATASTAR online - free to WRLS, others
charged.
HOLDINGS: 2,000 books;155 journal titles, 150 current journals;
20 Tape/slides; 10 videotapes (VHS)
SPECIAL COLLECTION: Orthopaedics (750 books, 24 current journals)
CLASSIFICATION: NLM
PUBLICATION: Current awareness lists: Orthopaedics, Aged
NETWORK: WRLIS

Amersham

7
AMERSHAM GENERAL HOSPITAL POSTGRADUATE CENTRE
Staff Library, Whielden St, Amersham, Bucks, HP7 0JD
Tel: 0494 734000
STAFF: Mrs A Flood BA ALA (part time)
FOUNDED: 1978 in present premises
TYPE: Multidisciplinary
HOURS: Mon-Wed 9.15-3, Fri 10.30-3.15. Key available at other times
READERS: Staff, others on introduction to Librarian
STOCK POLICY: Journals: some on exchange scheme. Books: superseded
editions discarded
LENDING: Books and journals. Photocopies provided
COMPUTER DATA RETRIEVAL: Access to terminal
HOLDINGS: 900 books; 48 journals, 36 current
CLASSIFICATION: NLM
NETWORK: Oxford Regional Library & Information Service

Ashford, Kent

8
WILLIAM HARVEY HOSPITAL. EDUCATION CENTRE LIBRARY
Kennington Road, Willesborough, Ashford, Kent TN24 0LZ
Tel:0233 33331 x260
STAFF: Mr A Booth, BA DipLib, 3 other (part-time) staff
TYPE: Multidisciplinary
HOURS: Mon-Fri 9-5 (Access outside these hours to card holders)
READERS: Staff and others
STOCK POLICY: Books discarded following Regional policy
LENDING: Books and journals; photocopies provided
COMPUTER DATA RETRIEVAL: DATASTAR online - free. CD-ROM available
HOLDINGS: 8500 books; 120 journals, 102 current.
CLASSIFICATION: NLM
SPECIAL COLLECTION: William Harvey Historical Collection (20 vols)
PUBLICATION: Library guide
NETWORK: SE Thames Regional Library and Information Service

Ashford, Middlesex

9
ASHFORD POSTGRADUATE MEDICAL CENTRE
Ashford Hospital, Ashford, Middlesex TW15 3AA
Tel: 0784 251188
FOUNDED: 1967
TYPE: Medical
HOURS: Mon-Thurs 11-5. Key available at all times.
READERS: All medical staff, GP's and allied professions
STOCK POLICY: Journals kept, books discarded after 10 years
LENDING: Books lent; photocopies provided.
COMPUTER DATA RETRIEVAL: Inhouse terminal.
CD-ROM: From 1983 : end-user
HOLDINGS: 1000 books ; 50 journal titles, 30 current .
CLASSIFICATION: NLM
NETWORK: NW Thames Regional Library and Information Service

10
WEST THAMES SCHOOL OF NURSING
Ashford Hospital, Ashford, Middlesex TW15 3AA
Tel: 0784 251188 ext 4182
STAFF: J Knight BLS ALA, Librarian/Media Resource Officer
TYPE: Multidisciplinary
HOURS: Mon-Fri 8.45-4.30
READERS: Staff and other users
STOCK POLICY: Books discarded after 10 years
LENDING: Books , videocassettes, audiocassettes
COMPUTER DATA RETRIEVAL: DATASTAR online - charged full cost.
CD-ROM available
HOLDINGS: 10,000 books ; 175 journals,165 current; 35 tape/slides,
  250 videotapes (VHS), 100 audiocassettes
CLASSIFICATION: modified DDC 19
SPECIAL COLLECTION: Patient's Library (2000 vols)
PUBLICATION: Library guide, bibliographies, AV catalogue
NETWORK: NW Thames Regional Library Service

Ashington

11
NORTHUMBRIA COLLEGE OF NURSING, NURSE EDUCATION LIBRARY
Ashington Hospital, West View, Ashington, Northumberland, NE63 0SA
Tel: 0670 812541 x2314
STAFF: Mrs CM Smith MA DipLib ALA (part time)
TYPE: Nursing
HOURS: Mon-Fri 8-4. Staffed 6 hours per week
READERS: Staff, other users on application to Librarian
STOCK POLICY: Books discarded at varying intervals
LENDING: Books, videos. Photocopies provided
HOLDINGS: 2,000 books; 26 journals, 18 current titles; various
    videotapes
CLASSIFICATION: DDC 19
PUBLICATION: Current contents
NETWORK: NRAHSL

12
WANSBECK POSTGRADUATE MEDICAL CENTRE
Ashington Hospital, Ashington, Northumberland NE63 0SA
Tel: 0670 812541
STAFF: Ms S Abernethy, BA DipLib ALA (part-time)
TYPE: Medical
HOURS: Always open, staffed Mon-Fri 9-12.
READERS: Staff and other users
STOCK POLICY: Journals over 10 years old discarded
LENDING: Books and journals; photocopies provided
COMPUTER DATA RETRIEVAL: Access to terminal - DATASTAR online.
HOLDINGS: 1200 books, 70 current journals.
CLASSIFICATION: DDC
NETWORK: Northern Regional Association of Health Service
Librarians

Ashton-under-Lyne

13
TAMESIDE GENERAL HOSPITAL POSTGRADUATE MEDICAL CENTRE LIBRARY
Ashton-under-Lyne, Lancashire, OL6 9RW
Tel: 061 330 8373
STAFF: Mrs S Harrison C&G Lib Asst Cert
FOUNDED: 1969
TYPE: Multidisciplinary
HOURS: Mon-Fri 9-5. Access at other times
READERS: Staff only
STOCK POLICY: Books and journals discarded
LENDING: Books & Journals only lent internally. Photocopies provided
HOLDINGS: 3000 books; 100 journals, 58 current; 20 tape/slides,
    videotapes (1 Betamax, 119 VHS)
CLASSIFICATION: Own scheme
PUBLICATION: New book list

14
BUCKINGHAMSHIRE COLLEGE OF NURSING LIBRARY
Vale of Aylesbury School of Nursing,
Stoke Mandeville Hospital, Aylesbury, Bucks HP21 8AL
Tel: 0296 84111 x3056
STAFF: Mrs K Evans (part-time), Mrs J Thomas
FOUNDED: early 1970s
TYPE: Nursing
HOURS: Always open. Staffed Mon-Fri 9-3.30
READERS: Staff only
STOCK POLICY: Books discarded after 10 years
LENDING: Books only; photocopies provided
COMPUTER DATA RETRIEVAL: DATASTAR online - free
HOLDINGS: 4,000 books; 30 journals
CLASSIFICATION: NLM
NETWORK: ORLIS, ULNJ

15
MINISTRY OF DEFENCE MEDICAL, DENTAL AND NURSING LIBRARY
Building 115, Royal Air Force Halton, Aylesbury, Bucks HP22 5PG
Tel: 0296 623535 x7616
STAFF: K Hollywood BA (Hons) Dip Lib Stud ALA
TYPE: Multidisciplinary
HOURS: Staffed Mon-Fri 8.30-5.30
READERS: Staff only
STOCK POLICY: Books discarded after 10 years
LENDING: Books only· photocopies provided
COMPUTER DATA RETRIEVAL: DATASTAR,DIALOG online - free
CD-ROM: From 1989
HOLDINGS: 230 journal titles, 180 current.
CLASSIFICATION: NLM

16
SAINT JOHN'S HOSPITAL MEDICAL LIBRARY
Stone, Aylesbury, Bucks HP17 8PP
Tel: 0296 748383 ext 293
STAFF: Mrs J Pearson ALA (part-time)
TYPE: Medical, psychiatric
HOURS: Always open. Staffed Mon-Thurs 10-2
READERS: Staff, other users with permission
STOCK POLICY: Books and journals discarded at librarian's discretion
LENDING: Books and journals; photocopies provided
COMPUTER DATA RETRIEVAL: Access to terminal, Datastar online.
        Charged .
HOLDINGS: 1,500 books, 40 journals
CLASSIFICATION: Own
SPECIAL COLLECTION: Psychiatry, Psychology
PUBLICATIONS: Library News
NETWORK: Oxford Region Library and Information Service; PLCS

Cooperation Scheme
BRANCHES: Manor House Hospital, Aylesbury (Mental handicap)

17
WILFRED STOKES MEDICAL LIBRARY
Stoke Mandeville Hospital Postgraduate Centre, Mandeville
Road, Aylesbury, Bucks. HP21 8AL
Tel: 0296 84111 x3294
STAFF: Mrs D Gulland ALA
FOUNDED: 1962
TYPE: Multidisciplinary
HOURS: Mon-Fri 8.30-5
READERS: Staff, other users by appointment
STOCK POLICY: Journals discarded after 20 years, books discarded
        after 10 years
LENDING: Books and journals to staff of organisation only
COMPUTER DATA RETRIEVAL: DATASTAR online - free
HOLDINGS: 3000 books, 144 journals, 115 current; 130 tape/slides
SPECIAL COLLECTION: Spinal cord injuries (70 vols)
CLASSIFICATION: NLM
PUBLICATIONS: Library guide; How to Use Index Medicus;
        Quoting References; bibliographies on spinal cord injury
NETWORK: Oxford Region Library and Information Service; Bucks
        Information Exchange; BBI; Orthopaedic Librarians Group

Banbury

18
TERENCE MORTIMER POSTGRADUATE EDUCATION CENTRE
Horton General Hospital, Banbury, Oxon OX16 9AL
Tel:0295 264521 x310
STAFF: Mrs CA Mortimer AIMLS (part-time)
FOUNDED: 1975
TYPE: Multidisciplinary
HOURS: Mon-Fri 9-4.00. Staffed only part of the time.
READERS: Staff and other users
STOCK POLICY: Out of date textbooks discarded
LENDING: Books, journals and bones.Photocopies provided.
COMPUTER DATA RETRIEVAL: DATASTAR online - free
HOLDINGS: 3,000 books, 75 journals , 71 current.
SPECIAL COLLECTION: Frank Bevan (100 vols)
CLASSIFICATION: NLM
NETWORK: Oxford Regional Library and Information Service

Bangor

19

MULTIDISCIPLINARY TRAINING UNIT LIBRARY
Ysbyty Gwynedd District General Hospital, Penrhosgarnedd, Bangor,
Gwynedd LL57 2PW
Tel:0248 370007 ext 4191
STAFF: AH Williams BA DipLib ALA, Mrs ME Morris-Jones
FOUNDED: 1984 by amalgamation of School of Nursing Library and
  Postraduate Medical Library
TYPE: Multidisciplinary
HOURS: Mon-Thu 9-5, Fri 9-4.30
READERS: Staff only.
STOCK POLICY: Books discarded after 10 years
LENDING: Books and cassettes only. Photocopies provided
COMPUTER DATA RETRIEVAL: DATASTAR online - free
HOLDINGS: 170 journals, 160 current; 35 mm slides, 38 videos (VHS)
CLASSIFICATION: NLM
BRANCHES: Schools of Nursing at Llandudno, Llanfairfechan, Glanador
NETWORK: AWHILES

Barking

20
BARKING HOSPITAL LIBRARY
Upney Lane, Barking, Essex, IG11 9LX
Tel: 081 594 3898 x4163
Staff: Librarian post vacant
FOUNDED: 1967
TYPE: Medical
HOURS: Mon-Fri 10-6. Key available at other times
READERS: Staff, other users for reference only
STOCK POLICY: Books discarded after 15 years, some discontinued
         journal titles offered to other libraries
LENDING: Books and back copies of journals to staff only.
         Photocopies provided
COMPUTER DATA RETRIEVAL: Access to DATASTAR online.
HOLDINGS: 600 books; 35 journals, 30 current titles
CLASSIFICATION: NLM
NETWORKS: NETRLS; Redbridge DHA Library Service

Barnet

21
BARNET DEPARTMENT OF NURSING STUDIES
Barnet General Hospital, Wellhouse Lane, Barnet, Herts
 EN5 3DJ
Tel: 01 440 5111 x4767
STAFF: Miss JM Nelson BEd DipLib ALA
TYPE: Nursing
HOURS: Mon-Fri 8.30-4.30
READERS: Student and pupil nurses, and other users within
 Area Health Authority
STOCK POLICY: Books discarded after 10 years
LENDING: Books and AV material only. photocopies provided
HOLDINGS: 17900 books, 110 journals; 104 current
 journals. 20 tape/slides, videotapes (40 U-matic, 40 VHS),

20 learning packages.
CLASSIFICATION: Own
PUBLICATIONS: Monthly accession list
NETWORK: NW Thames Regional Nursing Libraries
BRANCHES: Edgware General Hospital; Napsbury Psychiatric
Hospital (Nurses' Reading Room)

22
BARNET POST GRADUATE MEDICAL CENTRE
Barnet General Hospital, Wellhouse Lane, Barnet, Herts
EN5 3DJ
Tel: 01 440 5111 x4834
STAFF: Mrs M Davies (part-time)
FOUNDED: 1972
TYPE: Dental, Medical, Psychiatric
HOURS: Mon-Fri 8-5. Staffed Mon-Fri 8-12
READERS: Staff and other users
STOCK POLICY: Journals discarded after 10 years.
LENDING: Books, AV material, Videos only
COMPUTER DATA RETRIEVAL: Access to terminal - charged.
  CD-ROM: From 1990
HOLDINGS: 4,000 books; 84 journals; 200 videotapes (VHS)
CLASSIFICATION: UDC adapted
PUBLICATIONS: Information leaflet
NETWORK: HERTIS; NW Thames Regional Library and Information
Service

Barnsley
23
BARNSLEY POSTGRADUATE CENTRE
Barnsley District General Hospital, Cawber Road, Barnsley
S75 2EP
Tel: 0226 86122
No further information available

Barnstaple

24
NORTH DEVON DISTRICT HOSPITAL
Raleigh Park, Barnstaple, Devon EX31 4JB
Tel:0271 22363
STAFF: Mrs A Housley BA DipLib ALA
FOUNDED: 1978
TYPE: Multidisciplinary
HOURS: Mon-Fri 9-5. Keys available at other times
READERS: Staff, other users by special permission
STOCK POLICY: Some material discarded (no set policy)
LENDING: Books and journals (except current issues). Photocopies
        provided.
COMPUTER DATA RETRIEVAL: Inhouse online terminal
HOLDINGS: c.8000 books; c140 current journals
SPECIAL COLLECTION: General practice (c650 vols)
CLASSIFICATION: NLM
PUBLICATION: New accessions lists
NETWORK: SWEHSLinC, Devon Library Services

25
EDUCATION CENTRE LIBRARY, FURNESS GENERAL HOSPITAL
Dalton Lane, Barrow-in-Furness, Cumbria LA14 4LF
Tel:0229 32020 x2127
STAFF: Mrs P Rigden BEd (Hons) PG DipLib
FOUNDED: 1966 as medical library, becoming multidisciplinary in 1985
TYPE: Multidisciplinary
HOURS: Always open. Staffed Mon-Fri 9-5
READERS: Staff , others at librarian's discretion
STOCK POLICY: Journals discarded after 15 years, books at
    librarian's discretion
LENDING: Books , journals and videocassettes to staff only.
    Photocopies provided.
COMPUTER DATA RETRIEVAL: Access to DATASTAR online - free
HOLDINGS: 7683 books; 160 journals, 140 current
CLASSIFICATION: DDC
PUBLICATION: Guide to library services
BRANCHES: School of Nursing Library, Westmorland County Hospital,
    Kendal
NETWORK: Northern Regional Association of Health Service
    Librarians; Newcastle polytechnic Library.

Basildon

26
BASILDON AND THURROCK HEALTH AUTHORITY, DISTRICT MEDICAL LIBRARY
Postgraduate Centre, Basildon Hospital, Nethermayne, Basildon,
Essex SS16 5NL
Tel: 0268 533911 x3594
STAFF: Mrs MA Dunsford ALA (District Medical Librarian)
TYPE: Multidisciplinary
HOURS: Mon-Fri 8.30-4.30
READERS: Staff only
STOCK POLICY: No stock discarded
LENDING: Books only
COMPUTER DATA RETRIEVAL: Access to terminal. Free
HOLDINGS: 2,000 books; 197 journals, 112 current titles
CLASSIFICATION: NLM
NETWORK: NE Thames Regional Library and Information Service

Basingstoke

27
BASINGSTOKE AND NORTH HAMPSHIRE HEALTH AUTHORITY
Basingstoke District Hospital, Acute Unit, Aldermaston Road,
 Basingstoke, Hampshire RG24 9NA
Tel: 0256 473202 x3166
STAFF: Miss BM Goddard ALA
TYPE: Multidisciplinary
HOURS: Mon-Fri 9-5
READERS: Staff, other users for limited use

STOCK POLICY: Out of date editions of books discarded.   Out
    of date journals discarded as file length dictated by space
    available
LENDING: Books only
COMPUTER DATA RETRIEVAL: In-house terminal.   Free
HOLDINGS: 9,841 books, 4,000 bound journals; 159 current
        journals.   Tape/slides, videotapes (VHS)
CLASSIFICATION: NLM
PUBLICATIONS: Additions lists; bibliographies
NETWORK: HATRICS; WRLIS
BRANCHES: Nursing, Primary Care, Health Education and
    District Offices

Bath

28
BATH DISTRICT MEDICAL LIBRARY
Postgraduate Centre, Royal United Hospital, Bath BA1 3NG
Tel: 0225 428331
STAFF: DJ Rumsey BA ALA, Mrs D Baggage, Miss K Allen,
    Ms J Burnett BSc DipLib
TYPE: Multidisciplinary
HOURS: Key always available. Staffed Mon-Fri 9-5.30
READERS: Staff (except student nurses) and other users
STOCK POLICY: Stock discarded
LENDING: Books and journals
COMPUTER DATA RETRIEVAL: In-house terminal - free
HOLDINGS: c6,500 books; 219 current journals; tape/slides, 35 mm
        slides
SPECIAL COLLECTIONS: Rheumatology (960 vols); psychiatry, psychology
        (1,000 vols); hospital administration (1,280 vols)
CLASSIFICATION: NLM
BRANCHES: Royal National Hospital for Rheumatic Diseases, Bath;
        Saint Martin's Hospital, Bath; Roundway Hospital, Devizes

NETWORK: WRLIS

Bebington

29
WIRRAL POSTGRADUATE MEDICAL CENTRE
Clatterbridge Hospital, Bebington, Wirral L63 4JV
Tel:051 334 4000
STAFF: Ms S Swerdlow BA (Hons) 'part-time)
TYPE: Dental, Medical, Psychiatric
HOURS: Mon-Fri 9.30-5. Staffed 9.30-2
READERS: Postgraduate readers only
STOCK POLICY: Stock not discarded
LENDING: Books, journals and AV material. Photocopies provided
COMPUTER DATA RETRIEVAL: DATASTAR online - charged full cost
HOLDINGS: 70 journals, all current
CLASSIFICATION: Own

Beckenham

30
WELLCOME RESEARCH LABORATORIES
Langley Court, Beckenham, Kent BR3 3BS
Tel: 081 658 2211
STAFF: Mrs S Williams BA ALA
TYPE: Medical, pharmaceutical
HOURS: Mon-Fri 8.45-5.15
READERS: Staff only
STOCK POLICY: Books and journals discarded at variable intervals
LENDING: Books and journals. Photocopies supplied
COMPUTER DATA RETRIEVAL: In-house terminal - free. CD-ROM from
     1989. PRESTEL available
HOLDINGS: 50,000 books; 1,500 journals, 900 current titles
CLASSIFICATION: UDC

Belfast

31
NORTHERN IRELAND HEALTH AND SOCIAL SERVICES LIBRARY
QUEEN'S UNIVERSITY MEDICAL LIBRARY
Institute of Clinical Science, Grosvenor Road, Belfast,
     Northern Ireland BT12 6BJ
Tel:0232 322043 and 321487   Telex: 747578 (QUBMED G)
Electronic mail: EIIG 4886 @ U.K. AC. QUB. VI
STAFF: WD Linton BSc BLS MIBiol CBiol ALA ALAI, Vacancy (Deputy
     Librarian),Vacancy (Sub-Librarian,Acquisitions and Cataloguing),
     Miss GHE Creighton MA DipLibStud (Postgraduate Medical Education),
     SG O'Brien BA DipLibStud (Social Services), Mrs JM O'Connor BSc
     (Health Administration), Miss MM Saunders BA DipLibStud (Reader
     Service and Training), Miss PNY Watt BA DipLibStud (Nursing), Miss
     LW Green BSc DipLibStud ALA, Miss ME Patterson BA DipLibStud ALA,
     17 other (full-time), 1 (part-time) staff
FOUNDED: Medical branch of University Library opened 1954
TYPE: Multidisciplinary
HOURS: Mon-Fri 9-10 (9-5.30 in long vacation), Sat 9-12.30
READERS: Staff and other users
STOCK POLICY: Books discarded
LENDING: Books only; photocopies provided
COMPUTER DATA RETRIEVAL: Online to DATASTAR, BLAISE, DIALOG - free
          to faculty and HSS personnel. CD-ROM: Medline from 1983.
HOLDINGS: 120,000 books and bound journals; 2000 journals, 1200
     current titles; microfilms,16 mm cine films, tape/slides, video
     tapes (U-matic, VHS)
SPECIAL COLLECTIONS: Medical history; works by Northern Ireland doctors
CLASSIFICATION: LC
NETWORK: It is the centre for the Northern Ireland regional
     service
BRANCH: Biomedical Library, Belfast City Hospital: Dr K ap Rh Lewis
     BSc PhD DipLib MIBiol CBiol, 2 other (full-time) and 4 (part-time)
     staff.
     In its provincial role, the Northern Ireland Health and Social
Services Library has general oversight of the libraries in

postgraduate medical centres, district hospitals, schools of
nursing and social services units.

Betchworth

32
SMITHKLINE BEECHAM PHARMACEUTICAL RESEARCH DIVISION
Brockham Park, Betchworth, Surrey RH3 7AJ
Tel: 0737 364400
No furthur information available

Bexhill-on-Sea

33
THE HEALTH CARE PLANNING LIBRARY
South East Thames Regional Health Authority, Thrift House,
Collington Avenue, Bexhill-on-Sea, East Sussex TN39 3NQ
Tel: 0424 730073 x2271   Fax: 0424 730249
STAFF: JA Mills ALA
TYPE: Health administration
HOURS: Mon-Fri 8-7. Staffed Mon-Fri 9-5
READERS: Staff and other users
STOCK POLICY: Books discarded after 10-20 years
LENDING: Books and journals. Photocopies provided
COMPUTER DATA RETRIEVAL: DATASTAR, BLAISE online free.
     CD-ROM from 1989
HOLDINGS: 4,780 books; c200 journals; 140 current titles
SPECIAL COLLECTION: Regional Area and District Health plans
CLASSIFICATION: NLM (amended)
NETWORK: SE Thames Regional Library and Information Service

Birmingham

34
ALL SAINTS HOSPITAL PSYCHIATRIC EDUCATION CENTRE
Lodge Road, Birmingham, B18 5SD
Tel: 021 523 5151

All enquiries to District Medical Librarian, Dudley Road Hospital,
(No. 38)

35
BIRMINGHAM ACCIDENT HOSPITAL LIBRARY
Bath Row, Birmingham, B15 1NA
Tel: 021 643 7041
Mr PC Bewes (Honorary Librarian), Miss SM Hodge
TYPE: Medical
HOURS: Always open
READERS: Medical and other staff
STOCK POLICY: Reference only
COMPUTER DATA RETRIEVAL: Access to terminal.
HOLDINGS: 200 books; 50 current journals
CLASSIFICATION: LC

36
BIRMINGHAM AND MIDLAND EYE HOSPITAL
Church Street, Birmingham, B3 2NS
Tel:021 236 4911 x282   Electronic mail: BIRM.VAX1 MOSELEYMJ
STAFF: MJ Moseley PhD (Honorary)
FOUNDED: 1890
TYPE: Ophthalmology
HOURS: not staffed
READERS: Open to users by arrangement
STOCK POLICY: No stock discarded
LENDING: No lending. Photocopies provided
COMPUTER DATA RETRIEVAL: Access to DATASTAR online - free
HOLDINGS: 800 books; 20 journals, 15 current
SPECIAL COLLECTION: Historical (150 vols)

37
BIRMINGHAM CHILDREN'S HOSPITAL, BEN WOOD LIBRARY
Ladywood, Middleway, Birmingham B16 8ET
Tel:021 454 4851
STAFF: Ms E Furness BA ALA (part-time)
TYPE: Medical, paediatric
HOURS: Mon-Fri 9-5.30. Staffed Mon-Thu 9-2.30. Key available at
   other times
READERS: Staff, other users by arrangement
STOCK POLICY: Books kept, journals discarded at librarian's
   discretion
COMPUTER DATA RETRIEVAL: DATASTAR online - charged standard set
      charge
HOLDINGS: 1000 books; 98 journals, 94 current
CLASSIFICATION: LC
NETWORK: West Midlands Regional Health Libraries

38
DUDLEY POSTGRADUATE CENTRE, PETER GILROY BEVAN LIBRARY
Dudley Road Hospital, Dudley Road, Birmingham, B18 7QH
Tel: 021 554 3801 x4491
STAFF: Dr V. Melikian (Honorary), Mrs J Evans (District Medical
      Librarian)
TYPE: Medical
HOURS: Always open. Staffed Mon-Fri 8.30-5
READERS: Own staff only
STOCK POLICY: Books and journals discarded selectively
LENDING: Books only. Photocopies provided
COMPUTER DATA RETRIEVAL: DATASTAR, BLAISE online - charged
HOLDINGS: c.5500 books; 100 current journals
CLASSIFICATION: LC
PUBLICATIONS: Current awareness bulletin and service
NETWORK: West Midlands Regional Health Libraries

39
EAST BIRMINGHAM & SOLIHULL DEPT OF NURSE EDUCATION
LIBRARY & LEARNING RESOURCES DEPT
East Birmingham   Hospital, Bordesley Green East, Birmingham, B9 5ST

Tel: 021 766 6611 x4712
STAFF: A Beard B Ed(Hons) DipLib
FOUNDED: 1968
TYPE: Nursing, Psychiatric
HOURS: Mon & Thu 8.40-4.30,Tue & Wed 8.30-6, Fri 8.30-4
READERS: Staff and other users
STOCK POLICY: Books discarded
LENDING: Books, journals overnight only; Photocopies provided
COMPUTER FACILITIES: Inhouse terminal for catalogue & issue system
HOLDINGS: 78 journals, 46 current; 15 tape/slides; 70 35mm packages;
    videotapes (40 U-matic, 110 VHS)
CLASSIFICATION SCHEME: Own
SPECIAL COLLECTIONS: AIDS collection (100 vols) Spiritual care
    (50 vols)
PUBLICATIONS: Current awareness/Literature search
NETWORK: West Midland Regional Health Libraries, National Nursing
    Libraries

40
EAST BIRMINGHAM HOSPITAL MEDICAL REFERENCE LIBRARY
Postgraduate Medical Centre, East Birmingham Hospital,
Bordesley Green East, Birmingham, B9 5ST
Tel: 021 766 6611 x4790   Fax: (Hospital) 021 773 6736
STAFF: Mrs C Bell, BA DipLib ALA
TYPE: Medical
HOURS: Staffed Mon-Fri 9-5. Key available all other times
READERS: Staff, other users for Reference Only
STOCK POLICY: Out of date books discarded.
LENDING: Books only. Photocopies provided
COMPUTER DATA RETRIEVAL: DATASTAR online - charged set rate
HOLDINGS: 3000 books; 140 current journals.
CLASSIFICATION: LC
PUBLICATION: Library bulletin
NETWORK: West Midlands Regional Health Libraries
Birmingham (cont)

41
HIGHCROFT MEDICAL LIBRARY, HIGHCROFT HOSPITAL
Highcroft Road, Erdington, Birmingham B23 6AX
Tel:021 378 2211 x5122
STAFF: Mrs SV Brotherton (part-time)
FOUNDED: c.1974
TYPE: Psychiatric
HOURS: Normal working hours. Staffed Mon 9-3.15, Wed 9-12,
    Thurs 9-3.15
READERS: Professional staff
LENDING: Books and journals
COMPUTER DATA RETRIEVAL: Literature searches via University Library
HOLDINGS: 886 books; 32 journals, 25 current; videotapes (Betamax,
    VHS)
CLASSIFICATION: LC
NETWORK: West Midlands Regional Health Libraries

42
INSTITUTE OF CHILD HEALTH
Francis Road, Edgbaston, Birmingham B16 8ET
Tel:021 454 4851 x6008
STAFF: Ms E Furness BA ALA (part-time)
TYPE: Paediatric
HOURS: Mon-Fri 9-5. Unstaffed (Librarian at Children's
  Hospital)
READERS: Staff only
STOCK POLICY: Journals over 15 years old discarded
LENDING: Books and journals .Photocopies provided
COMPUTER DATA RETRIEVAL: Access to terminal
HOLDINGS: 640 books; 24 journals, 15 current
SPECIAL COLLECTION: Gastroenterology
CLASSIFICATION: LC
PUBLICATIONS: List of journals taken; accessions list
NETWORK: West Midlands Regional Health Libraries

43
JOHN CONOLLY HOSPITAL
Bristol Rd South, Rubery, Birmingham B45 9BD
Tel: 021 453 3771 x84
STAFF: Mrs D Hopker BA DipLib ALA (part time)
TYPE: Psychiatric
HOURS: Staffed Wednesday afternoons. Key available at other times
READERS: Staff only
STOCK POLICY: Books selectively discarded. General medical
  journals discarded
LENDING: Books only. Photocopies provided
COMPUTER DATA RETRIEVAL. Access to terminal.
HOLDINGS: 800 books; 26 journals, 15 current
CLASSIFICATION: LC
SPECIAL COLLECTIONS: Psychotherapy and child psychiatry
PUBLICATION: Current awareness bulletin
NETWORK: West Midlands Regional Health Libraries; Central
  Birmingham Mental Health Unit

44
MIDLAND NERVE HOSPITAL
Elvetham Road, Edgbaston, Birmingham, B15 2NJ
Tel: 021 440 3206
STAFF: Mrs D Hopker BA DipLib ALA (part-time). 1 other assistant
TYPE: Psychiatric
HOURS: Mon-Fri 9-5. Staffed Tue afternoon only
READERS: Own staff only
STOCK POLICY: Out of date books and journals selectively
          discarded
LENDING: Books only. photocopies provided
COMPUTER DATA RETRIEVAL: Access to DATASTAR online - free
HOLDINGS: 700 books; 27 journals, 15 current
CLASSIFICATION: LC
PUBLICATIONS: Current Awareness Bulletin

NETWORK: West Midlands Regional Health Libraries; Central
Birmingham Mental health Unit

45
PETER THOMAS NURSE EDUCATION CENTRE, COVENTRY & WARWICKSHIRE
COLLEGE OF NURSING
Chelmsley Hospital, Coleshill Rd, Marston Green, Birmingham, B37 7HL
Tel: 021 779 6981 x267
STAFF: Mrs M Wilson, ALA (part time)
TYPE: Multidisciplinary
HOURS: Mon-Fri 9-5 (Qualified librarian attends Tue & Thur 11-3)
READERS: Staff only
STOCK POLICY: No stock discarded
LENDING: No lending. Photocopies supplied
COMPUTER DATA RETRIEVAL: Access to terminal. Free
HOLDINGS: c. 4500 books; 45 journals, 19 current
CLASSIFICATION: modified RCN
NETWORK: West Midlands Regional Health Authority

46
QUEEN ELIZABETH SCHOOL OF NURSING
Queen Elizabeth Medical Centre, Edgbaston, Birmingham,B15 2TH
Tel:021 472 1311 x3469
STAFF: SP Gough BA (Hons)
TYPE: Nursing
HOURS: Mon 8.30-4.45,Tue 8.30-7,Wed 8.30-4.45,Thur 8.30-4.45,
    Fri 8.30-4
READERS: Staff and other users
STOCK POLICY: Books discarded at librarian's discretion
LENDING: Books only. Photocopies provided
COMPUTER DATA RETRIEVAL: DATASTAR online - charged computer time
HOLDINGS: 9500 books; 108 journals, 70 current
CLASSIFICATION: Own
PUBLICATIONS: *Writing Bibliographic References, Library Guide,*
    Journals Guide, and subject bibliographies
NETWORK: West Midlands Regional Health Libraries; UK Nursing
    Libraries

47
ROYAL ORTHOPAEDIC HOSPITAL, RESEARCH AND TEACHING CENTRE LIBRARY
The Woodlands, Bristol Road South, Northfield, Birmingham B31 2AP
Tel: 021 476 3111 x413
STAFF: Mrs J Dawson
TYPE: Medicine, orthopaedics
HOURS: Staffed Mon, Thu 9-1, Wed 3.45-7.30. Key available at other
        times
READERS: Staff only
COMPUTER DATA RETRIEVAL: Access to terminal
HOLDINGS: Small bookstock; 30 current journals; Slides, videotapes
CLASSIFICATION: NLM
NETWORK: West Midlands Regional Health Libraries

48
SAINT MARGARET'S HOSPITAL
Great Barr, Birmingham B43 7EZ
Tel: 021 360 7777
STAFF: Dr MW Imam MBBS MCCP MRCPsych DPM (Honorary Librarian), 1
       other (part-time) staff
HOURS: Mon-Fri 9-5
READERS: Medical staff
LENDING: Books only
HOLDINGS: 11 current journals

49
SELLY OAK HOSPITAL , MEDICAL EDUCATION CENTRE
Raddlebarn Road, Selly Oak, Birmingham, B28 0AA
Tel: 021 472 5313 x4154
STAFF: L Davies (Honorary Librarian), Mrs J Denning (Administrator)
FOUNDED: 1966
TYPE: Medical
HOURS: Always open.
READERS: Staff and other users
STOCK POLICY: Books and journals discarded after 15 years
LENDING: Books and journals. photocopies provided
COMPUTER DATA RETRIEVAL: Access to terminal.
HOLDINGS: 90+ current journals; Videotapes (U-matic, VHS)
NETWORK: West Midlands Regional Health Libraries

50
SISTER DORA SCHOOL OF NURSING LIBRARY
St Margaret's Hospital, Great Barr Park, Birmingham B43 7EZ
Tel: 021 360 7777 x265
STAFF: Mrs E Bradley
TYPE: Mental handicap
HOURS: Mon-Fri 12-5
READERS: Staff and students
HOLDINGS: 2,545 books; 4 current journals; tape/slides, video
          and audio tapes
CLASSIFICATION: DDC
NETWORK: West Midlands Regional Health Libraries

51
SKIN HOSPITAL
George Road, Birmingham, B15 1PR
021 455 7444
STAFF: Dr A Carmichael (Honorary Librarian)
TYPE: Dermatology
HOURS: Key available to hospital staff at all times
READERS: Staff only
LENDING: Reference only
COMPUTER DATA RETRIEVAL: Access to terminal
HOLDINGS: 431 books; 12 current journals
CLASSIFICATION: LC

52
SOUTH BIRMINGHAM HEALTH AUTHORITY, DISTRICT LIBRARY
Oak Tree Lane, Selly Oak, Birmingham B29 6JF
Tel: 021 472 1345
TYPE: Multidisciplinary
HOURS: 9 - 5
READERS: Staff only
STOCK POLICY: Journals discarded after 3-4 years, books discarded
    as space demands
LENDING: Books only
COMPUTER DATA RETRIEVAL: DATASTAR online - free. Prestel available
CLASSIFICATION SCHEME: Wessex

53
SOUTH BIRMINGHAM SCHOOL OF NURSING
Selly Oak Hospital, Raddlebarn Road, Selly Oak, Birmingham, B29 6JD
Tel:021 472 5313 x4622
Mrs A Charlton
FOUNDED: 1967
TYPE: Nursing
HOURS: Mon-Fri 8.30-4.30
READERS: Staff, other users for reference only
STOCK POLICY: Books over 5 years old discarded
LENDING: Books only. Photocopies provided
COMPUTER DATA RETRIEVAL: Access to DATASTAR
HOLDINGS: 10,000 books; 47 journals, 43 current
CLASSIFICATION: DDC (modified)
PUBLICATIONS: Journals digest; recent additions list (for
internal use only)
NETWORK: West Midlands Regional Health Libraries
BRANCHES: Birmingham Accident Hospital, Birmingham; Rubery
Hill Hospital, Birmingham; Monyhull Hospital, Birmingham;
Royal Orthopaedic Hospital, Birmingham; West Heath Hospital

54
UFFCULME AND CHARLES BURNS CLINICS
Queensbridge Road, Moseley, Birmingham, B13 8QD
Tel:021 449 4481
STAFF: Mrs D Hopker BA DipLib ALA (part-time) 1 other (part-time)
    staff
TYPE: Psychiatric
HOURS: Staffed Monday afternoons. Key available at other times
READERS: Own staff only
STOCK POLICY: Books selectively discarded. General medical
    journals discarded
LENDING: Books only. Photocopies provided
COMPUTER FACILITIES: Access to online terminal. Free
HOLDINGS: 1300 books; 60 journals, 37 current
CLASSIFICATION: LC
SPECIAL COLLECTIONS: Psychotherapy and child psychiatry
PUBLICATION: Current awareness bulletin
NETWORK: West Midlands Regional Health Libraries; Central
Birmingham Mental Health Unit

55
UNIVERSITY OF BIRMINGHAM, BARNES LIBRARY
Medical School, Vincent Drive, Birmingham, B15 2TJ
Tel:021 414 5862   Fax (Medical School): 021 414 4036
Electronic Mail: LANET - LLA 2069 ;
                 JANET - CLARIDJM @ UK. AC. BHAM IBM 3090
STAFF: Mrs JM Claridge BA FLA, SR Jenkins BA, Miss DJ Common BSc
        ALA, Mrs SC Lea BA, A Mickiewicz BA(Lib)
TYPE: Multidisciplinary
HOURS: Mon-Fri 9-9 (9-7 in vacation); Sat 9-12.30 (except
  in August)
READERS: Staff and other users
STOCK POLICY: Duplicate copies of superseded editions
LENDING: Books; journals on short loan only. Photocopies provided
COMPUTER DATA RETRIEVAL: In-house online terminal.Charged full cost
    of telephone, computer time. Reduced rates for own students.
  CD-ROM: Medline from 1983, SCI from 1987. Free to own readers ,
           others charged.
HOLDINGS: 66,000 books, 72,000 bound journals;3,000 journals 1,300
            current ;100 microfilms & tape/slides
SPECIAL COLLECTION: Plague (160 early vols)
CLASSIFICATION: LC
PUBLICATIONS: Library guide; periodicals holdings list; Union
    list of periodicals in the West Midlands Region; Directory of
    libraries in the West Midlands Region; Synapse (West Midlands
    Region Medical Libraries Network newsletter)
NETWORK: West Midlands Regional Health Libraries
BRANCH: University of Birmingham, Clinical Teaching Block
  Library

56
UNIVERSITY OF BIRMINGHAM, CLINICAL TEACHING BLOCK LIBRARY
General Hospital, Steelhouse Lane, Birmingham B4 6NH
021 236 8611 x5950/5951
Staff: Ms J Scott BA DipLib
TYPE: Dental, Medical, Nursing
HOURS: Mon-Fri 9-6
READERS: Staff, other users for reference only. Student nurses
          for reference only
STOCK POLICY: Duplicate copies of superseded editions
LENDING: Books; journals on short loan only.Photocopies provided
COMPUTER DATA RETRIEVAL: Datastar online. Charged full telephone
    and computer costs. Reduced rate for own students.
  CD-ROM: Medline from 1983 . Free to own readers,others charged
HOLDINGS: 6,500 books, 6,500 bound journals; 330 journals,
            140 current titles; videotapes - small collection for
            student use (VHS)
SPECIAL COLLECTIONS: Old and rare dental books (150 vols)
CLASSIFICATION: LC
PUBLICATIONS: Periodical holdings list; library guide
NETWORK: West Midlands Regional Health Libraries

57
UNIVERSITY OF BIRMINGHAM, HEALTH SERVICES MANAGEMENT CENTRE
Park House, 40 Edgbaston Park Road, Birmingham, B15 2RT
Tel:021 455 7511   Fax: 021 456 3592
STAFF: Mrs C Irving BA ALA (part-time)
TYPE: Health administration
HOURS: Mon-Fri 8.30-4.30
READERS: Staff, other users for reference only
STOCK POLICY:Books and journals discarded after variable no of years
LENDING: Books, videotapes, films, audiotapes . Photocopies provided
COMPUTER DATA RETRIEVAL: DATASTAR online. Free to HSMC users
HOLDINGS: 8000 books; 230 journals, 98 current; 3 35mm slides,
                20 tapes, 11 16mm films, 38 videotapes (VHS)
CLASSIFICATION: LC
PUBLICATIONS: Library accessions; Bibliography of health care in
                developing countries
NETWORK: West Midlands Regional Health Libraries; NHS Management
                Librarians' Group

58
WEST BIRMINGHAM DISTRICT EDUCATION CENTRE, DISTRICT NURSING LIBRARY
Arden House,Dudley Road Hospital, Birmingham, B18 7QH
Tel: 021 5230044 x313
STAFF: Mrs BEH Whitehouse, Ms J White
TYPE: Multidisciplinary
HOURS: Mon-Thurs 8.15-4.30, Fri 8.15-4
READERS: Staff and other users
STOCK POLICY: Books discarded after 10 years if appropriate
LENDING: Books and Distance Learning Packages only. Photocopies
    provided
COMPUTER DATA RETRIEVAL: Access to terminal.
HOLDINGS: 57 journals
CLASSIFICATION: Own
PUBLICATIONS: Monthly Bulletin of Journal Holdings
NETWORK: West Midlands Regional Health Libraries

59
WEST MIDLANDS REGIONAL HEALTH AUTHORITY LIBRARY
142 Hagley Road, Birmingham, B16 9PA
Tel: 021 456 1444   Telex 339973   Fax: 021 454 4406
STAFF: Mrs GH Giles BA ALA & Mrs AS Fry Smith BA ALA (job share),
        Miss L Allen BA, Mrs C Cushway
TYPE: Health administration
HOURS: Mon-Fri 9-5
READERS: Staff and other users
STOCK POLICY: Books and journals discarded after 5 years
LENDING: Books only. Photocopies supplied
COMPUTER DATA RETRIEVAL: DATASTAR, DIALOG online. Free
HOLDINGS: 6,000 books; 90 current journals
CLASSIFICATION: Bliss
PUBLICATIONS: Library guide; Current awareness bulletin; Library
        booklist; DHA abstracts
NETWORK: West Midlands Regional Health Libraries; West Midlands
        Regional Library services

60
WEST MIDLANDS REGIONAL HEALTH AUTHORITY, WORKS DEPARTMENT LIBRARY
1 Vernon Rd , Birmingham, B16 9SA
Tel: 021 455 7666 x2000
STAFF: Mrs M Hignell
TYPE: Technical publications, including manuals
HOURS: Mon-Fri 9-5
LENDING: Books only. Photocopies provided
HOLDINGS: 27 current journals
CLASSIFICATION: CI/SfB
NETWORK: West Midlands Regional Health Libraries

Bishop Auckland

61
BISHOP AUCKLAND GENERAL HOSPITAL MEDICAL LIBRARY
Bishop Auckland, Durham DL14 6AD
Tel: 0388 604040
STAFF: Mrs E Graham (part-time)
TYPE: Multidisciplinary
HOURS: Mon-Fri 830-530 (not always staffed)
READERS: Staff and other users
STOCK POLICY: Journals discarded after 10 years, books occasionally
               discarded
LENDING: Books, tape/slides only. photocopies provided
COMPUTER DATA RETRIEVAL: Access to terminal.
HOLDINGS: 1500 books; 60 journals; 10 Tape/slides
CLASSIFICATION: DDC
NETWORK: Northern Regional Health Authority

Bishop's Stortford

62
HERTS AND ESSEX GENERAL HOSPITAL MEDICAL LIBRARY
Bishop's Stortford, Herts CM23 5JH
Tel: 0279 655191
STAFF: Mrs BA Carter (part time), Mrs A Pullum BA (part-time)
TYPE: Medical
HOURS: Mon, Tues,Thurs 9.30-4, Wed, Fri 9.30-12.30
READERS: Staff and other users
STOCK POLICY: Books discarded after 10 years.
LENDING: Books only. Photocopies provided
COMPUTER DATA RETRIEVAL: Access to DATASTAR online - charged.
HOLDINGS: 1200 books; 60 journals, 30 current
CLASSIFICATION: NLM
NETWORK: NE Thames Regional Library and Information Service; EULOS

Blackburn

63
ROYAL INFIRMARY EDUCATION CENTRE LIBRARY
Royal Infirmary, Blackburn, Lancs BB2 3LR
Tel: 0254 63555 x380
STAFF: Mrs CL Riley.
TYPE: Multidisciplinary
HOURS: Mon-Fri 8.30-4.30
READERS: Staff, other users by special arrangement
STOCK POLICY: Books over 10 years old discarded. Selective
  discarding of journals
LENDING: Books and journals. Photocopies supplied.
HOLDINGS: 25000 books; 110 journals
CLASSIFICATION: DDC
NETWORK: NORWHSLA; North West Nursing Librarians Group
BRANCHES: 2 Schools of Nursing libraries staffed part time

Blackpool

64
VICTORIA HOSPITAL, POSTGRADUATE MEDICAL CENTRE
Whinney Heys Road, Blackpool FY3 8NR
Tel: 0253 34111 x559
STAFF: Mrs H Booth
TYPE: Medical
HOURS: Mon-Fri 9-5
READERS: Staff and other users
LENDING: Books only
HOLDINGS: 4,800 books and bound journals; 130 current
CLASSIFICATION: Own
PUBLICATIONS: Library users guide; recent additions
             booklist; periodicals guide
NETWORK: NORWHSLA
BRANCH: Wesham Park Hospital, Wesham

65
VICTORIA HOSPITAL, SCHOOL OF NURSING
Whinney Heys Road, Blackpool FY3 8NR
0253 303831
STAFF: Mrs B Cartmell (part-time), Mrs Sowerby (part-time),
       Mrs Whalley (part-time)
TYPE: Nursing, Psychiatric
HOURS: Mon-Thu 9-5, Fri 9-4
READERS: Nursing staff only
STOCK POLICY: Books over 10 years old discarded
LENDING: Books only. photocopies provided
HOLDINGS: 22 journals
CLASSIFICATION: DDC (modified)

66
BOLTON INSTITUTE OF HIGHER EDUCATION
Deane Road, Bolton BL3 5AB
Tel: 0204 28851   Fax: 0204 399074
STAFF: CH Bleasdale MA ALA AIRT, D. Rudd BSc ALA Cert Ed,
  AR Newell MEd BSc Cert Ed, Miss L Evans BA DipLib ALA,
  Mrs KW Senior BA ALA, Miss MJ Rowlands BA ALA, Miss CD Parry BA
   ALA L-es-L, Mrs VJ Poole BA ALA, Mrs L Berry BA ALA, A Jackson
   CM Hall BA ALA, Mrs J Parr BA ALA, Mrs W Carley MA ALA
TYPE: Multidisciplinary
HOURS: Mon-Fri 9.15-9
READERS: Staff and other users
STOCK POLICY: Books and journals discarded after varying periods
LENDING: Books only. Photocopies provided
COMPUTER DATA RETRIEVAL: DIALOG online - charged computer time
  only.CD-ROM from 1989. PRESTEL available
HOLDINGS: 103,000 books; 988 current journals; AV material
CLASSIFICATION: DDC
BRANCHES: Two
NETWORK: NWRLS

67
BOLTON & SALFORD COLLEGE OF MIDWIFERY AND NURSING
Bolton General Hospital, Farnworth, Bolton BL4 0JR
Tel: 0204 390754
STAFF: Mrs M Todd CGLI LibInfAssCert
FOUNDED: 1974
TYPE: Multidisciplinary
HOURS: Mon-Fri 8-4
READERS: Staff, paramedical staff
STOCK POLICY: Books discarded after 8-10 years.
LENDING: Books only. photocopies provided
HOLDINGS: 4,000 books; 27 journals, 16 current;
CLASSIFICATION: DDC
PUBLICATIONS: General information sheets
NETWORK: NW Nursing Librarians Group

68
PILGRIM HOSPITAL STAFF LIBRARY
Sibsey Road, Boston, Lincolnshire PE21 9QS
Tel: 0205 64801 x2272
STAFF: Miss AL Willis ALA (District Librarian), Miss M Thomas BA
  ALA (Hospital Librarian)
TYPE: Multidisciplinary
HOURS: Key available. Staffed Mon-Fri 9-5
READERS: All staff in district, other bona fide users for
                  reference only
STOCK POLICY: Journals over 8 years old discarded, with exceptions;
              Books discarded selectively
LENDING: Books and journals;Photocopies provided
COMPUTER DATA RETRIEVAL: Access to Datastar online. Free

HOLDINGS: 11000 books; 260 journals, 240 current
CLASSIFICATION: DDC
PUBLICATION: Additions to the library
BRANCHES: Grantham & Kesteven General Hospital Staff Library,
          Rauceby Hospital Staff Library
NETWORK: Base library of South Lincolnshire Health Authority
Library Service; Lincolnshire County Library

Boston Spa

69
BRITISH LIBRARY LENDING DIVISION
Boston Spa, Wetherby, West Yorkshire LS23 7BQ
Tel: 0937 546060 (General enquiries), 0937 843434
Telex: 557381
STAFF: D Bradbury BA ALA (Director), 149
(full-time), 2 (part-time) professional staff, 573
(full-time), 67 (part-time) non-professional staff
TYPE: Multidisciplinary
HOURS: Mon-Fri 9.15-4.30, bandwidth 7.30-6
READERS: Staff and other users
STOCK POLICY: Duplicate books and journals discarded
LENDING: Books and journals through BLDSC forms
COMPUTER DATA RETRIEVAL: In-house terminal. PRESTEL
available
HOLDINGS: 4.6 million books and journals; 54,000 current
journals. Tape/slides. 3.2 million documents in microform,
1,410 miles of microfilm
SPECIAL COLLECTIONS: Government publications; Cyrillic
material
CLASSIFICATION: None except for reading room

Bournemouth

70
EAST DORSET DISTRICT LIBRARY SERVICE
Bournemouth General Hospital, Castle Lane East, Bournemouth, BH7 7DW
Tel: 0202 303626
STAFF: Mrs S Dorey BSc ALA
FOUNDED: 1990
TYPE: Multidisciplinary
HOURS: Mon-Fri 9-5
READERS: Staff and other users
STOCK POLICY: Out of date books and journals discarded
LENDING: Books and journals. Photocopies provided
COMPUTER DATA RETRIEVAL: DATASTAR, BLAISE online. Flat rate
          contribution to cost.
HOLDINGS: 4,000 books ; 120 current journals; 20 tape/slides,
          10 videotapes (VHS)
CLASSIFICATION: NLM (Wessex modification)
NETWORK: WRLIS
BRANCHES: Royal Victoria Hospital, Bournemouth;
          Christchurch Hospital, Christchurch

71
BRADFORD HEALTH AUTHORITY LIBRARY SERVICE
Bradford Royal Infirmary, Duckworth Lane, Bradford, West
 Yorkshire BD9 6RJ
Tel: 0274 542200 x4130
STAFF.   IPG King BA ALA
TYPE: Multidisciplinary
HOURS: Always open. Staffed Mon-Fri 8.30-5.30
READERS: Staff and other users
STOCK POLICY: Out of date books discarded; Journals discarded
          after 10 years
LENDING: Books and journals. Photocopies provided
COMPUTER DATA RETRIEVAL: DATASTAR online - free
HOLDINGS: c.10000 books; 385 current journals.
CLASSIFICATION: NLM
PUBLICATION: Library guide
NETWORK: YRAHCLIS; Yorkshire Joint Medical Library Service
BRANCHES: Nursing/Medical Library, Saint Luke's Hospital, Bradford
          & 2 small subject collections

72
NURSING/MEDICAL LIBRARY, SCHOOL OF NURSING
Saint Luke's Hospital, Little Horton Lane, Bradford, West
 Yorkshire BD5 0JJ
Tel: 0274 734744 x5216
STAFF: Ms C Hardaker BA ALA
FOUNDED: 1976
TYPE: Multidisciplinary
HOURS: Mon-Wed 8.30-9pm Thurs 8.30-8pm, Fri 8.30-9pm
 Staffed Mon-Wed 8.30-5,Thurs 1.30-8, Fri 8.30-4.30
READERS: Staff. Other users at Librarian's discretion
STOCK POLICY: Books over 10 years old discarded.
LENDING: Books only. Photocopies provided
COMPUTER DATA RETRIEVAL: DATASTAR online at another library - free
HOLDINGS: 10,000 books; 46 current journals; tape/slides
CLASSIFICATION: NLM
PUBLICATION: New accessions list;Ethnic Minorities Health Current
          Awareness Bulletin
NETWORK: YRAHCLIS; Yorkshire Nursing Librarians Group
BRANCHES: Lynfield Mount Hospital, Bradford; Westwood
 Hospital, Bradford; Woodlands Orthopaedic Hospital

Brechin

73
STRACATHRO HOSPITAL
Brechin, Angus DD9 7QA
Tel: 03564 7291
STAFF: Mrs M Gillespie MA (part-time)
TYPE: Medical
HOURS: Key available. Staffed 3.5 hours twice a week
READERS: Staff, students on electives
LENDING: Books and journals.
HOLDINGS: 700 books; 571 bound journals
CLASSIFICATION: DDC
BRANCH: Arbroath Infirmary, Arbroath

Brentford

74
SMITHKLINE BEECHAM HEADQUARTERS MEDICAL LIBRARY
Great West Road, Brentford, Middlesex TW8 9BD
Tel: 081 975 3009/3010   Telex: 935986 BEECHM
Fax: 081 975 4011 or 081 847 0830
STAFF: D Younghusband BSc(Hons), Mrs A Kerridge BA(Hons),
       Mrs J Connolly (part-time)
TYPE: Medical, pharmaceutical
HOURS: Mon-Fri 9-5.15
READERS: Staff only
STOCK POLICY: Journals discarded after 10 years
COMPUTER DATA RETRIEVAL: DATASTAR, DIALOG, ORBIT, BRS, DIMDI
        online. Free
HOLDINGS: 1000 books; 200 journals, 160 current;
CLASSIFICATION: UDC
NETWORK: Smithkline Beecham Research & Medical

Brentwood

75
AUBREY KEEP EDUCATION CENTRE, MEDICAL LIBRARY
Warley Hospital, Warley Hill, Brentwood, Essex CM14 5HQ
Tel: 0277 213241 x64
STAFF: Mrs MF Rouse
TYPE: Multidisciplinary
HOURS: Mon-Fri 9.30-4
READERS: Staff, other users at discretion of librarian
STOCK POLICY: Out of date journals BL gift and exchange
LENDING: Books only
COMPUTER DATA RETRIEVAL: Access to terminal. Free
HOLDINGS: 4,000 books; 60 current journals. 16mm cine
  films, tape/slides, 35mm slides, videotapes (U-matic, VHS)
CLASSIFICATION: RCP (modified)
PUBLICATIONS: Weekly current awareness list; monthly
  accessions list; library guide
NETWORK: PLCS

76
BRIDGEND POSTGRADUATE MEDICAL CENTRE LIBRARY
Princess of Wales Hospital, Coity Road, Bridgend,
 Mid-Glamorgan CF31 1JP
Tel: 0656 662166 x2531
STAFF: Mrs BL Paullada ALA (part-time)
FOUNDED: 1986
TYPE: Multidisciplinary
HOURS: Staffed 9-3. Key available at other times
READERS: Staff only
STOCK POLICY: No stock discarded
LENDING: Books, videos only. Photocopies provided
COMPUTER DATA RETRIEVAL: Access to terminal.
HOLDINGS: 2000 books; 1000 journals, 90 current; 20 videotapes (VHS)
CLASSIFICATION: DDC
NETWORK: AWHILES; University College of Wales network

77
POSTGRADUATE/NURSE EDUCATION CENTRE LIBRARY
Pen-y-fai Hospital, Bridgend, Mid-Glamorgan CF31 4LN
Tel: 0656 766100 x3763
STAFF: P Rawle BA DipLib
TYPE: Multidisciplinary
HOURS: Mon-Fri 8.30-4.30
READERS: Staff and other users
STOCK POLICY: Books discarded after 10 years
LENDING: Books only. Photocopies provided
COMPUTER DATA RETRIEVAL: Access to terminal. Free
HOLDINGS: 2000 books; 61 journals, 53 current; 40 cassettes
CLASSIFICATION: DDC 19
BRANCH: Hensol Hospital
NETWORK: AWHILES; PLCS

Brighton

78
SUSSEX POSTGRADUATE MEDICAL CENTRE, DISTRICT LIBRARY
Brighton General Hospital, Elm Grove, Brighton, Sussex
 BN2 3EW
Tel: 0273 696011 x3702/3704
STAFF: Mrs J Lehmann BA DipLib ALA (part-time), Mrs M Bush BA
 DipLib ALA (part-time), 3 other (part-time) staff
FOUNDED: 1967
TYPE: Multidisciplinary
HOURS: Mon-Fri 9-5. Key always available
READERS: Staff, other users at discretion of librarian
STOCK POLICY: Out of date editions of standard texts
 discarded
LENDING: Books only. Photocopies provided
COMPUTER DATA RETRIEVAL: DATASTAR online - free
HOLDINGS: 11000 books; 367 journal, 254 current ; 2000 35mm slides,

35 videotapes (VHS)
SPECIAL COLLECTION: Brighton and Sussex Medico-Chirurgical
Society (400 vols)
CLASSIFICATION: NLM
NETWORK: SE Thames Regional Library and Information Service

Bristol

79
AVON COLLEGE OF NURSING AND MIDWIFERY
Bristol Centre, Eugene St, Bristol BS2 8HW
Tel: 0272 282263/283074 Electronic mail: YCL046
STAFF: Mrs E Weeks ALA (part time), Mrs MA Paull ALA MIInfSc
    (part time)
TYPE: Nursing, midwifery, psychiatry
HOURS: Mon, Tue, Thu 8-4.15, Wed 8-6.30, Fri 8-3.45
READERS: Staff, other users for reference
STOCK POLICY: Books discarded after 10 years
LENDING: Books, AV material. Photocopies provided
COMPUTER DATA RETRIEVAL: Access to DATASTAR. Standard charge
CLASSIFICATION: DDC

80
AVON COLLEGE OF NURSING AND MIDWIFERY
Frenchay Centre, Frenchay Hospital, Bristol BS16 1LE
Tel: 0272 701010 x2611   Electronic mail: YCL050
STAFF: Librarian vacancy, Mrs E Trotter (part time)
TYPE: Nursing, midwifery, psychiatry
HOURS: Mon 9-4, Tue, Wed, Thu 9-5.15, Fri 9-3.30
READERS: Staff, other users for reference
STOCK POLICY: Books discarded after 10 years
LENDING: Books, AV material
COMPUTER DATA RETRIEVAL: Access to DATASTAR. Standard charge
CLASSIFICATION: DDC

81
AVON COLLEGE OF NURSING AND MIDWIFERY
Glenside Centre, Glenside Hospital, Blackberry Hill, Stapleton,
Bristol, BS16 1DD
Tel: 0272 653285 x400   Electronic mail: YCL040
STAFF: Mrs G Poole BA(Hons) (part time)
TYPE: Nursing, midwifery, psychiatry
HOURS: Mon-Fri 9-4
READERS: Staff, other users for reference
STOCK POLICY: Books discarded after 10 years
LENDING: Books, AV material
COMPUTER DATA RETRIEVAL: Access to DATASTAR. Standard charge
CLASSIFICATION: DDC

82
AVON COLLEGE OF NURSING AND MIDWIFERY
Southmead Centre, Southmead Hospital, Westbury-on-Trym, Bristol,
BS10 5NB
Tel: 0272 505050 x3507   Electronic mail: YCL048
STAFF: Mrs A Boulton ALA (part time)
TYPE: Nursing, midwifery, psychiatric
HOURS: Mon-Thu 8.30-4.30, Fri 8.30-4
READERS: Staff, other users for reference
STOCK POLICY: Books discarded after 10 years
LENDING: Books, AV material
COMPUTER DATA RETRIEVAL: Access to DATASTAR. Standard charge
CLASSIFICATION: DDC

83
AVON COLLEGE OF NURSING AND MIDWIFERY
Stoke Park Hospital, Stapleton, Bristol, BS16 1QU
Tel: 0272 655047 x250 Electronic mail; YCL047
STAFF: Ms A Lawrence ALA (Learning Resources Manager - Tel:
               0272 655261 x210), Mrs C Pegler (part time)
TYPE: Nursing, midwifery, psychiatry
HOURS: Mon-Fri 12.30-4
READERS: Staff, other users for reference
STOCK POLICY: Books discarded after 10 years
LENDING: Books, AV material. Photocopies provided
COMPUTER DATA RETRIEVAL: Access to DATASTAR. Standard charge
HOLDINGS: 32,780 books; 125 journals
CLASSIFICATION: DDC
PUBLICATION: What's new bulletin
BRANCHES: 11
NETWORK: SWEHSLinC

84
BRISTOL & WESTERN HEALTH PROMOTION & RESOURCES CENTRE
Central Health Clinic, Tower Hill, Bristol, BS2 0JD
Tel: 0272 291010
STAFF: Ms C Adamson BA ALA
FOUNDED: 1986 (in present form)
TYPE: Multidisciplinary
HOURS: Mon-Thu 8.30-5, Fri 8.30-4.30
READERS: Staff and other users
STOCK POLICY: Books discarded after 10 years, journals also
               discarded
LENDING: Books, journals and audiovisual material. Photocopies
               provided
HOLDINGS: 4,000 books; 55 journals; 50 35mm slides, 300 videotapes
               (VHS), 200 multi-media models
CLASSIFICATION: NLM (Wessex)
PUBLICATION: "Promoting Health"
NETWORK: SWEHSLinC
85
BRISTOL ROYAL INFIRMARY, HOSPITAL LIBRARY
Bristol BS2 8HW

Tel: 0272 282209 and 282142
STAFF: Miss J Dyer ALA and Mrs VA Singleton ALA (job share),
    Miss CE Jones ALA
FOUNDED: 1956
TYPE: Multidisciplinary
HOURS: Mon-Fri 9-5. Key available at other times
READERS: Staff only
STOCK POLICY: Books discarded (generally only current editions kept)
LENDING: Books and journals on inter-library loans only
COMPUTER DATA RETRIEVAL: Access to terminal
HOLDINGS: c.1000 books; 95 journals, 86 current
CLASSIFICATION: Cunningham
NETWORK: SWEHSLinC
BRANCHES: Bristol Maternity Hospital; Bristol General
Hospital; Radiotherapy Centre, Bristol

86
FRENCHAY HEALTH AUTHORITY LIBRARY & INFORMATION SERVICE
Postgraduate Centre, Frenchay Hospital, Bristol BS16 1LE
Tel: 0272 701212 x2634/7   Fax: 0272 701691
STAFF: Ms C Plaice BLib ALA, 2 others (1 part time)
TYPE: Multidisciplinary
HOURS: Mon-Fri 8.30-4.30. Key available at other times.
READERS: Staff only.
STOCK POLICY: Some books over 15 years old discarded
LENDING: Books and journals. photocopies provided
COMPUTER FACILITIES: Datastar online. Charged flat rate
HOLDINGS: 6000 books; 420 journals, 60 current
SPECIAL COLLECTIONS: Neurosciences (1000 vols)
CLASSIFICATION: NLM
PUBLICATION: Library bulletin
NETWORK: SWEHSLinC
BRANCHES: Burden Neurological Institute, Bristol;
 Glenside Hospital, Bristol; Manor Park
Hospital, Bristol; Stoke Park Hospital, Bristol

87
MIDWIVES INFORMATION AND RESOURCE SERVICE
Institute of Child Health, Royal Hospital for Sick Children,
St Michael's Hill , Bristol, BS2 8BJ
Tel: 0272 251791
STAFF: Ms S Hawkins BA DipLib, Ms R Goldstrom BSc DipLib, J Lloyd BA
FOUNDED: 1985
TYPE: Midwifery
READERS: Staff and other users
LENDING: Reference only. Photocopies provided
COMPUTER DATA RETRIEVAL: DATASTAR, DIALOG online - charged computer
            time only. CD-ROM: From 1985
HOLDINGS: 85 journals, 83 current
CLASSIFICATION: Own
PUBLICATIONS: Information Packs; Directory of Maternity
            Organisations; How To Find Out - Information Sources in
            Midwifery; Midwives Diary
NETWORK: SWEHSLinC

88
SOUTHMEAD MEDICAL INFORMATION & LIBRARY SERVICE
Southmead Hospital, Westbury-on-Trym, Bristol BS10 5NB
Tel: 0272 505050 x3810
STAFF: Miss J Oldershaw BA ALA , Mrs LB Greig ALA (part-time)
FOUNDED: 1961
TYPE: Multidisciplinary
HOURS: Mon-Fri 9-5.30. Key available at other times
READERS: Staff and other users
STOCK POLICY: Books before 1980 selectively discarded
LENDING: Books and journals. Photocopies provided
COMPUTER DATA RETRIEVAL: DATASTAR online - charged computer
      time only
HOLDINGS: 4000 books; 417 journals, 200 current
CLASSIFICATION: NLM
SPECIAL COLLECTION: Renal medicine (330 vols)
PUBLICATIONS: Quarterly Newsletter, Library guide
BRANCHES: Ham Green Hospital, Bristol & Brentry Hospital
NETWORK: SWEHSLinC
BRANCHES: Brentry Hospital, Bristol; Ham Green Hospital,
  Bristol; Hortham Hospital, Bristol

89
SOUTH WESTERN REGIONAL TRANSFUSION CENTRE, UK TRANSPLANT SERVICE
Southmead Hospital, Westbury-on-Trym, Bristol BS10 5ND
Tel: 0272 507777
STAFF: Miss J Oldershaw BA ALA, Miss LR Greig ALA (part time)
FOUNDED: 1967
TYPE: Medical, Blood Transfusion and Organ Transplantation
HOURS: 24 hour access: staffed MON, Wed, Fri 9.30-12.30, Tue 12.30-3.30
READERS: Staff and other users
STOCK POLICY: No stock discarded
LENDING: Books and journals. Photocopies provided
COMPUTER DATA RETRIEVAL: Access to DATASTAR online - charged
          computer time only
HOLDINGS: 475 books; 60 journals, 50 current
CLASSIFICATION: NLM
NETWORKS: SWEHSLinC, Southmead Medical Information & Library Service

90
UNIVERSITY OF BRISTOL COMMUNITY MEDICINE LIBRARY
Department of Community Medicine, Canynge Hall, Whiteladies Road,
  Bristol BS8 2PR
Tel: 0272 38262
STAFF: Mrs K Little (part time)
TYPE: Health administration, preventive medicine & public health
HOURS: Mon-Fri 9-6
READERS: Staff and other users
STOCK POLICY: Books discarded at librarian's discretion

LENDING: Books and journals. Photocopies provided
COMPUTER DATA RETRIEVAL: Access to terminal.
HOLDINGS: 4043 books ; 35 current journals
CLASSIFICATION: Cunningham
BRANCH of University of Bristol Medical Library

91
UNIVERSITY OF BRISTOL DENTAL LIBRARY
Bristol Dental Hospital, Lower Maudlin Street, Bristol
BS1 2LY
Tel: 0272 230050 x4419
STAFF: Mrs A Smith
TYPE: Dental
HOURS: Mon-Fri 9-6
READERS: Staff and other users
STOCK POLICY: Little used material transferred to Medical
Library for storage/disposal
LENDING: Books and journals. Photocopies provided
COMPUTER DATA RETRIEVAL: Access to terminal.
HOLDINGS: 4,000 books and bound journals; 100 current
journals; Tape/slides, 35mm slides, videotapes(VHS)
CLASSIFICATION: Own
BRANCH of University of Bristol Medical Library

92
UNIVERSITY OF BRISTOL MEDICAL LIBRARY
Medical School, University Walk, Bristol BS8 1TD
Tel: 0272 303455   Telex: 931210824
Electronic Mail: Telecom Gold - 79:LLA1028
              Janet - LIBRARY @ UK AC BRISTOL
STAFF: C Ward BA DipLib, Mrs S Davies BA ALA , M Wall BA ALA
TYPE: Multidisciplinary
HOURS: Mon-Fri 8.45-9 (8.45-7 in vacation) Sat 8.45-1
READERS: Staff and other users
STOCK POLICY: Duplicated editions of books discarded
LENDING: Books and journals. Photocopies provided
COMPUTER DATA RETRIEVAL: DATASTAR online - charged computer time
              only. CD-ROM from 1976
HOLDINGS: 118,395 books; 4147 journals, 887 current.
SPECIAL COLLECTIONS: Library of Caleb Hillier Parry (940
vols); mineral waters and spas (310 vols)
CLASSIFICATION: Cunningham
PUBLICATION: library guides and periodical lists
BRANCHES: University of Bristol Dental Library; University
of Bristol Veterinary Library; University of Bristol
Community Health Library

Bristol (cont)

93
UNIVERSITY OF BRISTOL SCHOOL OF VETERINARY SCIENCE
Langford House, Langford, Bristol BS18 7DU
Tel: 0934 852581
STAFF: Mrs E Weaver BA (part-time)
FOUNDED: 1950
TYPE: Veterinary
HOURS: Staffed (term time) Mon - Thurs 9.15-3.30, Fri 9.15-1.15
     (vacations) 9.00-3.45
READERS: Staff and other users
STOCK POLICY: Little used material transferred to Medical
Library for storage/disposal
LENDING: Books only. Photocopies provided
COMPUTER DATA RETRIEVAL: Access to terminal.
HOLDINGS: 9688 books ; 130 current journals
CLASSIFICATION: Barnard
BRANCH of University of Bristol Medical Library

Bromsgrove

94
BARNSLEY HALL HOSPITAL, MEDICAL LIBRARY
Stourbridge Rd, Bromsgrove, Worcs , B61 0EX
Tel: 0527 75252 x94
STAFF: Mrs S Lindley
TYPE: Medical, psychiatric
HOURS: Always open. Staffed Mon-Thu 9.30-1, Fri 9.30-12.30
READERS: Staff and other users
COMPUTER DATA RETRIEVAL: Access to terminal
HOLDINGS: 850 books; 25 current journals
CLASSIFICATION: Own
NETWORK: West Midlands Regional Health Libraries

Broxburn

95
BANGOUR GENERAL HOSPITAL POSTGRADUATE MEDICAL CENTRE
Broxburn, West Lothian EH52 6LR
0506 81334
No further information available

A   96
LOTHIAN COLLEGE OF NURSING AND MIDWIFERY
Bangour General Hospital, Broxburn, West Lothian EH52 6LR
Tel: 050 419666 x4260/4261
STAFF: Mrs EJ Patience BA ALA
TYPE: Midwifery, Nursing
HOURS: Mon-Thurs 9-5, Fri 9-4.30
READERS: Staff and other users
LENDING: Books only. Photocopies provided
HOLDINGS: 4,500 books; 60 current journals; 20 tape/slides,

40 videotapes (VHS)
CLASSIFICATION: NLMC

Burnley

97
BURNLEY GENERAL HOSPITAL EDUCATION CENTRE LIBRARY
Casterton Avenue, Burnley BB10 2PQ
Tel: 0282 25071 x2167   Electronic Mail: YCL 013
STAFF: Mrs A Baird (part time)
TYPE: Nursing
HOURS: 8.30-4.30 (staffed mornings only)
READERS: Staff only
LENDING: Books only. Photocopies provided
COMPUTER FACILITIES: In-house terminal. Prestel

98
MACKENZIE MEDICAL CENTRE
Burnley General Hospital, Burnley, Lancs. BB10 2PQ
Tel: 0282 25071 x2175/6
STAFF: Mrs A Eastwood, 1 other (part-time) staff
FOUNDED: 1966
TYPE: Multidisciplinary
HOURS: Mon-Fri 8.30-5. Key available at other times
READERS: Staff and other users
LENDING: Books and journals
COMPUTER DATA RETRIEVAL: In-house terminal. PRESTEL
HOLDINGS: 1,300 books; 120 current journals; c.150 tape/slides,
c.1000 35mm slides, c.50 videotapes (VHS)
CLASSIFICATION: NLM
PUBLICATIONS: New book lists

Burton-on-Trent

99
BURTON GRADUATE MEDICAL CENTRE LIBRARY
Burton District Hospital, Belvedere Road, Burton-on-Trent,
 Staffs DE13 0RB
Tel: 0283 66333 x2104
STAFF: Mrs MG Thomson Lathbury BA MLS ALA
FOUNDED: 1973
TYPE: Multidisciplinary
HOURS: Mon-Fri 9-6
READERS: Staff and other users
STOCK POLICY: Out of date editions of books discarded
LENDING: Books , journals and A/V material. Photocopies provided
COMPUTER DATA RETRIEVAL: DATASTAR online - charged
HOLDINGS: 7300 books; 154 current journals; microfilms,
 62 tape/slides, 52 videotapes (VHS)
CLASSIFICATION: LC
PUBLICATIONS: Current contents, Library bulletin
BRANCH: Burton General Hospital
NETWORK: West Midlands Regional Health Libraries

100
BURTON NURSE EDUCATION CENTRE
Burton District Hospital, Belvedere Rd, Burton on Trent, Staffs,
 DE13 0RB
Tel: 0283 66333 x2237
STAFF: Ms E Watson BA DipLib ALA
FOUNDED: 1987
TYPE: Midwifery, Nursing
HOURS: 8.30-4.30
READERS: Staff only
STOCK POLICY: No stock discarded
LENDING: Books only. Photocopies provided
COMPUTER DATA RETRIEVAL: Access to terminal
HOLDINGS: 6000 books; 44 journals, 30 current
CLASSIFICATION: LC
PUBLICATIONS: Current awareness
NETWORK: West Midlands Regional Library Network

Bury

101
BURY AND DISTRICT POSTGRADUATE MEDICAL INSTITUTE
Bury General Hospital, Walmersley Road, Bury, Lancashire BL9 6PG
Tel: 061 705 3258
STAFF: IM Mather BA ALA
FOUNDED: 1951
TYPE: Multidisciplinary
HOURS: Mon - Fri 9-5
READERS: Staff and other users
STOCK POLICY: Books discarded after 15 years
LENDING: Books , journals and AV material. Photocopies provided
COMPUTER DATA RETRIEVAL: In-house terminal - free. CD-ROM from 1983
HOLDINGS: 3250 books; 156 journals, 118 current; 2500 35mm slides,
          80 videotapes (VHS)
CLASSIFICATION: NLM
NETWORK: NORWHSLA; Psychiatric Libraries Cooperation Scheme
BRANCH: Fairfield General Hospital, Bury

102
BURY SCHOOL OF NURSING
Talbot Grove, Bury, Lancashire BL9 6PH
Tel: 061 764 3350
STAFF: J France
TYPE: Health Administration, Nursing
HOURS: Mon-Fri 8.30-4.30
READERS: Nursing staff and students
STOCK POLICY: Books discarded after 10 years

LENDING: Books only. Photocopies provided
COMPUTER DATA RETRIEVAL: Access to terminal
HOLDINGS: 3,500 books; 27 current journals.
CLASSIFICATION: RCN (but changing to DDC)

Bury St Edmunds

103
WEST SUFFOLK HOSPITAL EDUCATION CENTRE LIBRARY
Hardwick Lane, Bury St Edmunds, Suffolk IP33 2QZ
Tel: 0284 763131 x343
STAFF: Mrs J Hunter MA ALA (District Health Librarian)
FOUNDED: 1974
TYPE: Multidisciplinary
HOURS: Always open. Staffed Mon-Fri 8.30-5.
READERS: Staff and other users
STOCK POLICY: Books discarded after 10-15 years
LENDING: Books only. Photocopies provided
COMPUTER DATA RETRIEVAL: DATASTAR, BMA online - free
  CD-ROM: From 1985
HOLDINGS: 15,000 books; 188 journals, 180 current
CLASSIFICATION: NLM
PUBLICATIONS: Library guide; accessions list; current
  awareness list
NETWORK: E Anglian NHS Region; Nursing Libraries Interloan Network;
  SULIS; EULOS

Camberley

104
FRIMLEY PARK HOSPITAL, DISTRICT HEALTH SCIENCES LIBRARY
Portsmouth Road, Frimley, Camberley, Surrey GU16 5UJ
Tel: 0276 692777
STAFF: RJ Kiley BA(Hons) MSc
TYPE: Medical
HOURS: Mon-Fri 9-5
READERS: Staff only
STOCK POLICY: Books and journals discarded.
LENDING: Books and journals. photocopies provided
COMPUTER DATA RETRIEVAL: DATASTAR online.
HOLDINGS: 3,500 books; 150 journals, 110 current titles
CLASSIFICATION: NLM
PUBLICATIONS: Library guide; recent additions list
NETWORK: SW Thames Regional Library and Information Service

105
AGRICULTURAL AND FOOD RESEARCH COUNCIL
Institute of Animal Physiology and Genetics Research, Babraham,
  Cambridge CB2 4AT
Tel: 0223 832312   Fax: 0223 833676
STAFF: Miss WM Reynolds , D Anderson BA
FOUNDED: 1948
TYPE: Multidisciplinary
HOURS: Mon-Thurs 9-5.30, Fri 9-5
READERS: Staff, other users by arrangement
STOCK POLICY: Books discarded after about 30 years
LENDING: Theses lent to approved libraries. Photocopies provided
COMPUTER DATA RETRIEVAL: BLAISE, DIALOG online - charged full cost
HOLDINGS: 7,000 books; c.500 journals, 327 current
CLASSIFICATION: UDC
PUBLICATION: List of periodicals held in library
NETWORK: AFRC Institute libraries

106
CAMBRIDGESHIRE HEALTH AUTHORITY INFORMATION SERVICES UNIT
Fulbourn Hospital, Cambridge, CB1 5EF
Tel: 0223 248074   Fax: 0223 410471
STAFF: Ms G Andrews ALA FRSA
TYPE: Health administration, health services management
HOURS: Mon-Fri 10-4
READERS: Staff, other users by arrangement
STOCK POLICY: Out of date books and journals discarded
LENDING: Books only. Photocopies provided
COMPUTER DATA RETRIEVAL: In-house terminal (catalogue)
HOLDINGS: 5,082 books ; 85 current journals; 2,479 DHSS/DOH
           circulars
PUBLICATIONS: Monthly bulletins: DOH circulars, recent additions

107
EAST ANGLIAN REGIONAL HEALTH AUTHORITY
Union Lane, Chesterton, Cambridge CB4 1RF
Tel: 0223 61212 x270 FAX: 0223 353209
STAFF: Miss MC Cawthorne BA ALA
TYPE: Health administration
HOURS: Mon-Thurs 8.30-5, Fri 8.30-4
READERS: Staff, other users on application
STOCK POLICY: Books and journals discarded at Librarian's discretion
LENDING: Books. Journals only lent internally. Photocopies provided
COMPUTER DATA RETRIEVAL: Access to terminal.
HOLDINGS: 3000 books; 90 journals, 37 current ; microfiche
CLASSIFICATION: Bliss (modified)
PUBLICATIONS: Guide to services; accessions lists

108
FULBOURN HOSPITAL MEDICAL LIBRARY
Fulbourn Hospital, Cambridge CB1 5EF
Tel: 0223 248074 x5330
STAFF: MJ Todd-Jones ALA (part-time)
FOUNDED: 1970
TYPE: Psychiatric
HOURS: Mon-Fri 9.30-3.30 (Tue till 5, Fri till 4.30). Key
   available at other times
READERS: Staff and other users
STOCK POLICY: Books and journals discarded after 10 years
LENDING: Books , AV material. Photocopies provided
COMPUTER DATA RETRIEVAL: Access to terminal and CD-ROM
   from 1983
HOLDINGS: c3,000 books; 164 journals, 83 current titles;
   12 Tape/slides, 3 16mm films, 26 videotapes (VHS)
CLASSIFICATION: NLM
SPECIAL COLLECTION: Fulbourn Hospital archival/related papers
   (15 vols/reports, 200 articles/theses)
PUBLICATION: Quarterly committee minutes and reports
BRANCHES: Child and Family Psychiatry Clinic, Cambridge;
   Ida Darwin Hospital, Cambridge
NETWORKS: East Anglian Region; PLCS

109
MEDICAL RESEARCH COUNCIL, DUNN NUTRITION UNIT
Downhams Lane, Milton Road, Cambridge CB4 1XJ
Tel: 0223 426356   Telex: 818448 DUNNUK   Fax: 0223 426617
STAFF: Miss AA Paul BSc (Hon Librarian), Mrs RE Sewell (part-time)
FOUNDED: 1927
TYPE: Multidisciplinary
HOURS: Outside enquiries 9 - 1
READERS: Staff and other users
STOCK POLICY: No stock discarded
LENDING: Books lent occasionally. Photocopies provided
COMPUTER DATA RETRIEVAL: Access to DATASTAR online
HOLDINGS: 1550 books; 146 journals, 106 current
SPECIAL COLLECTION: Dame Harriette Chick Collection of Reprints
CLASSIFICATION: DDC (modified)
NETWORK: Medical Research Council

110
MEDICAL RESEARCH COUNCIL, LABORATORY OF MOLECULAR BIOLOGY
University Postgraduate Medical School, Hills Road,
   Cambridge CB2 2QH
Tel: 0223 248011   Telex 81532
No furthur information available

111
ORGANON LABORATORIES LIMITED
Cambridge Science Park, Milton Road, Cambridge CB4 4FL
Tel: 0223 423445   Telex: 818866   Fax: 0223 61264
STAFF: B Clements ALA
FOUNDED: 1947
TYPE: Medical, Pharmaceutical
HOURS: Mon-Fri 9-5
READERS: Staff and other users
STOCK POLICY: Books and journals discarded after variable periods
LENDING: Reference only. Photocopies provided
COMPUTER DATA RETRIEVAL: DATASTAR online - free
HOLDINGS: 1,500 books; 25 journals,   22 current
CLASSIFICATION: Own
NETWORK: AKZO Group

112
UNIVERSITY OF CAMBRIDGE, COLMAN LIBRARY
Department of Biochemistry, Tennis Court Road, Cambridge, CB2 1QW
Tel: 0223 333613
STAFF: Dr CJR Thorne MA PHd (Honorary Librarian), Miss CD Osbourn
Founded: 1932
TYPE: Biochemistry
HOURS: Mon-Fri 9-5
READERS: Staff , other users with permission only
STOCK POLICY: No stock discarded
LENDING: Books only. Photocopies provided
COMPUTER DATA RETRIEVAL: DATASTAR online for internal use only
HOLDINGS: 2,500 books; 200 journals, 142 current titles
CLASSIFICATION: Own
NETWORK: Cambridge University

113
UNIVERSITY OF CAMBRIDGE, DEPARTMENT OF CLINICAL VETERINARY
  MEDICINE
Madingley Road, Cambridge CB3 0ES
Tel: 0223 55641 x238
No further information available

114
UNIVERSITY OF CAMBRIDGE, DEPARTMENT OF EXPERIMENTAL
  PSYCHOLOGY & MACCURDY PSYCHOPATHOLOGY LIBRARY
Downing Street, Cambridge CB2 3EB
Tel: 0223 333554
STAFF: Dr P Whittle MA PhD (Honorary Librarian), Mrs E Ingle
         (part time)
TYPE: Psychology
HOURS: Mon-Fri 9-5.30
READERS: Staff, other users by special permission
STOCK POLICY: Out of date books discarded
LENDING: Books to members of university only, journals to members

of Department only. Photocopies provided
COMPUTER DATA RETRIEVAL: Online to University system
HOLDINGS: c.10,000 books; 97 current journals
SPECIAL COLLECTION: Maccurdy library (3,000)
CLASSIFICATION: Own

115
UNIVERSITY OF CAMBRIDGE, MEDICAL LIBRARY
Addenbrooke's Hospital, Hills Road, Cambridge CB2 2QQ
Tel: 0223 336750 (enquiries)   Telex: 81240   Fax: 0223 336709
Electronic Mail: JANET - PBM2 @ UK.AC.CAM.PHX
STAFF: PB Morgan MA ALA, Mrs FW Roberts MA MSc MIInfSc ALA,
    SM Dale BA DipLib, Miss EJ Johnson MA BLib
FOUNDED: 1973
TYPE: Multidisciplinary
HOURS: Mon-Fri 8-10, Sat 9-9, Sun 2-6
READERS: Staff and other users
STOCK POLICY: No stock discarded
LENDING: Books only. Photocopies provided
COMPUTER DATA RETRIEVAL: DATASTAR, DIALOG online - charged
            computer time only. CD-ROM: From 1983
HOLDINGS: 22,000 books; 2200 journals, 900 current journals;
 270 microfilms, 300 tape/slides, 100 videotapes (VHS)
SPECIAL COLLECTION: Cambridge MD and M.Chir theses (1250 vols)
CLASSIFICATION: NLM
PUBLICATIONS: Medical Library bulletin; Guide to the medical
            library
BRANCH of Cambridge University Library
NETWORK: E Anglian NHS Region; CURL (through Cambridge University
            Library); Cambridgeshire LIP

116
UNIVERSITY OF CAMBRIDGE, PHYSIOLOGICAL LABORATORY
Downing Street, Cambridge CB2 3EG
Tel: 0223 333821
STAFF: Mrs ME Joyce
FOUNDED: On present site 1914
TYPE: Physiology
HOURS: Mon-Fri 8.30-5.30
READERS: Staff and other users
STOCK POLICY: Books and journals discarded
LENDING: No lending. Photocopies provided
COMPUTER DATA RETRIEVAL: In house terminal
HOLDINGS: 4078 Books; 210 journals, 124 current
CLASSIFICATION: Own scheme
NETWORK: University of Cambridge

117
UNIVERSITY OF CAMBRIDGE, WHIPPLE LIBRARY
Free School Lane, Cambridge CB2 3RH
Tel: 0223 358381 x383
STAFF: Miss R Youngman BA DipLib ALA
TYPE: History and philosophy of science and medicine
HOURS: Mon-Fri 9.30-5.30 (vacation Mon-Fri 9.30-5)
READERS: Staff and other users
LENDING: Books only
HOLDINGS: 16,000 books, 1,317 bound journals; 64 current
journals. Microcards
SPECIAL COLLECTION: 17th to 19th century books on
scientific instruments (1,000 vols)

Canterbury

118
KENT POSTGRADUATE MEDICAL CENTRE, LINACRE LIBRARY
Kent and Canterbury Hospital, Canterbury, Kent CT1 3NG
Tel: 0227 761849
STAFF: Mrs SE Cover ALA, 1 part time assistant
TYPE: Multidisciplinary
HOURS: Mon-Fri 8.30-5. Key available to members
READERS: Staff and other users
STOCK POLICY: Very out of date books discarded
LENDING: Books, journals, videos, tape/slides
COMPUTER DATA RETRIEVAL: DATASTAR online - free to members of Centre
HOLDINGS: 5,500 books ; 220 current journals. Tape/slides,
videotapes (VHS)
CLASSIFICATION: NLM
NETWORK: SE Thames Regional Library and Information Service

119
SAINT AUGUSTINE'S HOSPITAL
Chartham Down, near Canterbury, Kent CT4 7LL
Tel: 0227 738382 x259/346
STAFF: Ms J Sharman ALA (part time)
TYPE: Multidisciplinary
HOURS: Mon 9-5, Tue-Thu 9-3, Fri 9-4.30
READERS: Staff and other users
STOCK POLICY: Outdated and superseded books discarded, general
medical and nursing journals discarded
LENDING: Books only. Photocopies provided
HOLDINGS: 2,711 books; 60 journals, 56 current titles
CLASSIFICATION: DDC
NETWORKS: SETRLIS; PLCS; Kent County Library (for patients' service)

120
CARDIFF ROYAL INFIRMARY MEDICAL LIBRARY
Newport Road, Cardiff CF2 1SZ
Tel: 0222 492233 x478
STAFF: Ms R Soper BA DipLib ALA, Ms BM Vose BSc, Ms JA Bishop BA
TYPE: Multidisciplinary
HOURS: Mon-Fri 9-5
READERS: Staff, other users at librarian's discretion
STOCK POLICY: Discard non unique journals after 5 years
LENDING: Books and journals. Photocopies provided
COMPUTER DATA RETRIEVAL: DATASTAR online - free
HOLDINGS: 2000 books; 66 journals, 65 current
CLASSIFICATION: DDC 19
BRANCH of UWCM main library
NETWORK: AWHILES

121
HEALTH PROMOTION AUTHORITY FOR WALES
8th Floor, Brunel House, 2 Fitzalan Rd, Cardiff CF2 1EB
Tel: 0222 472472 x245   Fax: 0222 480851
STAFF: Ms S Thomas BA DipLib PGCE
FOUNDED: 1989
TYPE: Health Promotion
HOURS: Mon-Fri 9-5
READERS: Staff and other users
STOCK POLICY: No stock discarded
LENDING: Books, Publications catalogue, Information factsheets
COMPUTER DATA RETRIEVAL: DATASTAR online - free. Prestel
HOLDINGS: 100 current journals
CLASSIFICATION: NLM
PUBLICATIONS: Library guide, Journals list, Current awareness
               bulletin
NETWORK: AWHILES

122
UNIVERSITY HOSPITAL OF WALES COMBINED TRAINING INSTITUTE
Heath Park, Cardiff CF4 4XW
Tel: 0222 756431
STAFF: Mrs L Shewring BA DipLib ALA, Miss D Connell MA DipLib ALA
FOUNDED: 1972
TYPE: Multidisciplinary
HOURS: Mon, Wed, Fri 8.45-5, Tues, Thurs 8.45-8
READERS: Staff and students of the Institute. Other users
for reference only
STOCK POLICY: Out of date books discarded
LENDING: Books only. Photocopies provided
COMPUTER DATA RETRIEVAL: DIALOG online. CD-ROM from 1990
HOLDINGS: 23,000 books; 110 current journals; 108 Tape/slides,
             38 audiocassettes, 56 video-tapes (VHS)
CLASSIFICATION: DDC
PUBLICATIONS: Library Guide; subject guides
NETWORK: AWHILES

123
UNIVERSITY OF WALES COLLEGE OF MEDICINE, MAIN LIBRARY
University Hospital of Wales,Heath Park, Cardiff CF4 4XN
Tel: 0222 755944 x2874   Telex 498696   Fax: 0222 762208
STAFF: JM Lancaster MPhil ALA, SJ Pritchard BA ALA, Miss D Liepa
    BSc, MSc, S Baines BA DipLib, RL Somers BA DipLib, Ms R Soper BA
    DipLib ALA, Ms J Stevens BA ALA
FOUNDED: 1931
TYPE: Multidisciplinary
HOURS: Mon-Fri 9-9, Sat 9-5
READERS: Staff and other users
STOCK POLICY: Only obsolete or little used material discarded
LENDING: Books, videotapes only. Photocopies provided
COMPUTER DATA RETRIEVAL: DATASTAR, BLAISE, DIALOG online - free
    CD-ROM: MEDLINE from 1976.
HOLDINGS: 30,000 books; 1,000 journals, 700 current titles;
                100 videotapes (VHS)
SPECIAL COLLECTION: History of medicine (2,000 vols)
CLASSIFICATION: DDC
PUBLICATIONS: Guide; periodicals listings
BRANCHES: Dental Hospital library, Cardiff; Llandough Hospital;
                Cardiff Royal Infirmary
NETWORK: AWHILES

124
UNIVERSITY OF WALES COLLEGE OF MEDICINE, DENTAL LIBRARY
Dental Hospital,Heath Park, Cardiff CF4 4XY
Tel: 0222 755944 x2523/2525
STAFF: Miss J Stevens BA ALA
FOUNDED: 1965
TYPE: Dental
HOURS: Mon, Wed 9-6, Tues, Thurs, Fri 9-5.30
READERS: Staff and other users.
STOCK POLICY: Duplicates of superseded editions discarded.
LENDING: Books, theses only. Photocopies provided
COMPUTER DATA RETRIEVAL : Access to DATASTAR, BLAISE, DIALOG online
                - Free. PRESTEL available. CD-ROM: Medline from 1976
HOLDINGS: 5,000 books; 220 journals, 142 current; 15 microfilms,
                100 tape/slides, 37 videotapes (VHS)
SPECIAL COLLECTION: History of dentistry (c200 vols)
CLASSIFICATION: Own
PUBLICATIONS: Library guide; Guide to Reference Sources for Students

125
WHITCHURCH POSTGRADUATE MEDICAL CENTRE
Whitchurch Hospital, Cardiff CF4 7XB
Tel: 0222 693191
STAFF: Mrs J Walkden (part time), Mrs A Harris (part time)
FOUNDED: 1972?
TYPE: Medical, Psychiatric
HOURS: 9-5 (except Mon am)
READERS: Staff only
STOCK POLICY: Some unwanted book donations discarded
LENDING: Books only. Photocopies provided
COMPUTER DATA RETRIEVAL: DATASTAR online
HOLDINGS: c2000 books; 113 current journals
NETWORK: PLCS

Carlisle

126
CUMBERLAND INFIRMARY EDUCATION CENTRE LIBRARY
Newtown Road, Carlisle, Cumbria CA2 7HY
Tel: 0228 23444 x482
STAFF: Mrs P Goundry ALA , Mrs S Hughes ALA (part time)
FOUNDED: Multidisciplinary service at this site 1986
TYPE: Multidisciplinary
HOURS: Mon-Thurs 9 - 5, Fri 9-4.30
READERS: Staff, other users on application
STOCK POLICY: Books and journals over 15 years old discarded
LENDING: Books , journals and A/V material. photocopies provided
COMPUTER DATA RETRIEVAL: DATASTAR online - token charge.
HOLDINGS: 8,000 books; 135 journals, 130 current; 30 videotapes (VHS)
CLASSIFICATION: NLM
PUBLICATION: Library guides; List of journal holdings
NETWORK: Northern Regional Association of Health Service
 Librarians

127
GARLANDS HOSPITAL LIBRARY
Carlisle, Cumbria CA1 3SX
Tel: 0228 31081
STAFF: Ms V Bye ALA (part time)
FOUNDED: c1968
TYPE: Multidisciplinary
HOURS: Tue-Fri 9 - 4
READERS: Staff and other users
STOCK POLICY: Books and journals after 10 years
LENDING: Books, journals, slides, jigsaws, tapes, records
HOLDINGS: Medical - 500 books, 65 current journals; Patients: 4,000 vols
CLASSIFICATION: DDC
NETWORK: Northern regional Association of Health Service Librarians; PLCS

Carluke

128
LANARKSHIRE COLLEGE OF NURSING AND MIDWIFERY
Law Hospital, Carluke, Strathclyde ML8 5ER
Tel: 0698 355951 x2
STAFF: T Brown BSc DipLib ALA, Ms L Porch MA DipLib
FOUNDED: 1974
TYPE: Midwifery, Nursing
HOURS: 8.30-4.30
READERS: Staff and other users
STOCK POLICY: Books discarded selectively
LENDING: Books only. Photocopies provided
HOLDINGS: 60 journals, 57 current; 107 tape/slides, videotapes (44 U-mati
          72 Betamax, 115 VHS)
CLASSIFICATION: NLM
NETWORKS: ASHSL; Standing Conference of Nursing Librarians

129
LAW HOSPITAL, ALISTAIR MACKENZIE LIBRARY
Carluke, Lanarkshire ML8 5ER
Tel: 0698 351100 x256
STAFF: J Hodgson BMus ALA, Ms J Bryson (part-time)
TYPE: Multidisciplinary
HOURS: Always open to staff
READERS: Staff, other users by arrangement
STOCK POLICY: Books discarded after 10 years
LENDING: Books and journals. Photocopies provided
HOLDINGS: 4,800 books; 155 current journals; 7 tape/slides
CLASSIFICATION: NLM
PUBLICATIONS: Current awareness (monthly) Therapists; Child and family
 psychiatry;Addiction; Quarterly library bulletin
NETWORK: ASHSL
Carmarthen

130
WEST WALES GENERAL HOSPITAL
Glangwili, Carmarthen, Dyfed SA31 2AF
Tel: 0267 235151
STAFF: Mrs VE Bisnath ALA CHSM, Mrs FEC Wilde MA DipLib
FOUNDED: 1968
TYPE: Multidisciplinary
HOURS: Mon-Fri 9-5
READERS: Staff and other users
STOCK POLICY: Stock discarded
LENDING: Books and journals. Photocopies provided
COMPUTER DATA RETRIEVAL: Access to DATASTAR, BLAISE, DIALOG online
                        - free. PRESTEL available
HOLDINGS: 1,500 35mm slides
CLASSIFICATION: NLM
NETWORK: AWHILES

Carshalton

131
MEDICAL RESEARCH COUNCIL LABORATORIES
Woodmansterne Road, Carshalton, Surrey SM5 4EF
Tel:081 643 8000   FAX: 081 642 6538
STAFF: Miss JD Allen BA
TYPE: Medical
HOURS: Always open to staff. Staffed Mon-Thurs 9-5.15, Fri 9-5
READERS: Staff and other users
STOCK POLICY: Out of date books and journals discarded selectively
LENDING: Books and journals. photocopies provided
COMPUTER DATA RETRIEVAL: DATASTAR, BLAISE online - free
HOLDINGS: 2,300 books; 16,200 bound journals, 270 current
CLASSIFICATION: Barnard
NETWORK: Medical Research Council

132
SAINT HELIER HOSPITAL, HIRSON LIBRARY
Wrythe Lane, Carshalton, Surrey, SM2 5HQ
Tel: 081 644 4343 x2430
STAFF: Mrs R Cooke BA MLib
TYPE: Multidisciplinary
HOURS: Mon-Fri 9-5
READERS: All Health Authority staff in District
LENDING: Books and journals. Photocopies provided
COMPUTER DATA RETRIEVAL: In-house terminal. Free
HOLDINGS: 1,500 books; 144 current journals.
CLASSIFICATION: NLM
NETWORK: SW Thames Regional Library Service

Carstairs Junction

133
STATE HOSPITAL
Carstairs Junction, Lanark ML11 8RP
Tel: 0555 840293
STAFF: J Hodgson BMus ALA (part time)
TYPE: Forensic psychiatry, psychiatric nursing, psychology
HOURS: Key available 9-5
READERS: All hospital personnel
LENDING: Books , journals and offprints. Photocopies provided
HOLDINGS: 1,700 books; 40 current journals
CLASSIFICATION: RCP
PUBLICATION: Quarterly current awareness bulletin in
 forensic psychiatry
NETWORKS: ASHSL; PLCS

134
BROOMFIELD HOSPITAL MEDICAL LIBRARY
Medical Academic Unit, Broomfield Hospital, Chelmsford, Essex,
   CM1 5ET
Tel: 0245 440761   Fax: 0245 442140
STAFF: Librarian Vacancy, Mrs E Davis (part time clerical),
          Mrs P Kewell (part time
          clerical)
FOUNDED: 1966
TYPE: Dental, Medical
HOURS: Mon-Fri 9-5
READERS: Staff and other users
STOCK POLICY: Books discarded
LENDING: Books only. Photocopies provided
COMPUTER DATA RETRIEVAL: DATASTAR online - free
HOLDINGS: 2,500 books; 85 current journals
CLASSIFICATION: NLM
BRANCHES: St Johns Hospital
NETWORK: NE Thames Regional Library Service; Essex Libraries

135
GRAVES MEDICAL AUDIOVISUAL LIBRARY
Holly House, 220 New London Road, Chelmsford, Essex CM2 9BJ
0245 283351   Telex: 94012063 GMAL G Fax: 0245 354710
FOUNDED: 1977
TYPE: Multidisciplinary
HOURS: Postal only
LENDING: Audiovisual only
HOLDINGS: 10.000 35mm slides (National Medical Slide Bank);
          800 tapes/slides, 1 videodisc, 200 videotapes (all titles
          available in all formats)
PUBLICATION: Catalogue

136
MID & WEST ESSEX DEPARTMENT OF NURSING & MIDWIFERY EDUCATION
Broomfield, Chelmsford, Essex, CM1 5LG
Tel: 0245 440761 x4213
STAFF: Ms M Purry HCO, M Wakeham MA ALA (Anglia Higher Education
          College - Faculty Library)
FOUNDED: 1981
TYPE: Midwifery, Nursing
HOURS: Mon, Tue, Thu, Fri 8.30-4.30, Wed 8.30-6.30
READERS: All nursing staff
STOCK POLICY: Journals discarded after 5 years, books after 10 years
LENDING: Books only. Photocopies provided
COMPUTER DATA RETRIEVAL: Access to DHSS, CINAHL & MEDLINE - free
HOLDINGS: 10,000 books; 33 journals, 32 current
CLASSIFICATION: NLM
BRANCHES: three
NETWORK: This library is part of Anglia Higher Education College

137
CHELTENHAM GENERAL HOSPITAL, POSTGRADUATE MEDICAL CENTRE
2 College Lawn, Cheltenham, Gloucestershire GL53 7AG
Tel: 0242 222222
STAFF: Mrs P Beck BSc DipLib (part time)
TYPE: Dental, Medical
HOURS: Mon-Fri 9-5 (staffed 18½ hours)
READERS: Staff and other users
STOCK POLICY: Books discarded after 10 years
LENDING: Books and journals. Photocopies provided
COMPUTER DATA RETRIEVAL : DATASTAR online - free
HOLDINGS: 1450 books; 80 journals, 72 current;Index Medicus 1983-7
          on microfilm
CLASSIFICATION: Own
SPECIAL COLLECTIONS: Surgery, General Practitioner
NETWORK: SWEHSLinC

138
GLOUCESTERSHIRE COLLEGE OF NURSING AND MIDWIFERY (ADULT BRANCH)
Nurse Education Centre, College Lawn, Cheltenham, GL53 7AN
Tel: 0242 222222 x3188
STAFF: Mrs MB Burgess HCO
FOUNDED: 1972
TYPE: Multidisciplinary
HOURS: Mon-Fri 8.30-4.30
READERS: Staff and other users
STOCK POLICY: Journals discarded after 15 years, books after 10
             years
LENDING: Books only. photocopies provided
HOLDINGS: approx 5,000 books; 34 journals, 32 current
CLASSIFICATION: RCN
BRANCHES: Foundation Branch at Gloucester, Adult Branch at
          Cheltenham
NETWORK: SWEHSLinC
Chester

139
WEST CHESHIRE POSTGRADUATE MEDICAL CENTRE
Countess of Chester Hospital, Liverpool Road, Chester CH2 1BQ
Tel: 0244 383676
STAFF: Mrs ER Fletcher C&G LibInfServCert, 1 part time staff
TYPE: Medical & dental
HOURS: Mon-Fri 9-8
READERS: Staff only
STOCK POLICY: Journals discarded after 15 years
LENDING: Books & journals to staff only. Photocopies provided
HOLDINGS: c2,500 books; 159 current journals
CLASSIFICATION: LC
NETWORK: Mersey Region

Chesterfield

140
EDUCATION CENTRE LIBRARY
Chesterfield and North Derbyshire Royal Hospital, Calow,
Chesterfield, Derbyshire S44 5BL
Tel: 0246 277271
STAFF: DJ Rogers ALA
FOUNDED: 1984
TYPE: Multidisciplinary
HOURS: 8.30-6.30 . Key available at other times
READERS: Staff, other users on application to librarian
STOCK POLICY: Books and journals discarded after 10 years
LENDING: Books , journals and videos. Photocopies provided
COMPUTER DATA RETRIEVAL: DATASTAR online - free
HOLDINGS: 6,000 books; 200 current journals; videotapes
                    (32 Betamax, 67 VHS)
CLASSIFICATION: NLM
NETWORK: SINTO

Chichester

141
CHICHESTER POSTGRADUATE MEDICAL CENTRE
Saint Richard's Hospital, Spitalfield Lane, Chichester,
    West Sussex PO19 4SE
Tel: 0243 788122 x8119
STAFF: M Roddham BA(Hons) ALA
TYPE: Multidisciplinary
HOURS: Mon-Fri 9-5
READERS: Staff only
STOCK POLICY: Books selectively discarded
LENDING: Books ,journals and A/V material. Photocopies provided
COMPUTER DATA RETRIEVAL: DATASTAR, DIALOG online - free
HOLDINGS: 4,500 books; 220 journals, 183 current; 10 tape/slides,
            50 videotapes (VHS)
CLASSIFICATION: NLM
PUBLICATION: District documents database; Union list of journals
NETWORK: SW Thames Regional Library and Information Service; SASLIC

142
WEST SUSSEX COLLEGE OF NURSE EDUCATION LIBRARY
Bishop Otter College, College Lane, Chichester, West Sussex
    PO19 4PE
Tel: 0243 787911 x281
STAFF: Miss D Matrunola BLib ALA
TYPE: Nursing
HOURS: Mon-Thu 9-9, Fri 9-5.30, Sat 9.30-12.30 (Vacations Mon-Fri
    9-5)
READERS: Staff and other users
LENDING: Books, videodiscs only. Photocopies provided
COMPUTER DATA RETRIEVAL: DIALOG online - free. PRESTEL available
HOLDINGS: approx 9,000 books; 2,000 journals, 65 current;
            tape/slides, videotapes (VHS)
CLASSIFICATION: DDC

Chilton

143
MEDICAL RESEARCH COUNCIL, RADIOBIOLOGY UNIT
Chilton, Didcot, Oxon OX11 0RD
Tel:0235 834393   Fax: 0235 834918
STAFF: Mrs MJ Bulman ALA
FOUNDED: 1947
TYPE: Medical
HOURS: Mon-Thurs 8.30-5, Fri 8.30-4
READERS: Staff, other users at discretion of Librarian
STOCK POLICY: Superseded editions of books discarded.
Journals discarded as research emphasis changes
LENDING: Books and journals. Photocopies provided
COMPUTER DATA RETRIEVAL: DATASTAR, BLAISE online - free.
HOLDINGS: 5,000 books; 130 current journals
CLASSIFICATION: UDC
PUBLICATION: Accession list
NETWORK: Medical Research Council

Clonmel

144
SAINT JOSEPH'S HOSPITAL
Clonmel, Co Tipperary, Republic of Ireland
Tel: 010 353 52 21900
STAFF: Dr R Howard(Honorary Librarian)
TYPE: Medical
HOURS: Mon-Fri 9-10
READERS: Staff only
LENDING: Books only
HOLDINGS: 200 books, 35 bound journals; 20 current journals

Colchester

145
COLCHESTER POSTGRADUATE MEDICAL CENTRE
Essex County Hospital, Lexden Road, Colchester, Essex, CO3 3NB
Tel: 0206 853535 x4542
STAFF: Mrs M Parkinson (part-time)
FOUNDED: 1969
TYPE: Multidisciplinary
HOURS: Mon-Fri 9-9 Staffed Mon-Fri 1-5
READERS: Staff, other users on application
STOCK POLICY: Books and journals not discarded
LENDING: Books and journals. Photocopies provided
COMPUTER DATA RETRIEVAL: Access to DATASTAR - free
HOLDINGS: 1,000 books; 74 journals. 46 current
CLASSIFICATION: NLM
NETWORK: North East Thames Regional Library Service

51

146
SEVERALLS HOSPITAL , MEDICAL LIBRARY
Boxted Road, Colchester CO4 5HG
Tel: 0206 852271 x8607
STAFF: Mrs S Luck
TYPE: Psychiatric
HOURS: Mon, Tue, Wed, Fri 1.30-4, Thu 10-12.30
READERS: Staff only
HOLDINGS: 100 books; 14 journals
CLASSIFICATION: NLM
NETWORK: North East Thames Regional Library Service

Consett

147
SHOTLEY BRIDGE GENERAL HOSPITAL, POSTGRADUATE MEDICAL EDUCATION
   CENTRE LIBRARY
Consett, Co Durham DH8 0NB
Tel: 0207 503456
STAFF: Mrs FM Harris
FOUNDED: 1968
TYPE: Multidisciplinary
HOURS: Mon-Fri 8.30-5
READERS: Staff only
STOCK POLICY: Stock discarded when no furthur space available
LENDING: Books only. Photocopies provided
HOLDINGS: 1,391 books, papers, symposiums; 93 journals, 68 current
         titles
NETWORK: Northern Regional Health Libraries Association

Coulsdon

148
CANE HILL HOSPITAL, MEDICAL & PROFESSIONAL LIBRARY
Coulsdon, Surrey CR3 3YL
Tel; 07375 52221 x1
STAFF: Mrs S Tarbox ALA (part-time)
FOUNDED: 1977
TYPE: Multidisciplinary
HOURS: Always open (key system). Staffed Mon- Ws 9.30-3.30
READERS: Medical staff and heads of departments
STOCK POLICY: Books discarded after 15 years
LENDING: Books and AV material only. Photocopies provided
COMPUTER DATA RETRIEVAL: DATASTAR online - free
HOLDINGS: 1550 books; 40 journals, 35 current
CLASSIFICATION: NLM
PUBLICATION: Monthly bulletin
NETWORK: SE Thames Regional Library and Information Service; PLCS

149
NETHERNE HOSPITAL PROFESSIONAL LIBRARY
Netherne Hospital, Coulsdon, Surrey CR3 1YE
Tel: 07375 56700
STAFF: Ms B Hartley BA DipLib (part-time)
TYPE: Multidisciplinary
HOURS: Mon-Fri 9-5.
READERS: Staff and other users
STOCK POLICY: Books discarded after 10 years. Journals discarded
            selectively
LENDING: Books, journals and AV material. Photocopies provided
COMPUTER DATA RETRIEVAL: Access to DATASTAR online - free
HOLDINGS: 7,000 books; 60 journals, 40 current
CLASSIFICATION: NLM
PUBLICATIONS: Accessions lists; library guide
NETWORK: SW Thames Regional Library and Information Service

Coventry

150
COVENTRY SCHOOL OF NURSING
Walsgrave Hospital, Clifford Bridge Road, Coventry CV2 2DX
Tel: 0203 602020
STAFF: DA Guest, BA(Hons)
TYPE: Midwifery, Nursing
HOURS: Mon-Fri 8.30-4.30
READERS: Staff and other users
STOCK POLICY: Books discarded after 15 years
LENDING: Books and AV material only
HOLDINGS: 8,000 books; 30 journals, 28 current; 30 tape/slides,
                300 videotapes(VHS)
CLASSIFICATION: GNC
PUBLICATION: Guide to Literature Searching
NETWORK: West Midlands Regional Libraries

151
WARWICKSHIRE POSTGRADUATE MEDICAL CENTRE LIBRARY
Walsgrave Hospital, Clifford Bridge Road, Coventry CV2 2DX
Tel: 0203 602020 x8455
STAFF: Miss EM Edward BA ALA (part-time)
FOUNDED: 1988
TYPE: Multidisciplinary
HOURS: Mon-Fri 9-5
READERS: Medical staff if Members of PGMC and University of Warwick
STOCK POLICY: Out of date books discarded
LENDING: Books, tapes and slides only. Photocopies provided
COMPUTER DATA RETRIEVAL: Inhouse online terminal. Free
HOLDINGS: 2,500 books; 129 journals, 117 current; 15 tape/slides,
                50 35 mm slides
CLASSIFICATION: DDC, Own for psychiatry
PUBLICATIONS: Information leaflet, Newsletter
NETWORK: West Midland Regional Health Libraries; CADIG
BRANCH: Walsgrave Hospital Psychiatric Unit, Coventry

152
WARWICKSHIRE POSTGRADUATE MEDICAL CENTRE
Sir John Black Library, Stoney Stanton Road, Coventry, CV1 4FG
Tel: 0203 844120
STAFF: Miss EM Edward BA ALA (part-time) , Mrs J Wilkinson
FOUNDED: 1951
TYPE: Multidisciplinary
HOURS: Mon-Thurs 9-8, Fri 9-5, Sat 10-1
READERS: Medical staff if Members of PGMC and University of Warwick
LENDING: Books, tapes & slides only. Photocopies provided
COMPUTER DATA RETRIEVAL: DATASTAR online - free
HOLDINGS: 3,000 books; 92 journals, 61 current; 9,000 35mm slides,
           microscope slides, 6 videotapes (VHS)
CLASSIFICATION: DDC
NETWORK: West Midlands Regional Health Libraries; CADIG

Crewe

152
SOUTH CHESTER POSTGRADUATE MEDICAL CENTRE
Leighton Hospital, Middlewich Road, Crewe, Cheshire CW1 4QJ
Tel: 0270 255141 x2701
STAFF: Dr CS Hopkins (Honorary Librarian), Mrs GM Newall
       (Secretary/Librarian)
TYPE: Multidisciplinary
HOURS: Mon-Fri 8.30-5. Access available at all other times
READERS: Staff only
STOCK POLICY: Duplicate and unbound pre-1975 journals discarded
LENDING: Books and journals
HOLDINGS: c2.100 books; 94 current journals
CLASSIFICATION: Own
NETWORK: Mersey region; NORWHSLA

Crowthorne

154
BROADMOOR HOSPITAL STAFF LIBRARY
Broadmoor Hospital, Crowthorne, Berkshire RG11 7EG
Tel: 0344 773111 x4404/4400
STAFF: Mrs A Farrar ALA, Mrs J Phillips BA ALA (part time)
FOUNDED: 1975
TYPE: Multidisciplinary
HOURS: Mon-Fri 9-5
READERS: Staff, other users on application to Librarian
STOCK POLICY: Out of date editions of books discarded
LENDING: Books only. Photocopies provided
HOLDINGS: 7,000 books; 81 journals, 45 current; reprint collection;
           60 tape/slides
SPECIAL COLLECTIONS: Forensic psychiatry (275 vols)
CLASSIFICATION: DDC 19 (modified)
PUBLICATION: Monthly new books list
NETWORK: In co-operation with Oxford Region Library and
Information Service

155
CROYDON HEALTH EDUCATION LIBRARY
12-18 Lennard Road, Croydon, Surrey CR9 2RS
Tel: 081 680 2008 x263
STAFF: Mrs C Court BA (part time), Ms S Barnabas ALA
TYPE: Health education
HOURS: Mon 9-1, 1.30-3.30, Tue-Fri 9-1, 1.30-5
READERS: Staff and other users
STOCK POLICY: Out of date books discarded, journals discarded
                after 4 years
LENDING: Books, journals and teaching packs. Limited photocopying
HOLDINGS: 3,500 books; 40 current journals, 45 current Newsletters
SPECIAL COLLECTION: Teaching Packs (c180)
NETWORK: SW Thames Regional Library and Information Service;
            Croyden Health Information Providers (CHIPs)

156
CROYDON MEDICAL LIBRARY
Mayday Hospital, Mayday Road, Thornton Heath, Surrey CR4 8PA
Tel: 081 684 6999 x3272
STAFF: Miss PH Gaze BSc MSc ALA
FOUNDED: 1976
TYPE: Medical
HOURS: Mon-Fri 9-5.
READERS: Staff only
STOCK POLICY: Journals selectively discarded, books after 10 years
LENDING: Books and journals. photocopies provided
COMPUTER FACILITIES: DATASTAR online. Free
HOLDINGS: approx 2,000 books; 85 journals, 80 current;
            20 videotapes (VHS)
CLASSIFICATION: NLM
PUBLICATION: Introductory guide
BRANCHES: Saint Lawrence's Hospital, Caterham; Warlingham
 Park Hospital, Warlingham
NETWORKS: SW Thames Regional Library & Information Service;
            Croydon Health Information Providers (CHIPS)

Cupar

157
STRATHEDEN HOSPITAL MEDICAL LIBRARY
Cupar, Fife KY15 5RR
Tel: 0334 52611
STAFF: Ms C Sclater DipLib MIInfSc
TYPE: Psychiatric
HOURS: Staffed Tue-Thur 1-5
READERS: Medical staff only.
STOCK POLICY: Books discarded
LENDING: Books and journals. Photocopies provided
COMPUTER DATA RETRIEVAL: Access to DATASTAR and PRESTEL
HOLDINGS: 600 books; 70 journals, 50 current
NETWORK: ASHSL

158
RHÖNE - POULENC LIMITED
Rainham Rd South, Dagenham, Essex RM10 7XS
Tel: 081 592 3060 x2493   Fax: 081 593 2304
STAFF: Mrs E Elliott-Jay BA MIInfSc ALA, AG Clarke
TYPE: Pharmaceutical
HOURS: Mon-Fri 9-1, 2-5.30
READERS: Staff, bona fide enquirers by prior arrangement
STOCK POLICY: Out of date books and journals discarded
LENDING: Books, journals within organization only.
COMPUTER DATA RETRIEVAL: DIALOG, PROFILE, PFDS online - free
    CD-ROM: From 1989 for end users
HOLDINGS: 15,000 books; 450 current journals
SPECIAL COLLECTIONS: Papers by staff
CLASSIFICATION: UDC
PUBLICATIONS: Periodical holdings; Book acquisitions,
  various leaflets

Darlington

159
MEMORIAL HOSPITAL POSTGRADUATE MEDICAL EDUCATION CENTRE
Hollyhurst Road, Darlington, Co Durham DL3 6HX
Tel: 0325 380100
Mrs B Mais ALA, Mrs M Vasarheiyl ALA (part-time)
TYPE: Medical, psychiatric
HOURS: Always open. Staffed Mon-Fri 9.30-12.15, 1-5.15
READERS: Staff and other users
STOCK POLICY: Out of date books and ephemeral material discarded
LENDING: Books and journals
COMPUTER DATA RETRIEVAL: In-house terminal. Charged computer
                time only.   PRESTEL available
HOLDINGS: 2,000 books, 570 bound journals; 100 current journals
                Tape/slides, videotapes (U-matic)
SPECIAL COLLECTION: Psychiatry
CLASSIFICATION: DDC
PUBLICATION: Darlington postgraduate journal
NETWORK: Northern Regional Association of Health Service
  Librarians

Dartford

160
NORTH-WEST KENT POSTGRADUATE MEDICAL LIBRARY
Joyce Green Hospital, Dartford, Kent DA1 5PL
Tel: 0322 27242 x242/423
STAFF: Mrs CA Smith

TYPE: Multidisciplinary
HOURS: Mon-Fri 9-5. Key available after hours
READERS: Staff only
STOCK POLICY: Books discarded after 5 years
LENDING: Books and journals. Photocopies provided
COMPUTER DATA RETRIEVAL: DATASTAR online - free
HOLDINGS: 3,000 books; 160 journals, 130 current; tape/slides,
          20 videotapes (VHS)
CLASSIFICATION: NLM
PUBLICATIONS: 3 Current awareness bulletins; Library guide
NETWORK: SE Thames Regional Library and Information Service
BRANCHES: Gravesend and North Kent Hospital;
  Stone House Hospital, Dartford; West Hill Hospital, Dartford

Derby

161
DERBY CITY HOSPITAL MEDICAL LIBRARY
Uttoxeter Road, Derby DE3 3NE
Tel: 0332 40131
STAFF: Mrs JH Padmore BA MA ALA
TYPE: Medical
HOURS: Mon-Sun 7.00-midnight (Staffed Mon-Fri 9-5)
READERS: Medical and paramedical
STOCK POLICY: Books discarded after 10 years
LENDING: Books and journals. Photocopies provided
HOLDINGS: 1,500 books; 82 journals, 42 current titles
CLASSIFICATION: NLM

162
DERBY SCHOOL OF NURSING
Derbyshire Royal Infirmary, London Road, Derby DE1 2QY
Tel: 0332 47141 x2561
STAFF: Mrs C James BA ALA (part time)
FOUNDED: 1976
TYPE: Nursing
HOURS: Mon-Thurs 8.30-5, Fri 8.30-4
READERS: Only nurses in Health Authority
STOCK POLICY: Some books over 10 years old discarded
LENDING: Books only. Photocopies provided
HOLDINGS: c6,500 books; 42 journals 32 current titles; 50 tape/
  slides, 2,000 35mm slides, videotapes (20 U-matic, 50 VHS)
CLASSIFICATION: RCN
PUBLICATION: Monthly bulletin
BRANCHES: School of Nursing, Rykneld; School of Nursing,
                    Derbyshire Children's Hospital, Derby
NETWORK: Union list of nursing journals; TRAHCLIS

163
DERBY SCHOOL OF OCCUPATIONAL THERAPY
Highfield, 403 Burton Road, Derby DE3 6AN
Tel: 0332 43051
STAFF: Mrs K Carter BA ALA
TYPE: Paramedical
HOURS: Mon-Fri 9-5
READERS: Staff and students, other users by arrangement
STOCK POLICY: Out of date editions of books discarded
LENDING: Books only. Photocopies provided
HOLDINGS: 7,7500 books; 52 journals, 45 current titles;
                20 Tape/slides, 100 videotapes (VHS)
CLASSIFICATION: Own
PUBLICATIONS: Recent Additions List ; Library Guide
NETWORK: TRAHCLIS

164
DERBYSHIRE ROYAL INFIRMARY
District Medical Library, London Road, Derby DE1 2QY
Tel: 0332 47141 x2617
STAFF: Miss C Hough BA MA DipLib ALA
FOUNDED: 1974
TYPE: Medical
HOURS: 7.00 am-midnight. Staffed Mon-Fri 9-5
READERS: Staff only
STOCK POLICY: Books discarded
LENDING: Books and journals. Photocopies provided
HOLDINGS: 4,000 books; 200 journals, 125 current titles
CLASSIFICATION: NLM
PUBLICATIONS: Recent additions list; library guide
BRANCHES: Derby City Hospital, Derby; Derbyshire Childrens
 Hospital, Derby

Dewsbury

165
DEWSBURY POSTGRADUATE MEDICAL CENTRE
Dewsbury General Hospital, Moorlands Road, Dewsbury, West
 Yorkshire WF13 2LE
Tel: 0924 465111 x2283/2285
STAFF: K Conway BA ALA
FOUNDED: 1973
TYPE: Multidisciplinary
HOURS: Mon-Fri 9-5. Key available at other times
READERS: Staff and other users
LENDING: Books, journals and AV material. Photocopies provided
COMPUTER DATA RETRIEVAL: DATASTAR online - free
HOLDINGS: 6,500 books; 150 current journals; c2000 35mm slides,
                c200 other items
CLASSIFICATION: NLM
PUBLICATIONS: Accessions lists; Postgraduate bulletin
NETWORK: Yorkshire Joint Medical Library Service

166
DONCASTER ROYAL INFIRMARY, DEPARTMENT OF NURSE EDUCATION LIBRARY
C Block, Doncaster Royal Infirmary, Doncaster, South Yorkshire
  DN2 5LT
Tel: 0302 366666 x496
STAFF: Mrs B Johnson ALA
FOUNDED: 1986
TYPE: Multidisciplinary
HOURS: Mon-Thu 9-4.30, Fri 9-3.30
READERS: Staff only
STOCK POLICY: Journals discarded after 10 or 15 years, books after
              10 years
LENDING: Books, journals, AV material. Photocopies provided
COMPUTER DATA RETRIEVAL: In-house terminal. PRESTEL via Doncaster
                         Central Library
HOLDINGS: 6,500 books; 52 current journals; videotapes (VHS),
          Educational computer software models
CLASSIFICATION: NLM modified
PUBLICATIONS: Library guide
BRANCH: Nurse Teaching Unit, Loversall Hospital
NETWORKS: Yorkshire Joint Medical Library service; TRAHCLIS

167
DONCASTER ROYAL INFIRMARY, MEDICAL AND PROFESSIONAL LIBRARY
Armthorpe Road, Doncaster, South Yorkshire DN2 5LT
Tel: 0302 366666 x650
STAFF: Miss ME Evans ALA, 1 other (part time) staff
FOUNDED: 1968
TYPE: Multidisciplinary
HOURS: Mon-Fri 9-5. Key available at other times
READERS: Staff only.
STOCK POLICY: Books and journals discarded after 10-15 years
LENDING: Books and journals. Photocopies provided
COMPUTER DATA RETRIEVAL: DATASTAR online - free
HOLDINGS: 11,500 books; 172 current journals
CLASSIFICATION: NLM modified
PUBLICATION: Recent additions list; Library Guide
NETWORK: TRAHCLIS; Yorkshire Joint Medical Library Service

Dorchester

168
WEST DORSET HEALTH AUTHORITY POSTGRADUATE MEDICAL CENTRE
Dorset County Hospital, Princes Street, Dorchester, Dorset,
 DT2 7SE
Tel: 0305 263123
STAFF: Mrs AM Rampersad BA ALA LMIPP AMBPS, 1 other (full-time) and
               1 (part-time) staff
FOUNDED: 1967
TYPE: Multidisciplinary
HOURS: Staffed Mon-Fri 9-5 - can be used at other times
READERS: Staff, other users by arrangement
STOCK POLICY: Some books and journals discarded after 12-15 years
LENDING: Books, journals and AV material. Photocopies provided
COMPUTER DATA RETRIEVAL: Access to DATASTAR
HOLDINGS: c11,000 books; 130 journals, 103 current titles; c100
                   tape/slides, 2 videotapes (VHS)
CLASSIFICATION: NLM
PUBLICATIONS: Annual report
BRANCH: Herrison Hospital, Dorchester and small collections
                 elsewhere
NETWORK: WRLIS

Douglas

169
C.S. PANTIN MEMORIAL LIBRARY
Isle of Man Postgraduate Medical Centre, Noble's Hospital,
 Westmoreland Road, Douglas, Isle of Man
Tel: 0624 25516
STAFF: Mrs BA Jones
FOUNDED: 1968
TYPE: Multidisciplinary
HOURS: Always open
READERS: Staff only
STOCK POLICY: No stock discarded
LENDING: Books only
COMPUTER DATA RETRIEVAL: Access to terminal.
HOLDINGS: 2,000 books; 100 journals, 68 current titles;
          41 sets 35mm slides, videotapes
SPECIAL COLLECTION: The Barber-Lomax collection (history of
 medicine) (150 vols)
CLASSIFICATION: DDC

Droitwich

170
DROITWICH CENTRE FOR RHEUMATIC DISEASES
Highfield Hospital, Worcester Road, Droitwich, Worcs., WR9 8AP
Tel: 0905 794455
STAFF: Ms RM Clayton (part-time)
TYPE: Multidisciplinary
HOURS: Mon-Fri 9-5
READERS: Staff only
HOLDINGS: 530 books, 9 current journals
CLASSIFICATION: Own

Dublin

171
DUBLIN DENTAL HOSPITAL LIBRARY
Dunlop/Oriel House, Lincoln Place, Dublin 2, Republic of Ireland
Tel: 0001 794311 x205
STAFF: Ms AM O'Byrne DipInfStud
FOUNDED: 1968
TYPE: Medical, dental
HOURS: Mon-Fri 10-1, 2-5, 6-10, Sat 10-12.30 (term time),
 Mon-Fri 10-1, 2-5 (vacations)
READERS: Staff, others on written request to librarian
STOCK POLICY: No stock discarded
LENDING: No lendin. Photocopies provided (3LL system of payment)
COMPUTER DATA RETRIEVAL: Access to Medline only.
HOLDINGS: 12,500 books; 3,250 journals, 70 current; In process
         of acquiring AV facilities
SPECIAL COLLECTION: Sheldon Friel Memoralia (journal articles only)
CLASSIFICATION: Black's Medical and Dental classification
PUBLICATIONS: Library guide; Recent additions ; Current contents
         awareness service
NETWORK: SHIRL

172
MATER HOSPITAL MEDICAL LIBRARY
Eccles Street, Dublin 7, Republic of Ireland
Tel: 0001 301122 x312
STAFF: Miss P McCarthy, Sr de Lourdes Carney (part time)
FOUNDED: 1950s
TYPE: Multidisciplinary
HOURS: Staffed Mon-Fri 9-5. Reading room open 5-10
READERS: Staff only
STOCK POLICY: Books and journals discarded after 5 years
LENDING: Journals lent. Photocopies provided
COMPUTER DATA RETRIEVAL: Access to terminal. CD-ROM from1990
HOLDINGS: 662books; 44 journals; 103 audiotapes

173
ROYAL COLLEGE OF SURGEONS IN IRELAND
123 Saint Stephen's Green, Dublin 2, Republic of Ireland
Tel: 0001 780200 x248   Telex 30795 RCSI EI   Fax: 0001 780934
STAFF: Miss BM Doran BA DipLib, H Brazier MA DipLib ALA,
   Mrs KM Bishop BA
FOUNDED: 1784
TYPE: Medical, nursing, surgical
HOURS: Mon-Fri 9am-9.45pm, Sat 9-1245 (term),Mon-Fri 9-5 (vacation)
READRS: Staff, students and other users
STOCK POLICY: Out of date editions of textbooks discarded
LENDING: Books, videos, sudio tapes. Photocopies provided
COMPUTER DATA RETRIEVAL: DATASTAR, DIALOG online. Charged computer
            time only
HOLDINGS: 50,000 books; 800 journals, 500 current;
            1500 35mm slides, 50 tape/slides, 220 videotapes (VHS)
CLASSIFICATION: DDC
SPECIAL COLLECTIONS: Arthur Jacob Library (3,000 vols);
  Butcher-Wheeler Library (500 vols); William Doolin (380
  vols); Logan collection (500 vols); medical instruments
PUBLICATIONS: Library guides; Recent acquisitions; Periodicals list

174
SAINT VINCENT'S HOSPITAL MEDICAL LIBRARY
Elm Park, Dublin 4, Republic of Ireland
Tel: 0001 839444 x210
STAFF: Mrs HJ Beckett MA DipLIS ALAI, Ms G Doyle BA DipLIS
          (part time)
FOUNDED: 1970
TYPE: Medical, Nursing, Paramedical
HOURS: Mon-Fri 9.15-5.15, Mon, Tue, Wed until 9pm
READERS: Staff and other users
STOCK POLICY: Books discarded after 10 years
LENDING: Books, tape/slides, videos only. photocopies provided
COMPUTER DATA RETRIEVAL: BLAISE online. Charged computer time only
HOLDINGS: c 2,000 books; 73 journals, 66 current; 434 tapes,
           1484 slides, videotapes (6 U-matic, 58 VHS)
CLASSIFICATION: DDC
PUBLICATION: Library News

175
UNIVERSITY COLLEGE DUBLIN LIBRARY
Earlsfort Terrace, Dublin 2, Republic of Ireland
Tel: 0001 693244
STAFF: Ms S Murphy BA DipLib, P Murphy BA MLIS, Miss M
  Grace BA DipLib, Mrs M O'Sullivan MA (part-time), 8 other
  (full-time), 6 (part-time) staff
TYPE: Multidisciplinary
HOURS: Mon-Fri 9.30-10 (long vacation 9.30-5.30) Sat 9.30-1
READERS: Staff and other users
STOCK POLICY: Stock discarded ocassionaly
LENDING: Books only. photocopies provided
COMPUTER DATA RETRIEVAL: DIALOG, ESA, ORBIT online - non UCD

staff or students charged
HOLDINGS: 30,000 books, 27,000 bound journals; 1,150 current
titles;microfilms, tape/slides, VHS videotapes
CLASSIFICATION: DDC and UDC (Engineering only)
PUBLICATIONS: Library guides, accessions lists

176
UNIVERSITY COLLEGE DUBLIN, VETERINARY MEDICINE LIBRARY
Veterinary College, Ballsbridge, Dublin 4, Republic of Ireland
Tel: 0001 687988   Fax: 0001 687878
STAFF: Mrs M McErlean BComm DipLib, Mrs A Hastings BA DipLib,
Mrs E Doherty BA DipLibInfSt, DipInfSt
FOUNDED: 1968
TYPE: Veterinary science and related disciplines
HOURS: Mon-Fri 9.30-9.30, Sat 9.30-12.30 (term time), Mon-Fri
9.30-5.30 (long vacation)
READERS: Staff and other users.
STOCK POLICY: No stock discarded
LENDING: Books only. Photocopies provided
COMPUTER DATA RETRIEVAL: DIALOG, ESA online - charged computer
time plus handling charge
HOLDINGS: 15,000 books; 670 journals, 490 current titles;
Tape/slides, videotapes (U-matic and VHS)
CLASSIFICATION: DDC
PUBLICATIONS: Library guides; accessions bulletins

Dudley

177
DUDLEY AND STOURBRIDGE SCHOOL OF NURSING
Guest Hospital, Tipton Road, Dudley, West Midlands DY1 4SE
Tel: 0384 56966 x359
STAFF: Mrs G Williamson (part-time)
TYPE: Nursing
HOURS: Open Mon-Fri 9-4.30. Staffed Mon-Fri 9-1
READERS: Nursing staff
LENDING: Books only
HOLDINGS: 6,000 books; 20 current journals. 35mm slides,
videotapes (U-matic)
CLASSIFICATION: RCN
BRANCHES: Corbett School of Nursing, Stourbridge
NETWORK: West Midlands Regional Health Libraries

178
DUDLEY HEALTH AUTHORITY, LIBRARY INFORMATION ROOM
12 Bull Street, Dudley, West Midlands, DY1v 2DD
Tel: 0384 56911 x248
STAFF: I McGregor (Information Officer), Mrs L Peeler (Statistics
Officer)
TYPE: Health administration
HOURS: Mon-Fri 8.45-5
READERS: NHS District staff
COMPUTER DATA RETRIEVAL: In-house terminal
HOLDINGS: 2,000 books; 20 current journals

179
RUSSELLS HALL HOSPITAL MULTIDISCIPLINARY LIBRARY
Busheyfields Road, Dudley, West Midlands DY1 2HQ
Tel: 0384 456111
STAFF: Mrs BA Bolton ALA (part-time)
FOUNDED: 1985
TYPE: Multidisciplinary
HOURS: 9-5
READERS: All staff in Health District, other health professionals for
         reference upon application
STOCK POLICY: Books discarded after 10 years
LENDING: Books and AV material only. Photocopies provided
COMPUTER DATA RETRIEVAL: Access to terminal
HOLDINGS: 3,000 books; 67 current journals; 26 videotapes (VHS)
CLASSIFICATION: NLM
SPECIAL COLLECTION: ENB course reference books
PUBLICATIONS: 3 current awareness bulletins; Accessions list
NETWORK: West Midland Region

Dumfries

180
DUMFRIES AND GALLOWAY COLLEGE OF NURSING AND MIDWIFERY
Crichton Hall, Glencaple Road, Dumfries DG1 4TG
Tel: 0387 55301
STAFF: Ms J Anderson MA DpH-WU ALA
TYPE: Midwifery, Nursing
HOURS: Mon-Thurs 8.30-5, Fri 8.30-4.30
READERS: Nurses working for Health Board
STOCK POLICY: Stock discarded
LENDING: Books , some AV material only. Photocopies provided
HOLDINGS: 8,000 books; 60 journals; 40 tape/slides, 40 computer
           discs, 12 35mm slides, videotapes (125 U-matic, 75 VHS)
CLASSIFICATION: DDC
PUBLICATIONS: Library bulletin; Library guide

181
DUMFRIES & GALLOWAY ROYAL INFIRMARY , MEDICAL LIBRARY
Bankend Road, Dumfries, DG1 4AF
Tel: 0387 53151
STAFF: Dr JR Lawrence (Honorary Librarian), Miss AP Glencross
FOUNDED: 1975
TYPE: Multidisciplinary
HOURS: Mon-Fri 9-5.15
READERS: Staff, other users by arrangement
STOCK POLICY: No stock discarded
LENDING: Books and journals. Photocopies provided
COMPUTER DATA RETRIEVAL: Access to terminal. PRESTEL available
HOLDINGS: 80 journals; 20 35mm slide sets, 12 videotapes (VHS)
CLASSIFICATION: Barnard

182
DUNDEE AND ANGUS COLLEGE OF NURSING AND MIDWIFERY
Ninewells Hospital, Ninewells, Dundee DD1 9SY
Tel: 0382 60111 x2012
STAFF: N Sandeman MA(Hons) DipLib ALA, Mrs Phyllis McGurk BA DipLib
    (part-time)
FOUNDED: 1967
TYPE: Midwifery, Nursing
HOURS: Mon-Thurs 8.30-5, Fri 8.30-4
READERS: Staff and other users
STOCK POLICY: Books and journals discarded at various times
LENDING: Books only. photocopies provided
HOLDINGS: Approx 15,000 books; 79 journals, 61 current;
           153 Tape/slides, 750 35mm slides
CLASSIFICATION: DDC modified
PUBLICATIONS: Accessions list
BRANCHES: Stracathro Hospital, Brechin; Sunnyside Hospital,
              Montrose

183
UNIVERSITY OF DUNDEE, NINEWELLS MEDICAL LIBRARY
Ninewells Hospital and Medical School, Dundee, DD1 9SY
Tel: 0382 60111 x2515/2519
  Electronic mail: Library G UK.AC.DUNDEE.PRIMEB
STAFF: DA Orrock MA, Mrs MJ Franklin BSc MSc ALA (part time)
FOUNDED: 1974
TYPE: Multidisciplinary
HOURS: Mon-Fri 9-10, Sat 9-12 (long vacation Mon-Fri 9-5)
READERS: University and Tayside HB, other users by subscription
STOCK POLICY: No stock discarded
LENDING: Books , journals normally overnight only, photocopies
             provided by arrangement
COMPUTER DATA RETRIEVAL: DIALOG online. Charged
    CD-ROM: Medline from 1982 for end users
HOLDINGS: 22,000 books; c2,000journals, c574 current
CLASSIFICATION: NLM modified

Dunfermline
184
DUNFERMLINE AND WEST FIFE HOSPITAL POSTGRADUATE MEDICAL
 CENTRE
Reid Street, Dunfermline, Fife KY12 7EZ
Tel: 0383 737777
STAFF: Ms MC Smith BA ALA, Ms I Cowan
TYPE: Medical
HOURS: Always open
READERS: Staff, and other users
STOCK POLICY: Books and journals discarded at varying periods
LENDING: Books only. Photocopies provided
COMPUTER DATA RETRIEVAL: DATASTAR online - charged
HOLDINGS: 1,077 books: 64 journals, 43 current titles; 150
             cassettes, 12 videotapes (VHS)
CLASSIFICATION: Own
NETWORK: ASHSL

185
LYNEBANK HOSPITAL MEDICAL LIBRARY
Halbeath Road, Dunfermline, Fife KY11 4UW
Tel: 0383 737777
STAFF: Ms C Sclater DipLib MIInfSc (part-time)
TYPE: Mental handicap, psychiatric
HOURS: Always open. Staffed one afternoon per week
READERS: Medical staff and other users
LENDING: Books only. Photocopies provided
COMPUTER DATA RETRIEVAL: Access to DATASTAR, PRESTEL
HOLDINGS: 220 books; 30 current journals
SPECIAL COLLECTION: Mental handicap
CLASSIFICATION: NLM
NETWORK: ASHSL

East Grinstead

186
QUEEN VICTORIA HOSPITAL MEDICAL LIBRARY
Holtye Road, East Grinstead, West Sussex RH19 3DZ
Tel: 0342 410210
STAFF: Mrs C Beddard (part-time)
FOUNDED: 1946
TYPE: Medical
HOURS: Mon-Fri 9.30-1
READERS: Staff only
STOCK POLICY: Books and journals discarded
LENDING: Books and journals. Photocopies provided
COMPUTER DATA RETRIEVAL: DATASTAR online - free
HOLDINGS: 900 books; 52 journals, 50 current
CLASSIFICATION: NLM
NETWORK: South East Thames interlending scheme

Eastbourne

187
BURLEY MEDICAL LIBRARY
Eastbourne Postgraduate Medical Centre, District General
 Hospital, Kings Drive, Eastbourne, East Sussex BN21 2UD
Tel: 0323 21351 x4047
STAFF: Mrs J Blackburn BA PGCE DipLib (part-time)
FOUNDED: 1966
TYPE: Medical, psychiatric
HOURS: Always open. Staffed Mon-Thurs 9-5, Fri 9-3
READERS: Staff, other users with prior permission
LENDING: Books, back issues of journals . Photocopies provided
COMPUTER DATA RETRIEVAL: Access to DATASTAR online - free

HOLDINGS: (including Psychiatric library) 4225 books; 142 journals,
            106 current titles; 70 videotapes (VHS)
CLASSIFICATION: NLM
BRANCH: Psychiatric library, Dept of Psychiatry
NETWORK: SE Thames Regional Library and Information Service
Eastbourne (cont)

188
RORER HEALTH CARE LTD
Saint Leonard's Road, Eastbourne, East Sussex, BN20 8DL
Tel: 0323 21422   Telex 878205 RORER G   Fax: 0323 411606
STAFF: Miss J Edwards BA(Hons) DipPA (Information Officer)
FOUNDED: 1980
TYPE: PHARMACEUTICAL
HOURS: Mon-Fri 8.45-5.15 (Fridays 4)
READERS: Staff only
STOCK POLICY: Stock discarded according to space
LENDING: Books only. Photocopies provided
COMPUTER DATA RETRIEVAL: Online databases: DATASTAR, BLAISE,
            DIALOG, QUESTEL, IMSMARQ, DEPENDS
HOLDINGS: 400- 500 books ; 80-90 current journals
CLASSIFICATION: Own
SPECIAL COLLECTION: In-house database of over 8,000 papers
CLASSIFICATION: NLM

189
SUSSEX DOWNS SCHOOL OF NURSING LIBRARY
District General Hospital, Kings Drive, Eastbourne, East
 Sussex BN21 2UD
Tel: 0323 21351 x4048
STAFF: Ms S Hardwick BA DipLib ALA (District Librarian)
FOUNDED: 1976
TYPE: Nursing
HOURS: Mon, Tue, Thu 8.30-5, Wed 8.30-8, Fri 8.30-4.30
READERS: Staff only.
STOCK POLICY: Books discarded after 10 years
LENDING: Books only. Photocopies provided
COMPUTER DATA RETRIEVAL: DATASTAR online - free
HOLDINGS: 5,000 books; 40 current journals
CLASSIFICATION: NLM
BRANCH: Psychiatric library, Hellingly Hospital, Hailsham
NETWORK: SE Thames Regional Library and Information Service

Edgware

190
BARNET DEPARTMENT OF NURSING STUDIES
Edgware General Hospital, Edgware, Middlesex HA8 0AD
Tel: 081 952 2381 x605
No furthur information available

191
EDGWARE GENERAL HOSPITAL POSTGRADUATE MEDICAL CENTRE
Edgware, Middlesex HA8 0AD
Tel: 081 952 2381
STAFF: Mrs E Packter
TYPE: Multidisciplinary
HOURS: Mon-Fri 9-5. Key available after hours
READERS: Staff, local GP's, health visitors, social workers
STOCK POLICY: Books over 10 years old, journals over 15
 years old discarded
LENDING: Books only
COMPUTER DATA RETRIEVAL: Access to terminal. Free/charged
 depending on enquirer
HOLDINGS: 900 books, 2,200 bound journals; 96 current
 journals
CLASSIFICATION: NLM

Edinburgh

192
ANIMAL DISEASES RESEARCH ASSOCIATION
Moredun Research Institute, 408 Gilmerton Road, Edinburgh, EH17 7JH
Tel: 031 664 3262
STAFF: Ms D Donaldson BSc MSc MIInfSc
FOUNDED: 1920s
TYPE: Veterinary
HOURS: Mon-Fri 8.50-5.15
READERS: Staff, other users by appointment
LENDING: Books only. Photocopies provided
COMPUTER DATA RETRIEVAL: DATASTAR, DIALOG online - free
HOLDINGS: 2,500 books; c150 journals, c100 current titles
CLASSIFICATION: Barnard
PUBLICATIONS: Weekly current awareness list; Journals holdings list
NETWORK: Scottish Agricultural Librarians Group; Agricultural and
              Food Research Service

193
INSTITUTE OF OCCUPATIONAL MEDICINE
Roxburgh Place, Edinburgh EH8 9SU
Tel: 031 667 5131   Telex: 9312100237=TDG   Fax: 031 667 0136
STAFF: Mrs B McGovern BA MIInfSc ALA
FOUNDED: 1969

TYPE: Occupational health and hygiene
HOURS: Mon-Fri 8.45-5.15
READERS: Staff, other users by arrangement
STOCK POLICY: Selective discarding of books and journals
LENDING: Books and journals
COMPUTER DATA RETRIEVAL: DIALTECH/DIALOG online - external users
        charged full cost CD-ROM: OSH-ROM
HOLDINGS: 5,000 books; 60 current journals
CLASSIFICATION: UDC
PUBLICATIONS: Annual report; research reports

194
LOTHIAN COLLEGE OF NURSING AND MIDWIFERY, NORTH DIVISION
13 Crewe Road, Edinburgh EH4 2LD
Tel: 031 343 2654
STAFF: Mrs J. White MA ALA, Ms S Moffat BSc MSc MIInfSc
FOUNDED: 1969
TYPE: Nursing
HOURS: Mon-Tue 8.15-7.20, Wed-Fri 8.45-4.30
READERS: Staff and nurses only
STOCK POLICY. Books discarded after 10 years
LENDING: Books videos CAL programmes for College only
COMPUTER DATA RETRIEVAL: In-house terminal
HOLDINGS: 4,000 books ; 100 current journals; 600 35mm slides,
        128 tape/slides, 118 videotapes (VHS)
CLASSIFICATION: NLM
PUBLICATION: List of recent additions
NETWORK: ASHSL

195
LOTHIAN COLLEGE OF NURSING AND MIDWIFERY, SOUTH DIVISION
23 Chalmers Street, Edinburgh EH3 9EW
Tel: 031 229 2477 x4617
STAFF: GC Haldane BD DipLib ALA, 2 library assistants (1 part time)
FOUNDED: 1976, Royal Infirmary School of Nursing Library founded in
        19th century
TYPE: Midwifery, Nursing
HOURS: Mon-Fri 8.30-4.30
READERS: Staff , trained nursing staff, paramedicals in area
STOCK POLICY: Out of date editions of books discarded
LENDING: Books only. Photocopies provided
COMPUTER DATA RETRIEVAL: Access to terminal - free
HOLDINGS: c 10,000 books; c130 journals, c115 current;microfilms,
        35mm slides, 300 videotapes (mainly VHS)
CLASSIFICATION: RCN (converting to NLM)
PUBLICATIONS: Information retrieval guide; Library guide
BRANCH: Paediatric and Mental Handicap Area, 10 Chalmers
Crescent, Edinburgh EH9 1TS
NETWORK: ASHSL; Scottish Colleges of Nursing & Midwifery Libraries

196
LOTHIAN HEALTH BOARD
11 Drumsheugh Gardens, Edinburgh EH3 7QQ
Tel: 031 225 1341 x2281
STAFF: Ms A Aliaga BSc DipLib
FOUNDED: 1974
TYPE: Health administration
HOURS: Mon-Fri 9-4.30
READERS: Staff and other users. Bona fide enquirers
 welcome
STOCK POLICY: Books, Journals over 5 years old discarded
LENDING: Books only. photocopies provided
COMPUTER DATA RETRIEVAL: DATASTAR online - free
HOLDINGS: 11,500 books; 150 journals, 139 current titles
CLASSIFICATION: Bliss
NETWORK: ASHSL

197
MACFARLAN SMITH LTD
Wheatfield Road, Edinburgh EH11 2QA
Tel: 031 337 2434 Telex 727271
STAFF: Mrs MR Wells
TYPE: Industrial
READERS: Staff only
STOCK POLICY: Journals discarded after 4 years
LENDING: Books and journals. Photocopies provided
COMPUTER DATA RETRIEVAL: CAS ONLINE -STN
HOLDINGS: 2,500 books; 5C current journals
CLASSIFICATION: UDC
SPECIAL COLLECTION: Alkaloids (100 vols)

198
MEDICAL RESEARCH COUNCIL, HUMAN GENETICS LIBRARY
Western General Hospital, Crewe Road, Edinburgh EH4 2XU
Tel: 031 332 2471   Fax: 031 343 2620
 Electronic Mail: LIBRARY @ UK.AC.ED.MRCVAX
STAFF: Miss SM Mould Scot Cert Inf Sci, ALA MIInfSc
FOUNDED: 1974
TYPE: Medical
HOURS: Mon-Fri 8.50-5
READERS: Staff and other users
STOCK POLICY: Journals discarded
LENDING: Books only. Photocopies provided
COMPUTER DATA RETRIEVAL: DATASTAR online - other libraries charged
                computer time only
HOLDINGS: 3,000 books; 110 current journals
CLASSIFICATION: UDC
PUBLICATIONS: Library News (6 per year); Annual report; Guide to
         library services; Journal holdings; Subject index
NETWORKS: Medical Research Council; ASHSL; Scottish Union Catalogue
          of Books

199
QUEEN MARGARET COLLEGE
Clerwood Terrace, Edinburgh, EH12 8TS
Tel: 031 339 8111
STAFF: Miss J Playfair MA DipLib, Mrs P Aitken BA ALAA,
    Miss M Myles MA ALA
FOUNDED: 1962
TYPE: Multidisciplinary
HOURS: Mon-Thu 9-9, Fri 9-5 (Vacation Mon-Thu 9-4.30, Fri 9-4)
READERS: Staff and other users
STOCK POLICY: Books and journals discarded at varying intervals
LENDING: Books only. Photocopies only
COMPUTER DATA RETRIEVAL: DATASTAR online - free. CD-ROM
HOLDINGS: 732 current journals; 1168 items of AV material
CLASSIFICATION: DDC
PUBLICATION: Accession list

200
ROYAL COLLEGE OF PHYSICIANS OF EDINBURGH
9 Queen Street, Edinburgh EH2 1JQ
Tel: 031 225 7324   Fax: 031 220 3939
STAFF: Miss JPS Ferguson MA ALA, IA Milne ALA
FOUNDED: 1681
TYPE: Medical
HOURS: Mon-Fri 9-5
READERS: Staff and other users
STOCK POLICY: Duplicate books and journals discarded
LENDING: Books, journals under special circumstances. Photocopies
                provided
COMPUTER DATA RETRIEVAL: DATASTAR, BLAISE online - standard charge
HOLDINGS: 250,000 books and bound journals; 104 current
                journals. Tape/slides, 35mm slides, microfilms
SPECIAL COLLECTIONS: JW Ballantyne - foetal pathology; JY
                Simpson - gynaecology and obstetrics
CLASSIFICATION: Barnard
PUBLICATIONS: Annual report; BIRD, D (comp). Catalogue of 18th
            century books in Edinburgh libraries

201
ROYAL COLLEGE OF SURGEONS OF EDINBURGH
18 Nicolson Street, Edinburgh EH8 9DW
Tel: 031 556 6206   Fax: 031 557 6406
STAFF: AA Gunn FRCSEd (Honorary Librarian), Dr AHB Masson
    FFARCS Eng (Honorary Archivist), Miss AM Stevenson BA DipLib
    ALA, Ms M Smith ALA
FOUNDED: 1845
TYPE: Dental, Medical, Surgical History of Medicine
HOURS: Mon-Fri 9-5
READERS: Fellows of the College ; Bona fide researchers at the
    discretion of the Honorary Librarian, journals not available
    elsewhere may be consulted at the discretion of the Assistant
    Librarian
STOCK POLICY: Middle editions of textbooks not always kept
LENDING: Books and journals to Fellows. Photocopies provided
COMPUTER DATA RETRIEVAL: DATASTAR online - standard charge
HOLDINGS: 32,000 books and bound journals; 123 current journals;
                12 videotapes (U-matic)
CLASSIFICATION: Fixed location pressmark
PUBLICATION: Library guide

202
ROYAL PHARMACEUTICAL SOCIETY OF GREAT BRITAIN (SCOTTISH DEPT)
36 York Place, Edinburgh EH1 3HU
Tel: 031 556 4386
STAFF: Dr LC Howden (Assistant Secretary), 1 other (part-time)
            staff
TYPE: Pharmacy
HOURS: Mon-Fri 9-5 (Closed for lunch 1-2)
READERS: Staff only
LENDING: Books only
HOLDINGS: 2,000 books, 1,000 bound journals; 25 current titles
SPECIAL COLLECTIONS: Pharmacopoeias and early herbals
CLASSIFICATION: UDC

203
SCOTTISH HEALTH EDUCATION GROUP, LIBRARY & INFORMATION SERVICES
Woodburn House, Canaan Lane, Edinburgh EH10 4SG
Tel: 031 447 8044   Fax: 031 452 8140
STAFF: Mrs IC Coltart Fil Kand DipLib ALA, M Adamson MA DipLib,
    K Donaldson MA DipLib
FOUNDED: 1968
TYPE: Multidisciplinary
HOURS: Mon-Thurs 9-4.30, Fri 9-4
READERS: Staff and other users
LENDING: Books only. Photocopies provided
COMPUTER DATA RETRIEVAL: DATASTAR online - free
HOLDINGS: 12,000 books and bound journals; 270 current journals
CLASSIFICATION: UDC (modified)
SPECIAL COLLECTION: Health education/promotion

PUBLICATIONS: Information bulletin (monthly)
NETWORK: ASHSL

204
SCOTTISH HEALTH SERVICE CENTRE
Scottish Health Service Management Development Group,
Crewe Road South, Edinburgh EH4 2LF
Tel: 031 332 2335 x25   Fax: 031 315 2369
STTAFF: Mrs JM Payne BA ALA, Mrs M Thom BA DipLib
FOUNDED: 1965
TYPE: Multidisciplinary
HOURS: Mon-Thurs 9-5, Fri 9-4.30
READERS: Staff, other users on application to Librarian
STOCK POLICY: Books and journals discarded selectively
LENDING: Books only. Photocopies provided
COMPUTER DATA RETRIEVAL: DATASTAR online - free
HOLDINGS: c 15,000 books; 231 journals, 202 current titles
CLASSIFICATION: Bliss (amended)
PUBLICATIONS: Library bulletin; periodicals list

205
SCOTTISH HEALTH SERVICE COMMON SERVICES AGENCY
B044 Trinity Park House, South Trinity Road, Edinburgh EH5 3SE
Tel: 031 551 8775/8087   Fax: 031 552 8651
STAFF: AH Jamieson MA DipLib ALA
FOUNDED: 1976
TYPE: Health administration
HOURS: Mon-Fri 9-5
READERS: Staff and other users
STOCK POLICY: Books and journals discarded selectively
LENDING: Books only. Photocopies provided
COMPUTER DATA RETRIEVAL: DATASTAR, BLAISE online - free
HOLDINGS: 8,000 books; 205 journals, 152 current titles; microfiche
SPECIAL COLLECTION: Health statistics (3,000 vols)
CLASSIFICATION: BC 1
PUBLICATIONS: Serials list; library guide
NETWORK: ASHSL

206
SCOTTISH OFFICE LIBRARY
Room 047, Saint Andrews House, Regent Road, Edinburgh, EH1 3DH
Tel: 031 244 2619
STAFF:Miss JM Smith BA ALA, Ms EM Macdonald ALA,Miss PM St Aubyn ALA
TYPE: Multidisciplinary
HOURS: Mon-Fri 9-5
READERS: Staff, other users by arrangement
STOCK POLICY: Books and journals discarded at Librarian's discretion
LENDING: Books and journals. Photocopies provided
COMPUTER DATA RETRIEVAL: DIALOG online - free. CD-ROM from 1990
HOLDINGS: 310 current journals
CLASSIFICATION: UDC

207
SCOTTISH SCIENCE LIBRARY
National Library of Scotland, 33 Salisbury Place, Edinburgh EH9 1SL
Tel: 031 226 4531   Telex: 76238 NLSEDI G   Fax: 031 226 4531 x3513
STAFF: Ms AJ Bunch MA FLA MBIM MIInfSc (Director), Ms E Boak BA ALA,
Ms C Booth MA ALA (part time), J Coll BA DipLib, Ms F McGrath BA
DipLib, Ms L Macdonald MA DipLib, Ms M Nisbet BSc DipLib,
Ms J Scott MA DipLib (part time), J Wintrip BA MSc ALA MIInfSc
FOUNDED: 1989
TYPE: All Science, including Medicine
HOURS: Mon, Tue, Thu, Fri 9.30-5, Wed 9.30-8.30
READERS: Staff and other users
STOCK POLICY: No stock discarded
LENDING: No lending. Photocopies supplied
COMPUTER DATA RETRIEVAL: DATASTAR, DIALOG, ORBIT, ESA-IRS, TEXTLINE,
    PFDS online. Charged cost plus handling charge.CD-ROM from 1989
HOLDINGS: 5,000 current journals; microfilms
CLASSIFICATION: DDC
PUBLICATION: Guides

208
UNIVERSITY OF EDINBURGH, CENTRE FOR TROPICAL VETERINARY MEDICINE
Field Station, Easter Bush, Roslin, Edinburgh, Midlothian
Tel: 031 445 2001 x210
STAFF: Mrs S Smyth BMus DipLib ALA
TYPE: Tropical veterinary medicine
HOURS: Mon-Fri 9-5
READERS: Staff, other users at external users rates
STOCK POLICY: No stock discarded
LENDING: Books and journals. Photocopies provided
HOLDINGS: 150 current titles
CLASSIFICATION: Barnard
NETWORK: University of Edinburgh

209
UNIVERSITY OF EDINBURGH, CITY HOSPITAL LIBRARY
New Medical Block, City Hospital, Greenbank Drive, Edinburgh,
    EH10 5SB
Tel: 031 447 1001 x3316
STAFF: Mrs C Humphries BA (part time)
TYPE: Medical
HOURS: Access by key. Staffed Wed 2-5
READERS: Staff and and students of University and Hospital
STOCK POLICY: Journals discarded after 10 years
LENDING: Reference only. Photocopies provided
COMPUTER DATA RETRIEVAL: Access to terminal. Free to
 University and local Health Board personnel
HOLDINGS: 600 books; 1,100 bound journals, 55 current titles
CLASSIFICATION: NLM
NETWORK: University of Edinburgh

210
UNIVERSITY OF EDINBURGH, DEPARTMENT OF PSYCHIATRY
Royal Edinburgh Hospital, Morningside Park, Edinburgh, EH10 5HF
Tel: 031 447 2011 x4285   Fax: 031 667 9780
STAFF: Mrs M Nicholson
TYPE: Psychiatric
HOURS: Mon-Fri 9-5, Sat 9.30-12 (Closed lunchtime 12.45-2
and Sat during vacation)
READERS: Staff and students of University and Hospital
STOCK POLICY: No stock discarded
LENDING: Books only. photocopies provided
COMPUTER DATA RETRIEVAL: In-house terminal - external users
          charged full cost. CD-ROM: Medline from 1976
HOLDINGS: 7,700 books; 112 current journals
SPECIAL COLLECTION: Fairbairn collection on Psychoanalysis and
          Psychotherapy
CLASSIFICATION: NLM
NETWORK: University of Edinburgh

211
UNIVERSITY OF EDINBURGH, ERSKINE MEDICAL LIBRARY
Hugh Robson Building, George Square, Edinburgh EH8 9XE
Tel: 031 667 1011 x2258   Telex 727442   Fax: 031 667 9780
Electronic mail: JANET S CANNELL @ UK.AC.EDINBURGH
STAFF: Mrs SE Cannell MA ALA, Miss J Adams MA ALA, Mrs A McAlpin MA
ALA (part time), Mrs P Gilchrist BA ALA
TYPE: Biomedical sciences, dental, medical
HOURS: Mon-Thurs 9-10, Fri 9-5, Sat 9-1 (Vacation Mon-Thu
9-7, Fri 9-5, Sat 10-1)
READERS: Staff and Lothian Health Board, and other users at
          external rate
STOCK POLICY: Earlier than pre-current books discarded.
LENDING: Textbooks, journals over 7 years old lent overnight only.
COMPUTER DATA RETRIEVAL: DATASTAR, BLAISE, DIALOG online - external
          users charged full cost. CD-ROM: Medline from 1976,
          SCI from 1988, and other databases
HOLDINGS: 43,000 books; 58,000 bound journals, 950 current titles;
          400 microfilms
CLASSIFICATION: NLM
PUBLICATION: Accessions list
BRANCHES: University of Edinburgh Western General Hospital
(see 214); University of Edinburgh City Hospital (see 208);
University of Edinburgh Psychiatry Library (see 209)
NETWORK: University of Edinburgh

212
UNIVERSITY OF EDINBURGH, ROYAL (DICK) SCHOOL OF VETERINARY STUDIES
Summerhall, Edinburgh EH9 1QH
Tel: 031 667 1011 x5275   Fax: 031 667 9780
Electronic mail: JANET A.KENNETT @ UK.AC.EDINBURGH
STAFF: Mrs MAR Kennett BA ALA
TYPE: Veterinary, biomedical sciences
HOURS: Mon-Thu 9-10, Fri 9-5 , Sat 9.30-12.30 (Vacation Mon-Fri 9-5)
READERS: Staff, other users at external users rate
STOCK POLICY: No stock discarded
LENDING: Books and journals. Photocopies provided
COMPUTER DATA RETRIEVAL: In-house terminal. CD-ROM: Medline from
        1976, CABI from 1990 - external users charged full cost
HOLDINGS: 33, 260 books; 26,300 bound journals, 356 current titles;
            705 microfilms
CLASSIFICATION: Barnard
BRANCHES: University of Edinburgh Field Station Library (see 213);
        University of Edinburgh Centre for Tropical Veterinary
        Medicine (see 208)
NETWORK: University of Edinburgh

213
UNIVERSITY OF EDINBURGH, VETERINARY FIELD STATION LIBRARY
Field Station, Easter Bush, Roslin, Midlothian
Tel: 031 445 2001 x205
STAFF: Mrs H London
TYPE: Veterinary
HOURS: Mon-Fri 9-5
READERS: Staff, other users at external rates
STOCK POLICY: No stock discarded
LENDING: Books and journals. Photocopies provided
COMPUTER DATA RETRIEVAL: In-house terminal
HOLDINGS: 136 current titles
CLASSIFICATION: Barnard
NETWORK: University of Edinburgh Library Network

214
UNIVERSITY OF EDINBURGH, WESTERN GENERAL HOSPITAL MEDICAL
 LIBRARY
Crewe Road South, Edinburgh EH4 2XU
Tel: 031 332 2525 x4125   Fax: 031 667 9780
STAFF: Mrs D Walker ALA
TYPE: Medical
HOURS: Mon-Fri 9-9, Sat 9-1
READERS: Staff and students of University and Hospital
STOCK POLICY: No stock discarded
LENDING: Books and journals (overnight only). Photocopies provided

COMPUTER DATA RETRIEVAL: In-house terminal. CD-ROM: Medline from
                1976 - external users charged
HOLDINGS: 3,300 books; 5,100 bound journals, 248 current titles;
                26 microfilms, 128 other items
CLASSIFICATION: NLM
PUBLICATIONS: Newsletter; accessions list
NETWORK: University of Edinburgh

Elstree

215
BLOOD PRODUCTS LABORATORY
Dagger Lane, Elstree, Borehamwood, Herts WD6 3BX
Tel: 081 953 6191   Fax: 081 207 6220
STAFF: Ms C Padley BA DipLib
FOUNDED: 1980
TYPE: Biomedical
HOURS: Mon-Fri 9-5.30 (Staffed 10.30-1 & 2-5.30)
READERS: Staff, other users by prior arrangement
STOCK POLICY: Books and journals discarded selectively
LENDING: Books and journals. Photocopies provided
COMPUTER DATA RETRIEVAL: CD-ROM from 1988
HOLDINGS: 900 books; 75 current journals
CLASSIFICATION: own

Enfield

216
CHACE POSTGRADUATE MEDICAL CENTRE
Chase Farm Hospital, The Ridgeway, Enfield, Middlesex, EN2 8JL
Tel: 081 366 6600 x5500
STAFF: Mrs ME Butler (part-time)
FOUNDED: 1967
TYPE: Medical, psychiatric
HOURS:Key always available. Staffed - Librarian 9-2,secretaries 9-4
READERS: Staff and local general practitioners, other users on
                application to Librarian
STOCK POLICY: Selected journals discarded after 10 years
LENDING: Books and pre-current journals. Photocopies provided
COMPUTER FACILITIES: Access to terminal.
HOLDINGS: 1200 books; 80 journals, 70 current
CLASSIFICATION: NLM
PUBLICATION: Enfield medical gazette
NETWORK: NE Thames Regional Library and Information Service; PLCS

217

MID AND WEST ESSEX DEPARTMENT OF NURSING AND MIDWIFERY EDUCATION
Saint Margaret's Hospital, Epping, Essex CM16 6TN
Tel: 0378 561666
STAFF: Mrs L MacAvoy, Mrs J Blake (part-time)
TYPE: Multidisciplinary
HOURS: Mon-Fri 8.30-5.30
READERS: Staff and other users
STOCK POLICY: Books discarded after 7 years
LENDING: Books only. Photocopies provided
COMPUTER DATA RETRIEVAL: CAMPUS 2000 & TTNS online
HOLDINGS: 12,000 books; 45 journals, 43 current titles;
          tape/slides, videotapes (VHS)
CLASSIFICATION: DDC
PUBLICATION: Library guide
BRANCHES: Princess Alexandra Hospital, Harlow; Herts and
 Essex General Hospital, Bishop's Stortford
NETWORKS: NE Thames Regional Library & Information Service; Essex
          County Technical Library Service

218
WEST ESSEX MEDICAL CENTRE
Saint Margaret's Hospital, Epping, Essex CM16 6TN
Tel: 0378 561666
STAFF: Mr s JA Bixby (part time), Mrs E Holloway (part time)
TYPE: Medical
HOURS: Always open. Staffed Mon-Fri 9-3
READERS: Staff, GP's, medical students, NHS staff
STOCK POLICY: No stock discarded
LENDING: Books only. Photocopies supplied
COMPUTER DATA RETRIEVAL: Access to terminal.
HOLDINGS: 1,400 books; 105 journals, 63 current titles
 journals. 16mm cine films, tapes/slides, videotapes (VHS)
CLASSIFICATION: NLM
NETWORK: NE Thames Regional Library and Information Service

Epsom

219
EPSOM DISTRICT HOSPITAL, SALLY HOWELL LIBRARY
Bradbury Centre, Dorking Road, Epsom, Surrey KT18 7EG
Tel: 03727 726100 x429
STAFF: GHR Smith BA ALA
FOUNDED: 1940s, Bradbury Centre opened 1980
TYPE: Medical
HOURS: Staffed Mon-Fri 8.45-4.45. Access by key at other times
READERS: Medical staff only
STOCK POLICY: Out of date books discarded
LENDING: Books and journals. Photocopies provided
COMPUTER DATA RETRIEVAL: DATASTAR online - free
HOLDINGS: 1,600 books; 80 journals, 70 current titles; 15 videotapes
          (VHS)

CLASSIFICATION: NLM
NETWORK: SW Thames Regional Library Service

220
LONG GROVE PSYCHIATRIC HOSPITAL
Horton Lane, Epsom, Surrey KT19 8PU
Tel: 0372 726200 x279
STAFF: Mrs P East BA ALA (part time)
TYPE: Psychiatric
HOURS: Mon-Thu 10-2.30
READERS: Staff and other users
STOCK POLICY: Out of date books discarded
LENDING: Books and journals. Photocopies provided
HOLDINGS: Approx 500 books; approx 55 journals, 42 current titles
CLASSIFICATION: NLM
NETWORKS: SW Thames Regional Library Service; PLCS

221
SMITHKLINE BEECHAM PHARMACEUTICALS RESEARCH DIVISION
Great Burgh, Yew Tree Bottom Road, Epsom, Surrey KT18 5XQ
Tel: 0737 364089   Fax: 0737 364079
STAFF: P Hamilton ALA
FOUNDED: 1978
TYPE: Pharmaceutical
HOURS: Mon-Fri 9-5.15
READERS: Staff , other users at discretion of Librarian
STOCK POLICY: Books and journals discarded after 10 years
LENDING: Books and journals. photocopies provided
COMPUTER DATA RETRIEVAL: In-house terminal - free. CD-ROM
HOLDINGS: 280 journals (40 titles on microfiche), 200 current titles
CLASSIFICATION: UDC
PUBLICATION: Weekly internal information bulletin

222
WEST PARK HOSPITAL, DEPARTMENT OF EDUCATION & TRAINING
Horton Lane, Epsom, Surrey, KT19 8PB
Tel: 0372 720308
STAFF: CC Ruffle ALA
TYPE: Midwifery, Nursing, Paramedical
HOURS: Mon-Fri 8.30-4.30
READERS: Staff and other users
STOCK POLICY: Books and journals discarded after 10 years
LENDING: Books, AV material. Photocopies provided
COMPUTER DATA RETRIEVAL: DATASTAR online. Free
HOLDINGS: Approx 7,400 books; 70 journals, 66 current titles;
          10 tape/slides, 120 videotapes (VHS)
CLASSIFICATION: NLM
SPECIAL COLLECTION: Local History - West Park Hospital
BRANCHES: 3 School of Nursing libraries
NETWORK: SW Thames Regional Library Service

223
NORTH EAST SURREY COLLEGE OF TECHNOLOGY
Reigate Road, Ewell, Surrey KT17 3DS
Tel: 081 394 3174   Fax: 081 394 3030
STAFF: Mrs J Upson BSc DipLib ALA, Mrs J Reid MA (Hons) MA ALA;
 B Robertson BA (Hons) DipLib ALA
TYPE: Multidisciplinary
HOURS: Mon-Thurs 8.30-8.30, Fri 8.30-6 (vacation Mon-Fri 9-4.30)
READERS: Staff, other users for reference only
STOCK POLICY: Out of date books and journals within NESCOT
LENDING: Books only. Photocopies provided
COMPUTER DATA RETRIEVAL: DIALOG online - charged. CD-ROM from 1989.
              PRESTEL available
HOLDINGS: 45,000 books and bound journals; 500 current journals;
 microfilms, tape/slides, 35mm slides, audio discs,videodiscs,
 videotapes (VHS), computer programmes
CLASSIFICATION: DDC
PUBLICATIONS: College library guide; guides for courses
NETWORK: SASLIC

Exeter

224
EXETER MEDICAL LIBRARY,
Postgraduate Medical Centre, Barrack Road, Wonford, Exeter EX2 5DW
Tel: 0392 403002
STAFF: Miss VB Newton BSc DipLib ALA, 1 other (part-time) staff
FOUNDED: 18th century ?
TYPE: Medical, dental
HOURS: Mon-Fri 9-5.30. Access at other times by special arrangement
READERS: Staff and other users
STOCK POLICY: Most books over 10 years old discarded
LENDING: Books and journals. Photocopies provided
COMPUTER DATA RETRIEVAL: DATASTAR online - charged standard rate
HOLDINGS: 35,800 books; 150 journals, 120 current; 35 tape/slides
SPECIAL COLLECTION: 17th and 18th century medical books in
 Exeter Cathedral library (1,200 vols)
CLASSIFICATION: NLM
NETWORK: SWEHSLinC; University of Exeter

225
EXETER SCHOOL OF NURSING LIBRARY
Butts Road, Heavitree, Exeter, Devon, EX
Tel:
No furthur information available

226
ST LOYE'S SCHOOL OF OCCUPATIONAL THERAPY
Millbrook Lane, Topsham Road, Exeter, Devon, EX2 6ES
Tel: 0392 219774
STAFF: G Barber BA ALA DipLib, Mrs R Warren BA ALA DipLib
TYPE: Paramedical
READERS: Staff and other users
STOCK POLICY: Journals discarded after 10 years, books discarded
        after 15 years
LENDING: Books only. Photocopies provided
COMPUTER DATA RETRIEVAL: DATASTAR, BLAISE, DIALOG. Charged computer
        time only
HOLDINGS: 151 journals, 114 current titles; 179 tape/slides, 26
        software programs, videotapes (70 U-matic, 81 VHS)
CLASSIFICATION: NLM
SPECIAL COLLECTION: Computer index to OT journal articles 1988-;
        Union list of OT journals database
PUBLICATIONS: Library guide; Guide to reference sources; Guide to
        information sources in occupational therapy; Guide to
        information sources in psychology/psychiatry; Writing
        bibliographic references; Online databases; Learning
        resources bulletin; Union list of OT journals
NETWORKS: SWEHSLinC; PLCS; Librarians in Occupational Therapy
        Schools Group

227
WONFORD HOUSE HOSPITAL
DRYDEN ROAD, EXETER, DEVON, EX
Tel:
No furthur information available

Falkirk

228
FORTH VALLEY COLLEGE OF NURSING AND MIDWIFERY
Westburn Avenue, Falkirk, Scotland, FK1 5ST
Tel: 0324 35091
STAFF: M Christie BA DipLib ALA, J Ingram SHNCLibInfSc
FOUNDED: 1975
TYPE: Multidisciplinary
HOURS: 8.45-4.15
READERS: Staff and other users
STOCK POLICY: Journals discarded after 4 years, books discarded
                after 5 years
LENDING: Books only
HOLDINGS: 9,000 books and bound journals, 130 current titles;
                150 tape/slides, 300 videotapes (VHS)
CLASSIFICATION: RCN

Fareham

229
WESSEX REGIONAL LIBRARY AND INFORMATION SERVICE
Education Centre, Knowle Hospital, Fareham, Hants PO17 5NA
Tel: 0329 832271
STAFF: Mrs CA Wilson ALA, Mrs D Campbell-Lendrum (part-time)
TYPE: Nursing, psychiatric
HOURS: Mon-Fri 8.30-4.30. Key available at other times
READERS: Staff, other users for reference only
STOCK POLICY: Books and journals discarded after a variable number
       of years
LENDING: Books, journals and AV material. Photocopies provided
COMPUTER DATA RETRIEVAL: DATASTAR, BLAISE online. Free
HOLDINGS: 4,000 books; 70 current journals; tape/slides,
       videotapes (VHS)
CLASSIFICATION: NLM
BRANCH: Moorgreen Hospital, Southampton
NETWORKS: WRLIS; PLCS

Farnborough

230
ROYAL AIR FORCE INSTITUTE OF AVIATION MEDICINE
Farnborough, Hants GU14 6SZ
Tel: 0252 24461 x3077
No furthur information available

Galway

231
UNIVERSITY COLLEGE HOSPITAL, MEDICAL LIBRARY
University College, Galway, Republic of Ireland
Tel: 010 353 91 24222 x296
STAFF: Ms A Downing MALS DipCompProg , Ms T Kennedy MA (part time),
 Ms E McDonald (part time), Ms A Madden BA H.DipEd (part time),
  Ms M O Haodha BA DipLibTrn (part time), Ms B Tomkins (part time)
FOUNDED: 1970
TYPE: Multidisciplinary
HOURS: Mon-Fri 9.15am-10pm
READERS: Staff and other users in medical field
STOCK POLICY: Books discarded after 10 years
LENDING: Books, journals, pamphlets, lecture notes. Photocopies
       provided
COMPUTER DATA RETRIEVAL: Access to terminal.
HOLDINGS: 102 current journals;
CLASSIFICATION: DDC
NETWORK: James Hardiman Library, University College Galway

Gateshead

232
GATESHEAD EDUCATION CENTRE LIBRARY
Queen Elizabeth Hospital, Sheriff Hill, Gateshead, Tyne and
 Wear NE9 6SX
Tel: 091 487 8989 x2103
STAFF: Mrs P Kerr C&G Lib Asst Cert, FE Teachers Cert,
 Mrs P Hutchinson, Mrs M Baggaley (part time)
FOUNDED: 1985
TYPE: Multidisciplinary
HOURS: Mon-Fri 8.30-5
READERS: Staff only
STOCK POLICY: Books and journals discarded after 10-15 years
LENDING: Books, Distance Learning Packs only. Photocopies provided
HOLDINGS: 10,000 books;
CLASSIFICATION: DDC 19th ed
PUBLICATIONS: Library Guide; Additions to stock
NETWORK: Northern Regional Association of Health Service
 Librarians

Gillingham

233
MEDWAY HEALTH AUTHORITY, DISTRICT LIBRARY SERVICE
Education Centre , Medway Hospital,Windmill Rd, Gillingham,
 Kent, ME7 5NY
Tel: 0634 407820   Fax: 0634 829470
STAFF: DC Stewart BA DipLib ALA
FOUNDED: 1970
TYPE: Multidisciplinary
HOURS: Mon-Fri 8.45-9
READERS: Staff, other users at the District Librarian's
 discretion
STOCK POLICY: Books discarded after 10 years
LENDING: Books only. Photocopies provided
COMPUTER DATA RETRIEVAL: DATASTAR, DIALOG online - free. CD-ROM
HOLDINGS: 10,000 books; 400 journals, 250 current titles
CLASSIFICATION: NLM
PUBLICATIONS: Library Guide; Current Journals
NETWORK: SE Thames Regional Library and Information Service
BRANCHES: Saint Bartholomew's Hospital, Rochester; All
 Saints Hospital, Chatham; Sheppey Hospital, Minster; Keycol
 Hospital, Sittingbourne

234
COMMON SERVICES AGENCY BUILDING DIVISION
Clifton House, Clifton Place, Glasgow G3 7YY
Tel: 041 332 7030   Fax: 041 331 2481
STAFF: DN Macdonald BA DipLib
FOUNDED: 1974
TYPE: Health service building & estate management
HOURS: Non-Thu 10-4.45, Fri 10-1.45
READERS: Staff and other users
STOCK POLICY: Stock discarded
LENDING: Books, journals, AV material, maps. Photocopies provided
COMPUTER DATA RETRIEVAL: In-house terminal
HOLDINGS: 5,000 books; 100 journals, c90 current titles;
          microfilms, 35mm slides, 10 videotapes (VHS)
CLASSIFICATION: C1/SfB
PUBLICATIONS: Additions List; List of health building design
          guidance publications
BRANCHES: Edinburgh, Dundee, Aberdeen, Inverness
NETWORK: Scottish Health Service Common Services Agency

235
GLASGOW EASTERN COLLEGE OF NURSING AND MIDWIFERY
110 St James Road, Glasgow G4 0PS
Tel: 041 552 1562 x2148   Fax: 041 552 0040
STAFF: Mrs S Gillespie ALA, Miss A Jones BA(Hons)
FOUNDED: 1969
TYPE: Midwifery, Nursing, Psychiatric
HOURS: Mon-Fri 8.15-4
READERS: Staff, nurses in training and qualified staff
STOCK POLICY: Current and pre-current editions of books
 kept. Journals reviewed each year and discarded depending
 on use and cost.
LENDING: Books only. Photocopies supplied
COMPUTER DATA RETRIEVAL: CD-ROM from 1989
HOLDINGS: 20,000 books; 200 current journals; 220 tape/slides,
          230 videotapes (VHS)
CLASSIFICATION: RCN
PUBLICATIONS: Accessions list; Library guide; Journal holdings;
          Information Sheets 1-16
NETWORK: ASHSL

GLASGOW NORTHERN COLLEGE OF NURSING AND MIDWIFERY
300 Balgrayhill Road, Glasgow G21 3UR
Tel: 041 557 3448
STAFF: Ms FG McLeod MA DipLib ALA, Mrs A Illingworth MA DipLib ALA,
    V Anglim BA DipInfTech, Mrs S Dickie MA DipLib ALA (part time)
FOUNDED: 1976
TYPE: Nurse education
HOURS: Mon-Fri 8.30-4.30, Tue & Thu evenings to 7.45
READERS: Staff and other users
STOCK POLICY: Stock discarded at Librarian's discretion
LENDING: Books only. Photocopies provided
HOLDINGS: c20,000 books; c140 journals, c130 current titles;
    35 mm slides, tape/slides, videotapes (VHS), CAL software
CLASSIFICATION: RCN (modified)
PUBLICATIONS: Leaflets for users
BRANCH: Lennox Castle Hospital, Glasgow; Woodilee Hospital, Glasgow

237
GLASGOW ROYAL INFIRMARY, MEDICAL LIBRARY
8-16 Alexandra Parade, Glasgow, G31 2ER
Tel: 041 552 3535 x5464
STAFF: Miss D Lindsay MA DipLib ALA, Mrs AMT Davis ALA (GGHB
    librarian)
    part time)
FOUNDED: In present accomodation since 1982
TYPE: Multidisciplinary
HOURS: Mon-Fri 9.30-5.30
READERS: Staff, other users on application to the Librarian
STOCK POLICY: Out of date editions of standard works and
duplicate journals discarded
LENDING: Books, reports & pamphlet literature. Photocopies provided
COMPUTER DATA RETRIEVAL: BLAISE online - charged telecommunications
    and computer output only. CD-ROM under review
HOLDINGS: 12,000 books,pamphlets & reports; 335 journals,
    180 current titles; 225 tape/slides, 25 videotapes (VHS)
CLASSIFICATION: NLM (medical), Bliss (administrative literature)
SPECIAL COLLECTIONS: Elias Jones (bacteriology, public health &
    hygiene)
PUBLICATIONS: Guides ; bulletins; bibliographies

238
GLASGOW SOUTH COLLEGE OF NURSING AND MIDWIFERY
517 Langside Road, Glasgow G42 9LF
Tel: 041 649 4545 x5161
STAFF: Librarian vacancy, Ms M McGarry MA DipLib
TYPE: Nursing
HOURS: Mon-Thu 8.30-4.30, Fir 8.30-4
READERS: Staff only
STOCK POLICY: Stock discarded
LENDING: Books only. Photocopies provided
HOLDINGS: 10,500 books; 100 journals, 60 current titles;
    Tape/slides, videotapes (VHS)
CLASSIFICATION: RCN
BRANCH: SE branch of Glasgow South College of Nursing (see 239)

239
GLASGOW SOUTH COLLEGE OF NURSING AND MIDWIFERY
Southern General Hospital, Govan Road, Glasgow G51 4TF
Tel: 041 445 2466
STAFF: Librarian vacancy, Ms M McGarry MA DipLib
FOUNDED: 1979
TYPE: Nursing
HOURS: Mon-Thurs 8.30-4.30, Fri 8.40-4.
READERS: Staff and students only
STOCK POLICY: Out of date books and journals discarded
LENDING: Books only. Photocopies provided
HOLDINGS: 12,500 books; 106 journals, 60 current titles;
            160 tape/slides, 197 35mm slides
CLASSIFICATION: RCN

240
GLASGOW WESTERN COLLEGE OF NURSING AND MIDWIFERY
120 University Place, Glasgow G11
Tel: 041 339 8822
STAFF: Ms J Howden MA DipLib ALA
FOUNDED: 1975
TYPE: Midwifery, Nursing
HOURS: Mon-Fri 8.30-4.30
READERS: Staff, other users on application to Librarian
STOCK POLICY: Books and journals discarded
LENDING: Books only. Photocopies provided
HOLDINGS: 20,000 books; 70 current journals
CLASSIFICATION: RCN
PUBLICATIONS: Library and information skills guide
NETWORK: ASHSL

241
GLASGOW WESTERN INFIRMARY
Gardiner Institute of Medicine and Therapeutics, 44 Church Street,
Glasgow, G11 6NT
Tel: 041 339 8822 x4472
STAFF: Ms JA Russell MA DipLib ALA
TYPE: Medical
HOURS: Mon-Fri 9-5. Staffed Mon & Wed am, Tue & Thu all day, Fri pm
READERS: Staff and other users
STOCK POLICY: Books discarded after a variable number of years
LENDING: No lending. Photocopies supplied
COMPUTER DATA RETRIEVAL: DATASTAR online. Free
HOLDINGS: c1,500 books; 125 journals, 105 current
CLASSIFICATION: LC/NLM adaptation
PUBLICATION: Guide for readers
BRANCHES: Gartnavel General Hospital
NETWORK: ASHSL

ROYAL COLLEGE OF PHYSICIANS AND SURGEONS OF GLASGOW
234 Saint Vincent Street, Glasgow G2 5RJ
Tel: 041 221 6072   Fax: 041 221 1804
STAFF: AM Rodgers BA DipLib ALA
FOUNDED: 1690
TYPE: Medical, dental, psychiatric
HOURS: Mon-Fri 9.15-5
READERS: Staff and other users
STOCK POLICY: Books discarded after a variable period
LENDING: Books, slides, only. Photocopies provided
COMPUTER DATA RETRIEVAL: DATASTAR online - free. PRESTEL available
HOLDINGS:2,000 journals, 300 current;250 35mm slides,20 tape/slides
CLASSIFICATION: NLM
SPECIAL COLLECTIONS: MacEwen mss - surgery; Ross mss - tropical
 medicine; Mackenzie - ophthalmology (300 vols)
PUBLICATIONS: Journal holdings; Guide

243
SOUTHERN GENERAL HOSPITAL, CENTRAL MEDICAL LIBRARY
Southern General Hospital, Govan Road, Glasgow G51 4TF
Tel: 041 445 2466 x4012   Fax: 041 445 2466 x4334
STAFF: Mrs HN Williamson BSc MIInfSc, Mrs ME Robins HNC LibInfSc
                                                        (part time)
FOUNDED: 1979 (amalgamation of Medical Staff Library and Institute
                        of Neurological science Library)
TYPE: Multidisciplinary
HOURS: Mon, Wed, Thurs, Fri 9-4.45, Tues 9-6
READERS: Staff, other bona fide users for reference only
STOCK POLICY: Certain journals discarded after 2 years, books
            discarded after useful life
LENDING: Books and journals. Photocopies provided
COMPUTER DATA RETRIEVAL: Access to terminal. CD-ROM: CSA Medline
                from 1976 - charged stationery costs
HOLDINGS: 3,000 books; 265 journals, 145 current titles;
                 35mm slides, audiotapes, VHS videotapes
SPECIAL COLLECTION: Neurological sciences
CLASSIFICATION: NLM (modified)
PUBLICATION: Library guide
NETWORK: ASHSL; Greater Glasgow Health Board; PLCS

244
STOBHILL GENERAL HOSPITAL MEDICAL LIBRARY
Stobhill General Hospital, Glasgow G21 3UW
Tel: 041 558 0111 x5089
STAFF: Mrs EA Gordon BSc DipLib ALA
TYPE: Medical
HOURS: Mon-Fri 8.30-4.30
READERS: Staff, other users at discretion of librarian
STOCK POLICY: Books and journals discarded after variable periods
LENDING: Books and journals. Photocopies provided
COMPUTER DATA RETRIEVAL: DATASTAR online - charged full cost
HOLDINGS: 2,000 books; 230 journals, 110 current; videotapes (VHS)
CLASSIFICATION: NLM
NETWORK: ASHSL

245
UNIVERSITY OF GLASGOW LIBRARY
Hillhead Street, Glasgow G12 8QE
Tel: 041 330 4283   Telex 777070 UNIGLA
Electronic mail: JANET LIBRARY @ AC.GLASGOW.UME
STAFF: HJ Heaney MA FLA, DRH Adams BA DipLib (Principal Assistant
  Librarian, Sciences), RJ Diamond MSc MBA Senior Asst Librarian,
  Life Sciences), Ms AJ Faichney MA DipLib, GO Saunders BSc MB ChB
FOUNDED: 1451
TYPE: Multidisciplinary
HOURS: Mon-Thu 9-9.30 (9-5 in vacation), Fri 9-5, Sat 9-7.30,
  Sun 2-7.30
READERS: Open to teaching and research staff and students
  of the University; other users on application to the Librarian
STOCK POLICY: Unwanted duplicates and some superseded
  editions discarded
LENDING: Books and journals. photocopies provided
COMPUTER DATA RETRIEVAL: Online: DATASTAR, BLAISE, DIALOG, BRS and
  16 other host systems. Non-university readers charged
  computer time only.   CD-ROM available
HOLDINGS: Life Sciences Division: 28,000 books; 2,500 journals,
  1,100 current
SPECIAL COLLECTIONS: Hunterian (10,000 vols) rich in
  history of medicine; Ferguson (8,000 vols) mainly on
  history of chemistry
CLASSIFICATION: Own, based on LC, NLM (in medicine)
PUBLICATIONS: Reader's guide; directory of departmental
  libraries; Glasgow list of medical periodicals; exhibition
  catalogues
BRANCHES: Dental, Chemistry and Veterinary Medicine Branch
  libraries
NETWORKS: JANET, MEDIS

246
UNIVERSITY OF GLASGOW, DENTAL BRANCH LIBRARY
Glasgow Dental Hospital and School, 378 Sauchiehall Street,
  Glasgow G2 3JZ
Tel: 041 332 7020 x225
Electronic Mail: JANET H.MARLBOROUGH @ UK.AC.GLASGOW.VME
STAFF: Ms HS Marlborough MA DipEd ALA
FOUNDED: 1969
TYPE: Multidisciplinary
HOURS: Mon-Fri 9-5.30
READERS: Staff and other users
STOCK POLICY: No stock discarded
LENDING: Books, journals, AV material. Photocopies provided
COMPUTER DATA RETRIEVAL: DATASTAR online.Non-University,Non-Hospital
  users are charged. Access to CD-ROM from 1982
HOLDINGS: 5,500 books; 80 current journals; 44 tape/slides,
  videotapes (10 U-matic, 18 VHS)
SPECIAL COLLECTION: History of dentistry (c100 vols)
CLASSIFICATION: Own, based on LC

NETWORK: West of Scotland Postgraduate Dental Education Centre;
Glasgow university Library

247
UNIVERSITY OF GLASGOW, PATHOLOGY DEPARTMENT LIBRARY
Western Infirmary, Glasgow G11 6NT
Tel: 041 339 8822   Fax: 041 337 2494
STAFF: Mrs I Todd (Secretary - part time)
TYPE: Medical
HOURS: Mon-Fri 9-12.30
READERS: Staff and other users
STOCK POLICY: Stock discarded
LENDING: No lending
HOLDINGS: 38 current journals
CLASSIFICATION: Own

248
UNIVERSITY OF GLASGOW, VETERINARY BRANCH LIBRARY
Garscube Estate, Bearsden Road, Bearsden, Glasgow G61 1QH
Tel: 041 339 8855 x5708
STAFF: Mrs M Findlay ALA, Miss AJ Williams
TYPE: Medical, Veterinary
HOURS: Mon, Wed, Fri 8.45-5.30, Tue, Thu 8.45-7
READERS: Staff, students and other users
STOCK POLICY: Non-veterinary journals discarded after five years,
          books discarded after variable periods
LENDING: Books and journals
COMPUTER DATA RETRIEVAL: Access to terminal
HOLDINGS: 1,500 books; 150 journals, 140 current titles
SPECIAL COLLECTIONS: Veterinary science; agriculture;
 animal husbandry
CLASSIFICATION: Own, based on LC
NETWORK: Glasgow University Library

249
UNIVERSITY OF STRATHCLYDE, NATIONAL CENTRE FOR TRAINING AND
 EDUCATION IN PROSTHETICS AND ORTHOTICS
Curran Building, 131 St James' Road, Glasgow G4 0LS
Tel: 041 552 4400 x3814 Fax: 041 552 0775
STAFF: Ms H Smart BA(Hons) ALA MIInfSc
FOUNDED: 1978
TYPE: Multidisciplinary
HOURS: Mon-Fri 9-5
READERS: Staff, students, other users at discretion of
 Librarian
STOCK POLICY: Books discarded
LENDING: Books, journals and literature searches. Photocopies
          provided
COMPUTER DATA RETRIEVAL: In-house terminal.
HOLDINGS: 3,000 books; 200 journals, 115 current titles
CLASSIFICATION: NLM
PUBLICATIONS: RECAL abstracts, RECAL thesaurus

250
VICTORIA INFIRMARY, MEDICAL LIBRARY
Langside Road, Glasgow G42 9TY
Tel: 041 649 4545 x5760
STAFF: Mrs AM Clackson BMus DipLib
FOUNDED: 1943
TYPE: Medical, paramedical
HOURS: Mon-Fri 9-5
READERS: Staff and other users
STOCK POLICY: No stock discarded
LENDING: Books, journals, slides, videotapes. Photocopies provided
COMPUTER DATA RETRIEVAL: DATASTAR online - free
HOLDINGS: 770 books; 162 journals, 133 current titles;
           c12,000 35mm slides, 36 tape/slides, 44 videotapes (VHS)
CLASSIFICATION: Glasgow University Library: medicine
PUBLICATIONS: Newsletter, User guide

Glenrothes

251
FIFE HEALTH BOARD
Glenrothes House, North Street, Glenrothes KY7 5PB
Tel: 0592 754355   Fax: 0592 756552
STAFF: Ms C Sclater DipLibInfStud MIInfSc
TYPE: Multidisciplinary
HOURS: Mon-Fri 8.30-5.
READERS: Staff, other users for reference only
STOCK POLICY: Journals discarded after 5 years, books discarded
        after a variable number of years
LENDING: Books only. Photocopies provided
COMPUTER DATA RETRIEVAL: DATASTAR online - free
HOLDINGS: 5,000 books; 165 journals, 150 current titles;
        AV material (2,000 items)
CLASSIFICATION: DHSS Thesaurus
PUBLICATIONS: Library update (monthly)
NETWORK: ASHSL

Gloucester

252
CONEY HILL HOSPITAL POSTGRAUATE LIBRARY
Coney Hill, Gloucester GL4 7QJ
Tel: 0452 617033 x2271
STAFF: Ms AJ Perrett BA(Hons) DipLib ALA (part-time)
FOUNDED: 1981
TYPE: Psychiatry, patients
HOURS: Always open. Staffed 21 hours per week
READERS: Staff only
LENDING: Books only. Photocopies provided

HOLDINGS: 1650 books; 78 journals, 59 current titles
CLASSIFICATION: NLM
SPECIAL COLLECTION: Historical (60 vols)
PUBLICATION: Current awareness abstracts
NETWORK: PLCS; SWEHSLinC
BRANCH: Coney Hill Hospital Patients/Staff Library,
Gloucester

253
GLOUCESTERSHIRE COLLEGE OF NURSING AND MIDWIFERY
Gloucestershire Royal Hospital, Great Western Road,
Gloucester GL1 3NN
Tel: 0452 28555 x4410
STAFF: Mrs AM Colley BSocSci DipLib
TYPE: Nursing
HOURS: Mon 8-6, Tues-Fri 8-4.30
READERS: Staff, other users for reference only
STOCK POLICY: Books over 10 years old discarded
LENDING: Books only. photocopies provided
HOLDINGS: 6,000 books; 6,300 bound journals; 43 current titles
CLASSIFICATION: RCN
NETWORK: SWESHLinC

254
GLOUCESTERSHIRE ROYAL HOSPITAL MEDICAL LIBRARY
Great Western Road, Gloucester GL1 3NN
Tel: 0452 28555 x4495/4496/4170
Telex: +45 913 237 001 (Answerback: 913237 DMS CH)
Electronic Mail: DATAMAIL
STAFF: Miss HJ Perry BA(Hons) DipLib ALA
TYPE: Medical
HOURS: Access available at any time upon request. Staffed
Mon-Thurs 9-5.30, Fri 9-5
READERS: Staff, others by arrangement with Librarian
STOCK POLICY: Books discarded after 10 years
LENDING: Books only. Photocopies provided
COMPUTER DATA RETRIEVAL: DATASTAR online - charging policy
under review. PRESTEL available
HOLDINGS: 3,000 books; 350 journals, 85 current
CLASSIFICATION: NLM
PUBLICATION: General Practice Newsletter; Periodical holdings list;
Library guide
BRANCH: Standish Hospital, Stonehouse; Patients/Staff library.
(part of Glos County Library) - Ms D Arnold Assistant i/c
NETWORKS: SWEHSLinC; Gloucestershire County Library Arts & Museums
service; Gloucestershire Librarians Group

255
GRANTHAM AND KESTEVEN GENERAL HOSPITAL STAFF LIBRARY
Manthorpe Road, Grantham, Lincolnshire NG31 8DG
Tel: 0476 65232 x4321
STAFF: Miss AL Willis (District Librarian, based at Pilgrim
         Hospital), Mrs SJ Swain (Senior Library Assistant)
FOUNDED: 1981
TYPE: Multidisciplinary
HOURS: Key always available. Staffed Mon-Thu 9-5, Fri 8.30-4.30
READERS: All Health Service staff, other bona fide users
 for reference
STOCK POLICY: Journals discarded after 6 years, books discarded at
         Librarian's discretion
LENDING: Books and journals. Photocopies provided
HOLDINGS: 4,700 books; 124 journals, 109 current
CLASSIFICATION: DDC
NETWORK: South Lincolnshire Health District Library Service;
         Lincolnshire County Library

Grays

256
ANGLIA HIGHER EDUCATION COLLEGE, SOUTH ESSEX DEPT OF NURSING
AND MIDWIFERY EDUCATION, LEARNING RESOURCE SERVICE
Orsett Hospital, Grays, Essex RM16 3EU
Tel: 0375 891100 x2632
STAFF: SL Beard BA ALA
TYPE: Nursing, Midwifery
HOURS: Mon, Tue, Wed 8.30-4.30, Thu 8.30-7.30, Fri 8.30-4
READERS: Nursing staff, nursing students and other users
STOCK POLICY: Books discarded at librarian's discretion
LENDING: Books only. Photocopies provided
COMPUTER DATA RETRIEVAL: DATASTAR online. PRESTEL
HOLDINGS: 5,000 books ; 60 current journals; 200 videotapes (VHS)
CLASSIFICATION: NLM
PUBLICATIONS: Library guide
NETWORK: NE Thames Regional Library and Information Service;
         Anglia Higher Education College

Great Yarmouth

257
SIR JAMES PAGET LIBRARY
James Paget Hospital, Lowestoft Road, Gorleston, Great
 Yarmouth, Norfolk, NR31 6LA
Tel: 0493 653432
STAFF: Mrs C Thompson Cert Ed ALA, A Bullimore BA DipLib
TYPE: Multidisciplinary

HOURS: Mon-Fri 8-5, sat 8.30-12
READERS: Staff and other users
STOCK POLICY: Books discarded
LENDING: Books and journals. Photocopies provided
COMPUTER DATA RETRIEVAL: DATASTAR online - free
HOLDINGS: 6,000 books; 130 journals, 100 current titles
CLASSIFICATION: NLM
BRANCHES: Child & Family Centre, Northgate Hospital, Great
          Yarmouth; ; Saint Nicholas Psychiatric Hospital, Great
          Yarmouth ; Southwold Hospital; Beccles Hospital; Lowestoft
          Hospital
NETWORK: East Anglian NHS Region

Greenock

258
ARGYLL & CLYDE COLLEGE OF NURSING LIBRARY
Larkfield Road, Greenock, Renfrewshire, PA16 OXL
Tel: 0475 33777 x4582
STAFF: T McClymont ALA
FOUNDED: 1966
TYPE: Nursing, psychiatric
HOURS: Mon-Thu 8.30-5, Fri 8.30-4.30
READERS: Staff and students only
STOCK POLICY: Journals discarded after 10 years, books after 3 years
LENDING: Books only. photocopies provided
COMPUTER DATA RETRIEVAL: In-house terminal
HOLDINGS: 40 current journals
CLASSIFICATION: DDC 19th ed
PUBLICATIONS: Library Guide

259
ROBERT LAMB MEDICAL LIBRARY, INVERCLYDE ROYAL HOSPITAL
Larkfield Road, Greenock, Renfrewshire, PA16 OXN
Tel: 0475 33777 x4402
STAFF: Dr RC Brown FRCP (Honorary Librarian), Mrs M Wright
                                        (part-time)
FOUNDED: 1962 (1979 in present building)
TYPE: Medical, paramedical, pharmaceutical
HOURS: 24 hours . Staffed Mon-Wed 8-1, Thu-Fri 8-12
READERS: Staff, other users at Librarian's discretion
STOCK POLICY: Out of date editions of books given to other
          departments
LENDING: No lending. Photocopies supplied
HOLDINGS: 1,200 books; 103 journals, 80 current titles
CLASSIFICATION: DDC

Grimsby

260
ROTHERHAM MEMORIAL LIBRARY
Postgraduate Medical Education Centre, District General Hospital,
Grimsby, S Humberside, DN33 2BA
Tel: 0472 74111
STAFF: Dr S Moss MD FRCP (Honorary Librarian)
FOUNDED: 1948
TYPE: Medical, psychiatric
HOURS: Open 24 hours (not staffed at all times)
READERS: Medical staff, general practitioners and students
LENDING: Books, tape/slides, videotapes
COMPUTER DATA RETRIEVAL: Access to DATASTAR - charged
HOLDINGS: 1,500 books; 98 current journals; 30 tape/slides, 10
          videotapes (VHS)
CLASSIFICATION: Own
PUBLICATION: Acquisition list
NETWORK: HULTIS

Guildford

261
GUILDFORD EDUCATION CENTRE LIBRARY
Royal Surrey County Hospital, Egerton Rd, Guildford, Surrey GU2 5XX
Tel: 0483 571122 x4247   Fax: 0483 303691
STAFF: C Smith BSc ALA
TYPE: Multidisciplinary
HOURS: Mon-Fri 9- 5
READERS: Staff and other users
STOCK POLICY: Books over 10 years old selectively discarded
LENDING: Books , journals, videos, tape/slides. Photocopies
          provided
COMPUTER DATA RETRIEVAL: DATASTAR, BLAISE online. Free
HOLDINGS: 3,500 books; c200 journals, 130 current titles;
          tape/slides, videotapes (VHS)
CLASSIFICATION: NLM
PUBLICATION: Library bulletin (monthly)
NETWORK: SW Thames Regional Library and Information Service

262
SOUTH WEST THAMES REGIONAL LIBRARY SERVICE
Royal Surrey County Hospital, Egerton Road, Guildford,
 Surrey GU2 5XX
Tel:0483 37270   Fax: 0483 303691
Electronic Mail: DATAMAIL (SAWERS)
STAFF: MJ Carmel BA FLA, Miss HE Taylor BA ALA, Mrs C Sawers ALA
HOURS: Mon-Fri 9-5
COMPUTER DATA RETRIEVAL: DATASTAR, BLAISE, DIALOG online.   Free
          within Region. Charged on a consultancy basis outside region

PUBLICATIONS: Directory of libraries; Union list of serials
(not available outside region); 12 current awareness literature
services; checklists for libraries serving nurses; subject
cataloguing guide; library manual
NETWORK: SW Thames Regional Library and Information Service

263
STERLING WINTHROP GROUP LIMITED, LIBRARY SERVICES
Sterling Winthrop House, Onslow Street, Guildford, Surrey, GU1 4YS
Tel: 0483 505515   Fax: 0483 35432
STAFF: Mrs AK Johnson BSc DipLib
TYPE: Medical, pharmaceutical
HOURS: Mon-Thurs 9-5.15, Fri 9-4
READERS: Staff only
STOCK POLICY: Books and journals discarded selectively
LENDING: Books and journals to company staff only, except
in special circumstances. Photocopies provided
COMPUTER DATA RETRIEVAL: DATASTAR online
HOLDINGS: 2,000 books; 200 journals, 150 current titles; microforms
CLASSIFICATION: UDC
NETWORK: SASLIC

Halifax

264
HALIFAX POSTGRADUATE MEDICAL LIBRARY
Postgraduate Medical Education Centre, Halifax General
Hospital, Halifax HX3 0PW
Tel:0422 357171
No further information available

Harlow

265
MERCK SHARP & DOHME RESEARCH LABORATORIES, LITERATURE RESOURCES
CENTRE
Neuroscience Research Centre, Terlings Park, Eastwick Road,
Harlow, Essex, CM20 2QR
Tel: 0279 440131   Telex: 817905   Fax: 0279 440390
STAFF: J Ashenden BA(Lib) ALA
FOUNDED: 1985
TYPE: Neuroscience, pharmaceutical
HOURS: Mon-Fri 8.45-5
READERS: Staff only
STOCK POLICY: No stock discarded
LENDING: Reference only. Photocopies provided only occasionally
COMPUTER DATA RETRIEVAL: DATASTAR, DIALOG online - free to staff
HOLDINGS: 2,000 books; 240 journals, 215 current titles
CLASSIFICATION: NLM, LC
PUBLICATION: Journals holding list

266
PRINCESS ALEXANDRA HOSPITAL, MEDICAL LIBRARY
Pardin Hall, Hemstel Road, Harlow, Essex CM20 1QX
Tel: 0279 444455
STAFF: Mrs BA Carter (part time)
TYPE: Medical
HOURS: Mon-Fri 8-5
READERS: Staff, other users for reference if requested
STOCK POLICY: Books discarded after 15 years
LENDING: Books only. Photocopies provided
COMPUTER DATA RETRIEVAL: Access to DATASTAR - free
HOLDINGS: 1,000 books; 2,000 bound journals, 69 current titles
CLASSIFICATION: NLM
NETWORK: NE Thames Regional Library and Information Service;
                    EULOS

Harold Wood

267
HAROLD WOOD HOSPITAL POSTGRADUATE ACADEMIC CENTRE
Harold Wood Hospital, Gubbins Lane, Harold Wood, Essex
 RM3 0BE
Tel: 04023 45156
STAFF: Mrs MJ Harris (Administrator), Mrs S Gateson
             (Assistant/librarian)
FOUNDED: 1969
TYPE: Medical
HOURS: Mon-Fri 9-5.
READERS: Medical staff and local GP's
LENDING: Books only. photocopies provided
HOLDINGS: 1,000   books;   45   current   journals;   microfilms,
        tape/slides, 35 mm slides,   videotapes (VHS)
NETWORK: NE Thames Regional Library and Information Service

268
ROMFORD COLLEGE OF NURSING & MIDWIFERY
Gubbins Lane, Harold Wood, Essex, RM3 0BE
Tel: 04023 71716
STAFF: Ms E Hoey ALA, Mrs G Hylands, Miss C Thompson, Mrs A North,
         Mrs L Rothon, N Goodman (Media Resources Manager), G Jones
         (AV Technician)
FOUNDED: 1989, based on previous library founded c1969
TYPE: Midwifery, nursing, psychiatric
HOURS: Mon-Fri 8.30-5
READERS: Staff only
STOCK POLICY: Books discarded
LENDING: Books only. Photocopies provided
COMPUTER DATA RETRIEVAL: Access to DATASTAR. CD-ROM from late 1990

HOLDINGS: 20,800 books; 50 current journals; 144 tape/slides,
2 videodiscs, 64 packs of 35mm slides, 185 videotapes (VHS),
71 audiocassettes, 51 charts, 74 models, 37 teaching packs
CLASSIFICATION: NLM
BRANCHES: Oldchurch hospital, Warley hospital
NETWORK: NETRLS

Harrow

269
HARROW NURSE EDUCATION CENTRE, BRENT AND HARROW SCHOOL OF NURSING,
Northwick Park Hospital, Watford Road, Harrow, Middlesex, HA1 3UJ
Tel: 081 869 2348
STAFF: Ms JE Smith BA(Hons)
TYPE: Nursing
HOURS: Mon-Fri 8.30-4.30
READERS: Nursing staff, other users on request
STOCK POLICY: Books discarded after 10 years
LENDING: Books only. Photocopies provided
HOLDINGS: 7,000 books; 69 journals, 55 current titles
CLASSIFICATION: DDC
NETWORK: NW Thames Regional Library and Information Service
BRANCHES: Central Middlesex Hospital Nurse Education
Centre, London; Shenley Hospital Nurse Education Centre,
Shenley, Radlett

270
MEDICAL RESEARCH COUNCIL, CLINICAL RESEARCH CENTRE
John Squire Medical Library, Watford Road, Harrow, Middlesex
HA1 3UJ
Tel:081 869 3322 (enquiries) 081 869 3326 (Medical Librarian)
081 869 3331 (Head Librarian)
Telex: 923410   Electronic Mail: JANET LIBRARY @ UK.AC.CRC
STAFF: Miss J Wade BA ALA (Head Librarian), Mrs S Mason BSc ALA
(Medical Librarian), M Kendall BA DipLib, M Wheeler BA DipLib
FOUNDED: 1970
TYPE: Multidisciplinary
HOURS: Mon-Thurs 8.45-5.15, Fri 8.45-5
READERS: Staff, other users for reference only on written
application and at discretion of Librarian
STOCK POLICY: Books discarded after variable intervals
LENDING: Books only. Photocopies provided
COMPUTER DATA RETRIEVAL: DIALOG online - other libraries charged
full cost. CD-ROM from 1989
HOLDINGS: 19,000 books; c800 journals, 649 current titles
CLASSIFICATION: NLM/LC
PUBLICATIONS: Library bulletin (monthly)
NETWORK: Medical Research Council

Hartlepool

271
HARTLEPOOL GENERAL HOSPITAL, DISTRICT LIBRARY/RESOURCES CENTRE
The General Hospital, Holdforth Road, Hartlepool, TS24 9AH
Tel: 0429 266654 x2632
STAFF: Ms R O'Neill BA(Hons) DipLib ALA
TYPE: Multidisciplinary
HOURS: Mon-Thu 8.45-4.45, Fri 8.45-4.15
READERS: Staff, other users for reference upon application
STOCK POLICY: Some books discarded after 10 years
LENDING: Books and AV material. Photocopies provided
COMPUTER DATA RETRIEVAL: DATASTAR online - charged computer time
        only.
HOLDINGS: c5,000 books; c55 journals; 35mm slides, tape/slides,
        microfiche, videotapes (VHS)
CLASSIFICATION: DDC
PUBLICATIONS: Library guide, periodicals list, new additions
BRANCHES: Cameron Hospital
NETWORKS: Northern Regional Library Service; Northern Regional
        Association of Health Service Librarians

Hastings

272
HASTINGS POSTGRADUATE MEDICAL CENTRE LIBRARY
7 Holmesdale Gardens, Hastings, East Sussex TN34 1LY
Tel: 0424 434513 x320
STAFF: Miss J Turner BA (Hons)
FOUNDED: 1976
TYPE: Multidisciplinary
HOURS: Mon-Fri 9-5.
READERS: Staff only
STOCK POLICY: Superseded editions of books discarded.
LENDING: Books , journals and AV material
COMPUTER DATA RETRIEVAL: In-house terminal (DATASTAR online due)
HOLDINGS: 1,100 books; 110 journals, 80 current titles;
                20 videotapes (VHS)
CLASSIFICATION: NLM
NETWORK: SE Thames Regional Library and Information Service

Hatton

273
COVENTRY & WARWICKSHIRE COLLEGE OF NURSING
Central Hospital, Birmingham Rd, Hatton, Warks, CV35 7EE
Tel: 0926 49621 x2269
STAFF: Mrs L Alcock B App Sci(Lib Stud)

FOUNDED: early 1970s
TYPE: Multidisciplinary
HOURS: Mon-Fri 9-5. Staffed Mon, Thu 9.30-2.30
READERS: Staff and students only
STOCK POLICY: No stock discarded
LENDING: No lending. photocopies provided
COMPUTER FACILITIES: Access to terminal
HOLDINGS: c4,500 books; 45 journals, 19 current
CLASSIFICATION: RCN
BRANCHES: Nurse Education Centre, Leamington Spa; Nunscroft Nurse
        Education Centre, Nuneaton; Peter Thomas Nurse Education
        Centre, Marston Green
NETWORK: West Midlands Regional Health Authority

274
MEDICAL LIBRARY
Central Hospital, Birmingham Rd, Hatton, Warks, CV35 7EE
Tel: 0926 496241
STAFF: Mrs VA Dalton (part time)
TYPE: Psychiatric
HOURS: Access by key. Staffed Mon-Tue 10.45-1, Fri 9-12
READERS: Staff and GPs. Medical students for reference only
COMPUTER DATA RETRIEVAL: Access to terminal
HOLDINGS: 1250 books; 12 current journals
CLASSIFICATION: Own
NETWORK: West Midlands Regional Health Libraries

Haverfordwest

275
WITHYBUSH GENERAL HOSPITAL MEDICAL LIBRARY
Haverfordwest, Pembrokeshire, Dyfed, Wales SA61 2PZ
Tel: 0437 764545
STAFF: Ms A Wood BLib ALA
TYPE: Medical, Nursing
HOURS: Always open. Staffed Mon-Fri 9-5
READERS: Staff and other users in Pembokeshire Health Authority
STOCK POLICY: Some stock discarded
LENDING: Books only. Photocopies provided
CLASSIFICATION: NLM
NETWORK: Welsh Health Libraries Network

276
MID-SUSSEX POSTGRADUATE MEDICAL CENTRE
Cuckfield Hospital, Cuckfield, Haywards Heath, West Sussex
RH17 5HQ
Tel: 0444 459122
STAFF: Mrs JM Thorpe ALA , 1 other (part-time) staff
FOUNDED: 1976
TYPE: Multidisciplinary
HOURS: Mon-Fri 9-10. Staffed Mon - Thurs 9.30-3.30.
READERS: Staff, other users at discretion of librarian
STOCK POLICY: Books discarded after 10 years
LENDING: Books only. Photocopies provided
COMPUTER DATA RETRIEVAL: Access to DATASTAR - free. PRESTEL
 available
HOLDINGS: 800 books; 55 current journals; tape/slides,
                     35 mm slides, videotapes (VHS)
CLASSIFICATION: NLM
NETWORK: SW Thames Regional Library and Information Service
BRANCHES: Crawley Hospital, Crawley; Saint Francis (Psychiatric)
                  Hospital, Haywards Heath

Hemel Hempstead

277
HEMEL HEMPSTEAD HOSPITAL MEDICAL LIBRARY
Hemel Hempstead General Hospital, Hillfield Road, Hemel Hempstead,
Herts, HP2 4AD
Tel: 0442 3141
STAFF: Mrs KA Warden BA ALA (part time), 1 assistant (part time)
TYPE: Multidisciplinary
HOURS: Mon, Wed-Fri 8.30-5, Tue 2-7
READERS: All staff of NW Herts DHA
STOCK POLICY: Out of date editions discarded
LENDING: Books and non-current journals
COMPUTER DATA RETRIEVAL: In-house databases. CD-ROM
HOLDINGS: 1,150 books; 91 journals; some AV material
CLASSIFICATION: NLM
NETWORK: NW Thames RLIS

Hereford

278
JOHN ROSS POSTGRADUATE MEDICAL CENTRE
County Hospital, Hereford, HR1 2ER
Tel: 0432 355444 x5193/4   Fax: 0432 351006
STAFF: Dr JRS Rendall (Honorary Librarian), Mrs PM Rossi, Mrs J Ball
FOUNDED: Library moved to PMC in 1968
TYPE: Medical
HOURS: Mon-Fri 9-10. Staffed 9-5.
READERS: Hospital doctors, general practitioners, dentists
STOCK POLICY: Stock discarded as shelf space fills up
LENDING: Books lent occasionally to own users. Photocopies provided

COMPUTER DATA RETRIEVAL: Access to terminal.
HOLDINGS: 2,000 books; 40 current journals; 50 videotapes (VHS)
CLASSIFICATION: DDC
NETWORK: West Midlands Regional Health Libraries

279
SCHOOL OF NURSING LIBRARY
County Hospital, Hereford HR1 2ER
Tel: 0432 268161 x468
STAFF: Mrs S Jones BA DipLib (part time), Mrs E Radford
TYPE: Nursing
HOURS: Mon-Fri 8.30-5. Staffed Mon 9-1.30, Thurs 9-1.30
READERS: Staff, other users for reference only
STOCK POLICY: Some out of date books and journals over 5
 years old discarded
LENDING: Books only
HOLDINGS: 3,500 books; 20 current journals; 16mm cine films,
              tape/slides, 35 mm slides, videotapes (Betamax, VHS)
CLASSIFICATION: DDC
NETWORK: West Midlands Regional Health Libraries

280
VICTORIA EYE HOSPITAL
Eign Street, Hereford HR4 0AJ
Tel: 0432 265961
STAFF: MJ Lloyd (part time)
TYPE: Ophthalmology
HOURS: Mon-Fri 9-5. Access available to resident staff at
 other times
READERS: Staff only
STOCK POLICY: No stock discarded
LENDING: None

Hertford

281
HERTFORD COUNTY HOSPITAL POSTGRADUATE CENTRE LIBRARY
North Road, Hertford, Herts, SG14 1LP
Tel: 0707 328111 x3182
STAFF: Mrs A Poyner ALA (part time)
FOUNDED: 1975
TYPE: Multidisciplinary
HOURS: Mon-Fri 9-3
READERS: Staff and other users
STOCK POLICY: Journals discarded as space demands, books discarded
          after 10 years
LENDING: Books, limited lending of journals, AV material.
              Photocopies provided
COMPUTER DATA RETRIEVAL: DATASTAR online - free. CD-ROM from 1989
HOLDINGS: 33 journals, 29 current titles
CLASSIFICATION: NLM
PUBLICATION: Recent additions list
NETWORKS: NW Thames RLIS; E Herts District Health Authority;
          Herts County Library Service; Hospital Librarians' Group

282
RYDER POSTGRADUATE MEDICAL CENTRE LIBRARY
Hexham General Hospital, Hexham, Northumberland NE46 1QJ
Tel: 0434 606161
STAFF: M Benjamin ALA (part-time - contracted from County Library
Service)
FOUNDED: c1972
TYPE: Medical
HOURS: Mon-Fri 9-5. Staffed Mon, Fri 9-11
READERS: Staff and other users
STOCK POLICY: Journals discarded after 10 years, no set policy on
books.
LENDING: Books and journals. Photocopies provided
COMPUTER DATA RETRIEVAL: Access to terminal.
HOLDINGS: 300 books; 42 current journals
CLASSIFICATION: DDC
PUBLICATION: Introductory leaflet
NETWORK: Northern Regional Library Service

High Wycombe

283
BUCKINGHAMSHIRE COLLEGE OF NURSING & MIDWIFERY
Lovelock-Jones Nursing Education centre, Barracks Road, High
Wycombe, Bucks HP11 1QN
Tel: 0494 425137
STAFF: Mrs R Weston BLib ALA
FOUNDED: 1970
TYPE: Nursing
HOURS: Mon-Fri 8.15-5. Staffed Mon-Fri 9-5
READERS: Staff, other users at discretion of librarian
STOCK POLICY: Books and journals discarded after 10 years
LENDING: Books only. AV material for use in Centre only.
Photocopies provided
COMPUTER DATA RETRIEVAL: DATASTAR online - free
HOLDINGS: 3,000 books; 45 journals, 38 current titles;
42 microfilms, 99 tape/slides, videotapes (45 U-matic, 168 VHS)
CLASSIFICATION: NLM
PUBLICATION: Guide to services; searching journal indexes
NETWORK: Oxford Region Library and Information Service
BRANCH: Medical/Nursing Library, Amersham General Hospital

284
CHILTERN POSTGRADUATE MEDICAL CENTRE
Wycombe General Hospital, High Wycombe, Bucks HP11 2TT
Tel: 0494 425573
STAFF: Mrs LA Martyn
FOUNDED: 1965
TYPE: Multidisciplinary
HOURS: Mon-Fri 9-5.30. Key available at other times.
READERS: Staff, other users on application to Librarian

STOCK POLICY: Journals discarded after 20 years, books discarded
        after variable intervals
LENDING: Books and journals. Photocopies provided
COMPUTER DATA RETRIEVAL: DATASTAR, BLAISE, DIALOG online - free
HOLDINGS: 2,100 books; 94 journals, 72 current titles
CLASSIFICATION: NLM
PUBLICATIONS: Library guide; Union list of periodicals; Current
        awareness bulletins
NETWORK: Oxford Regional Library and Information Service
BRANCHES: Amersham General Hospital

Hoddesdon

285
MERCK SHARP AND DOHME LIBRARY & INFORMATION SERVICES
Hertford Road, Hoddesdon, Hertfordshire EN11 9BU
Tel: 0992 467272   Telex 261915   Fax: 0992 451669
STAFF: Mrs M Gordon ALAA BA(LibSci)
TYPE: Multidisciplinary
HOURS: Mon-Fri 8.30-5
READERS: Staff only
LENDING: Books and journals internally only
COMPUTER DATA RETRIEVAL: 15 different hosts online
HOLDINGS: 12,000 books; 800 journals
CLASSIFICATION: DDC

Huddersfield

286
HUDDERSFIELD HEALTH AUTHORITY LIBRARY SERVICE
Royal Infirmary, Lindley, Huddersfield, West Yorkshire HD3 3EA
Tel: 0484 422191
STAFF: RW Heywood BA ALA
FOUNDED: 1972
TYPE: Multidisciplinary
HOURS: Mon-Fri 9-5
READERS: Staff, other users for reference only
STOCK POLICY: Superseded editions of books discarded
LENDING: Books ,journals and AV material. photocopies supplied
COMPUTER DATA RETRIEVAL: DATASTAR online - free
HOLDINGS: 10,000 books; 200 current journals; 10 microfilms,
        120 tape/slides, 50 audiotapes, 30 videotapes (VHS)
CLASSIFICATION: NLM (adapted)
PUBLICATION: Library guide; resources list
NETWORK: Yorkshire Joint Medical Library Service

287
HULL MEDICAL LIBRARY
Postgraduate Education Centre, Hull Royal Infirmary, Anlaby Roa‹
   Hull HU3 2JZ
Tel: 0482 28541 x4337/4767
STAFF: DI Thompson ALA, Mrs S Johnson, Mrs P Clarke ALA (part tim‹
TYPE: Multidisciplinary
HOURS: Mon, Tues, Thurs, Fri 9-8, Wed 9-5.30, Sat 9-12
READERS: Staff and other users
STOCK POLICY: Books discarded at Librarian's discretion
LENDING: Books, journals, pamphlets, reports. Photocopies provide‹
COMPUTER DATA RETRIEVAL: DATASTAR online - free
HOLDINGS: 6,600 books; 197 journals, 186 current titles
CLASSIFICATION: DDC
SPECIAL COLLECTION: Medical history (150 vols)
PUBLICATIONS: Contents list of journals; New books list
NETWORK: HULTIS

288
RECKITT AND COLMAN PHARMACEUTICAL DIVISION, BUSINESS AND
   COMMERCIAL LIBRARY
Dansom Lane, Hull HU8 7DS
Tel: 0482 26151 x2910   Telex 592166   Fax: 0482 25322
STAFF: GE Stephenson ALA DMS, BE Robinson
FOUNDED: 1924
TYPE: Pharmaceutical, business, commercial, marketing
HOURS: Mon-Thurs 8.30-4.45, Fri 8.30-4
READERS: Staff, other users by arrangement
STOCK POLICY: Books and journals discarded at variable intervals
LENDING: Books only. Photocopies provided
COMPUTER DATA RETRIEVAL: DIALOG, REUTERS, FT PROFILE, etc, online
HOLDINGS: 8,000 books; 200 journals, 100 current titles; ?00
                35mm slides, videotapes (200 U-matic, 150 VHS)
CLASSIFICATION: UDC
SPECIAL COLLECTION: Corporate archives (1.000 vols)
PUBLICATIONS: Various current awareness bulletins
NETWORK: Hultis

Huntingdon

289
HINCHINGBROOKE HOSPITA¹ EDUCATION CENTRE LIBRARY
Huntingdon, Cambs, PE18 8NT
Tel: 0480 456131 x3114
STAFF: Ms TK Dorey BA DipLib ALA
TYPE: Medical, nursing, paramedical

HOURS: Mon-Thu 9-5.30, Fri 9-5. Key available after hours
READERS: Staff, other users in Huntingdon Health Authority
STOCK POLICY: Out of date or superseded editions discarded
LENDING: Books only. Photocopies provided
COMPUTER DATA RETRIEVAL: DATASTAR online - non-Health Authority
          users charged

HOLDINGS: 3,500 books; 135 journals, 110 current titles; VHS
          videotapes
CLASSIFICATION: NLM

Ilford

290
GOODMAYES HOSPITAL POSTGRADUATE CENTRE
Barley Lane, Ilford, Essex, IG3 6XJ
Tel: 081 590 6060 x2497
STAFF: Miss HA Jackson ALA (District Librarian)
FOUNDED: 1970
TYPE: Psychiatric
HOURS: Mornings 10-2 (Staffed Mon 10-6, Wed 10-1.30, Fri 2.30-6
READERS: Staff, other users on request
LENDING: Books and journals. Photocopies supplied
COMPUTER DATA RETRIEVAL: Access to terminal
HOLDINGS: 60 journals, 40 current titles
CLASSIFICATION: NLM
NETWORKS: NETRLS; Redbridge District Library Service

291
REDBRIDGE DISTRICT LIBRARY
King George Hospital, Newbury Park, Ilford, Essex, IG2 7RL
Tel: 081 554 8811 x3335
STAFF: Miss HA Jackson ALA (District Librarian)
FOUNDED: 1975
TYPE: Multidisciplinary
HOURS: 9.30-6 (Staffed Tue 10-6, Wed 2.30-6, Thu 10-6, Fri 10-1.30
STOCK POLICY: Old editions and short cancelled runs of journals
          discarded
LENDING: Books and journals. Photocopies provided
COMPUTER DATA RETRIEVAL: DATASTAR online - outside users charged
HOLDINGS: 55 journals, 45 current titles
CLASSIFICATION: NLM
PUBLICATION: District book catalogue
BRANCHES: Barking Hospital (see 20); Goodmayes Hospital (see 290)
NETWORKS: NETRLS ; Central library for Redbridge Health Authority

Inverness

292
HIGHLAND HEALTH SCIENCES LIBRARY
Raigmore Hospital, Inverness IV2 3UJ
Tel: 0463 234151
STAFF: Mrs RB Higgins ALA, Mrs D McGinley BSc ALA, Ms M Gilmour
              MA ALA (part time)
FOUNDED: 1973
TYPE: Multidisciplinary
HOURS: Mon-Fri 9-9, Sat 9-12
READERS: Staff and other related interest groups at a price
STOCK POLICY: Books discarded after 10 years (last 2 editions kept)
LENDING: Books, journals, AV material. Photocopies provided
COMPUTER DATA RETRIEVAL: DATASTAR online - free
HOLDINGS: 14,000 books; 350 journals, 330 current titles;
                    400 tape/slides, videotapes (100 U-matic, 150 VHS)
CLASSIFICATION: NLM
SPECIAL COLLECTION: Royal Northern Infirmary archives 1789- and
              pre-Health Board archives for the area
CLASSIFICATION: NLM
PUBLICATIONS: Library guide; video list; journals list
BRANCHES: Education Unit, Lewis Hospital, Stornoway; Craig
              Dunain Psychiatric Hospital, Inverness; Craig Pharig
          Mental Handicap Hospital, Inverness; Caithness General, Wick;
              Belford Hospital, Fort William
NETWORKS: ANSLICS; ASHSL; PLCS

Ipswich

293
DEPARTMENT OF NURSING STUDIES, IPSWICH HOSPITAL
Ipswich Hospital, Heath Road Wing, Ipswich, Suffolk IP4 5PD
Tel: 0473 712233 x4522
No furthur information available

294
IPSWICH MEDICAL LIBRARY
Education Centre, Ipswich Hospital, Heath Road, Ipswich IP1 5PD
Tel: 0473 712233 x4527/8
STAFF: Miss H McGlen BSc ALA, Mrs J Harvey
FOUNDED: 1953
TYPE: Multidisciplinary
HOURS: Always open. Staffed Mon-Fri 9-5
READERS: Staff, other users at discretion of librarian
STOCK POLICY: Bound journals kept, unbound journals discarded
              after 10 years; Out of date editions of books discarded
          kept. Ephemeral material discared after 1-2 years
LENDING: Books, bound journals and videos. Photocopies provided
COMPUTER DATA RETRIEVAL: DATASTAR online - free to E Suffolk HA
HOLDINGS: 6,000 books; 307 current journals; 50 videotapes (VHS)
CLASSIFICATION: NLM
SPECIAL COLLECTION: Historical (50 vols)
PUBLICATIONS: Library guide; district periodicals list; regional

periodicals list
NETWORK: E Anglian NHS Region
BRANCHES: Psychiatric Library, Saint Clements Hospital, Ipswich
(see 295); Radiotherapy Library, Ivry Street, Ipswich;
Administration Offices Library ESHA Foxhall Road, Ipswich;
Institute of Family Psychiatry Library, Ivry St, Ipswich

295
SAINT CLEMENT'S HOSPITAL PSYCHIATRIC DIVISION LIBRARY
Foxhall Road, Ipswich, Suffolk IP3 8LS
Tel: 0473 715111 x245
STAFF:Mrs J Harvey (part-time)
FOUNDED: 1975
TYPE: Multidisciplinary
HOURS: Open 24 hours. Staffed approx 3 hours each pm
READERS: Staff, other users at Librarian's discretion
STOCK POLICY: Unbound journals discarded after 5-10 years,
        out of date editions discarded
LENDING: Books and bound journals. Photocopies provided
COMPUTER DATA RETRIEVAL: Access to DATASTAR online - free to
        E Suffolk Health Authority
HOLDINGS: 2,000 books; 56 current journals
CLASSIFICATION: NLM
PUBLICATIONS: Journal holdings; library guide
NETWORK: E Anglian NHS Region; PLCS

Keighley

296
AIREDALE GENERAL HOSPITAL POSTGRADUATE MEDICAL CENTRE
Steeton, Keighley, W Yorks, BD20 6TD
Tel: 0535 52511 x556
STAFF: Mrs SM Thompson BA ALA, Mrs M Roach BA ALA (part-time)
FOUNDED: 1974
TYPE: Multidisciplinary
HOURS: Mon-Thurs 9-5, Fri 9-4. Access by key at other times
READERS: Staff and other users
STOCK POLICY: Books discarded after 10 years
LENDING: Books, journals and AV material. Photocopies provided
COMPUTER DATA RETRIEVAL: DATASTAR online - free
HOLDINGS: 8,000 books; 330 journals, 200 current titles
CLASSIFICATION: NLM
PUBLICATION: Recent accessions list; library guide
NETWORK: YRAHCLIS; NISG
BRANCH: Scalebor Park Hospital (Psychiatric), Ilkley

Kettering

297
PRINCE WILLIAM POSTGRADUATE MEDICAL EDUCATION CENTRE
General Hospital, Kettering, Northants NN16 8UZ
Tel: 0536 81141
No furthur information available

298
NURSE EDUCATION CENTRE LIBRARY
Kidderminster General Hospital, Bewdley Rd, Kidderminster, Worcs,
    DY11 6RJ
Tel: 0562 3424 x37
STAFF: Mrs P Simpson (part time)
TYPE: Nursing
READERS: Qualified nurses and nurses in training
HOURS: Mon - Fri 8.30-4.30. Staffed Thu only
COMPUTER DATA RETRIEVAL: Access to terminal
HOLDINGS: 800 books; 4 current journals
CLASSIFICATION: RCN
NETWORK: West Midlands Regional Health Libraries

299
KIDDERMINSTER POSTGRADUATE MEDICAL CENTRE
Bewdley Road, Kidderminster, Worcs DY11 6RJ
Tel: 0562 3424 x3199
STAFF: Mrs S Gallagher
TYPE: Medical
HOURS: Mon-Fri 8.30-5
READERS: Medical staff only
COMPUTER DATA RETRIEVAL: Access to terminal
HOLDINGS: 1021 books; 60 current journals; AV material
CLASSIFICATION: LC
NETWORK: West Midlands Regional Health Libraries

300
LEA CASTLE HOSPITAL LIBRARY
Wolverley, Kidderminster, Worcs DY10 3PP
Tel: 0562 850461
STAFF: Mrs K Roy BA (part-time)
TYPE: Mental Handicap, Psychiatric
HOURS: Mon-Fri 9-1
READERS: Staff and other users
STOCK POLICY: Bo stock discarded
LENDING: Books and journals. Photocopies supplied
COMPUTER DATA RETRIEVAL: Access to terminal.
HOLDINGS: 3,000 books; 80 journals, 60 current titles
CLASSIFICATION: Own
NETWORK: West Midlands Regional Health Libraries; PLCS

Kilkenny

301
SOUTH EASTERN HEALTH BOARD LIBRARY
Lacken, Dublin Road, Kilkenny, Republic of Ireland
Tel: 010 353 56 21702   Fax: 010 353 56 65270
STAFF: Mrs H Tuite BA DLIS NT, Ms M Ryan
FOUNDED: 1987
TYPE: Multidisciplinary
HOURS: Mon-Fri 9-5
READERS: Staff and other users
LENDING: Books and Government Acts. Photocopies provided
HOLDINGS: 3,800 books; 99 current journals
CLASSIFICATION: Bliss

Kilmarnock

302
AYRSHIRE & ARRAN HEALTH BOARD, AREA MEDICAL LIBRARY
Crosshouse Hospital, Kilmarnock, Ayrshire KA2 0LG
Tel: 0563 21133 x2092
STAFF: Ms U Brita-Carlsen BA DipLib ALA
TYPE: Medical, Psychiatric
HOURS: Access always available. Staffed Mon-Fri 10-4
READERS: Medical staff, other users at librarian's discretion
STOCK POLICY: Superseded editions of books discarded
LENDING: Books, journals and AV material. Photocopies provided
COMPUTER DATA RETRIEVAL: In-house terminal
HOLDINGS: 2,500 books; 230 journals, 212 current titles;
                90 videotapes (VHS)
CLASSIFICATION: NLM
NETWORK: Association of Scottish Health Sciences Librarians
BRANCHES: Ailsa Hospital, Ayr; Ayr County Hospital, Ayr;
Ayrshire Central Hospital, Irvine; Ballochmyle Hospital,
Mauchline; Heathfield Hospital, Ayr; Seafield Hospital,
Ayr; War Memorial Hospital, Lamlash, Arran

King's Lynn

303
KING'S LYNN HEALTH SCIENCE LIBRARY
Queen Elizabeth Hospital, Gayton Road, King's Lynn, Norfolk,
  PE30 4ET
Tel: 0553 766266 x2424
STAFF: Mrs AM Osborne
FOUNDED: 1975
TYPE: Multidisciplinary
HOURS: Always open. Staffed Mon-Fri 8.30-5.30
READERS: Staff only
STOCK POLICY: Books discarded at Librarian's discretion
LENDING: Books only. Photocopies provided
COMPUTER DATA RETRIEVAL: DATASTAR, BLAISE online - free
HOLDINGS: 9,000 books; 150 journals, 120 current titles
CLASSIFICATION: NLM
NETWORK: E Anglian NHS Region

304
KINGSTON POSTGRADUATE MEDICAL CENTRE
1 Galsworthy Road, Kingston-upon-Thames, Surrey, KT2 7BE
Tel: 081 546 7711
STAFF: Mrs G Lambe ALA (part time)
FOUNDED: 1965
TYPE: Medical
HOURS: Mon-Fri 9-5 (Staffed 9.30-1.30). Key available by arrangement
READERS: Doctors, dentists, general practitioners, physiotherapists,
              pharmacists, dieticians
STOCK POLICY: Books selectively discarded after 10 years
LENDING: Books, journals, AV material only to doctors, dentists.
              Photocopies provided
COMPUTER DATA RETRIEVAL: Access to terminal
HOLDINGS: 1,800 books ; 110 journals, 104 current titles; tape/
              slides, 40 videotapes (VHS)
CLASSIFICATION: NLM
PUBLICATION: Monthly bulletin
NETWORK: SWTRLS

Kirkcaldy

305
FIFE COLLEGE OF NURSING AND MIDWIFERY
Forth Avenue, Kirkcaldy KY2 5YS
Tel: 0592 268888
STAFF: Mrs JM Sanson BA(Hons) ALA, Mrs L Scade ONC (LibInfSc),
          Mrs M Ritchie (part time)
TYPE: Midwifery, Nursing, Psychiatric
HOURS: Mon, Tues, Thurs, Fri 8.45-4.30, Wed 8.45-7
READERS: Staff , other users for reference only
STOCK POLICY: Out of date editions of books discarded
LENDING: Books, AV material only. Photocopies provided
COMPUTER DATA RETRIEVAL: In-house terminal
HOLDINGS: 6,600 books; 70 journals; 45 current titles
CLASSIFICATION: RCN
PUBLICATION: Index to recent journal articles/current awareness
              service
BRANCHES: Stratheden Hospital, Cupar; Lynebank Hospital,
 Dunfermline; Dunfermline and West Fife Hospital,
 Dunfermline; Cameron Hospital, Leven; Forth Park Maternity
 Hospital, Kirkcaldy; Milesmark Hospital, Dunfermline

306
VICTORIA HOSPITAL POSTGRADUATE MEDICAL CENTRE
Hayfield Road, Kirkcaldy, Fife KY2 5AH
Tel: 0592 261155 x2614
STAFF: Miss M Smith (part time), Miss AH Hutchison (Postgraduate
                                        Secretary)
TYPE: Multidisciplinary
HOURS: Mon-Fri 9-5. Key available at other times
READERS: Staff only
STOCK POLICY: Stock discarded at Librarian's discretion

LENDING: Books and AV material only
COMPUTER DATA RETRIEVAL: DATASTAR online - other libraries charged
        full cost. CD-ROM
HOLDINGS: 700 books; c145 journals, c120 current titles;
        41 videotapes (VHS)
PUBLICATION: Postgraduate Newsletter (Annual)
NETWORK: ASHSL

Lancaster

307
LANCASTER POSTGRADUATE MEDICAL CENTRE
Ashton Road, Lancaster LA1 4RR
Tel: 0524 65944
STAFF: Dr DR Telford(Honorary Librarian), Mrs A Hamy BA
FOUNDED: 1966
TYPE: Medical
HOURS: Mon-Fri 10-6. Access at all other times
READERS: Medical Staff, other users with permission
STOCK POLICY: Books discarded
LENDING: Books only. Photocopies provided
COMPUTER DATA RETRIEVAL: Access to terminal.
HOLDINGS: 1,800 books; 60 current journals
CLASSIFICATION: NLM
PUBLICATIONS: Lancaster & Westmorland Medical Journal
NETWORK: NORWHSLA

Leamington Spa

308
COVENTRY & WARWICKSHIRE COLLEGE OF NURSING
Nurse Education Centre, St Mary's Lodge, 12 St Mary's Rd,
Leamington Spa, Warks, CV31 1JN
Tel: 0926 39218
STAFF: Mrs L Alcock B App Sc(Lib Stud) (part time)
TYPE: Multidisciplinary
HOURS: Mon-Fri 9-5 (Staffed Tue, Fri 9.30-2.30)
READERS: Staff only
BRANCH: This library is a branch of Central Hospital, Hatton

Leeds

309
CHAPEL ALLERTON HOSPITAL
Harehills Lane, Leeds LS7 4RB
Tel: 0532 623404
STAFF:Mrs M Lewin BSc ALA (part-time)
TYPE: Medical
HOURS: Always open. Staffed three mornings a week
READERS: Staff only
STOCK POLICY: Old editions of books discarded
LENDING: Books and journals. Photocopies provided
COMPUTER DATA RETRIEVAL: Access to terminal. Charged full cost
HOLDINGS: 500 books; 31 journals, 25 current titles
CLASSIFICATION: NLM

310
LEEDS COLLEGE OF NURSING
Saint James's University Hospital, Beckett Street, Leeds, LS9 7TF
Tel: 0532 433144
STAFF: Mrs J Gilroy BA ALA , Ms K Jarvis
TYPE: Nursing
HOURS: Mon- Thu 8.45-5, Fri 8.45-4.30
READERS: Nursing staff
STOCK POLICY:Journals discarded after 5 years, books after 10 years
LENDING: Books only. Photocopies provided
COMPUTER DATA RETRIEVAL: Access to terminal
HOLDINGS: 2,000 books; 35 current journals; 160 tape/slides,
        80 videotapes (VHS)
CLASSIFICATION: DDC
PUBLICATIONS: New accessions list; current awareness bulletin
BRANCH: Meanwood Park School of Nursing, Leeds
  NETWORK: YRAHCLIS; NISG

311
REGIONAL RADIOTHERAPY CENTRE MEDICAL LIBRARY
Cookridge Hospital, Leeds LS16 6QB
Tel: 0532 673411 x293
STAFF: Dr ME Carver MB ChB DipLib (part-time)
FOUNDED: 1971
TYPE: Medical, oncology
HOURS: Always open. Staffed 18.5 hours per week
READERS: Staff, other users for limited use by arrangement
STOCK POLICY: Older books to stack or historical collection
LENDING: Books and journals. Photocopies provided
COMPUTER DATA RETRIEVAL: Access to terminal - free
HOLDINGS: 1,400 books; 89 journals, 72 current titles
CLASSIFICATION: Own, changing to NLM
PUBLICATION: List of recent additions; Library guide

312
SEACROFT HOSPITAL MEDICAL LIBRARY
York Road, Leeds LS14 6UH
Tel: 0532 648164
STAFF: Ms F Norton BA Dip NZLS MA(Lib Man), Ms C Walley BA
                                                    (part time)
TYPE: Multidisciplinary
HOURS: Always open. Staffed Mon-Fri 8.30-5
READERS: Staff and other users   .
STOCK POLICY: Books discarded after 5-8 years
LENDING: Books and journals. photocopies provided
COMPUTER DATA RETRIEVAL: DATASTAR online - free
HOLDINGS: 3,000 books; 190 journals, 134 current titles
CLASSIFICATION: NLM
BRANCHES: Killingbeck Hospital, Leeds; Meanwood Park
 Hospital, Leeds; Leeds Chest Clinic, Leeds
NETWORK: University of Leeds

313
UNIVERSITY OF LEEDS MEDICAL AND DENTAL LIBRARY
University of Leeds, Leeds LS2 9JT
Tel: 0532 335549   Fax: 0532 334381
STAFF: Mrs AMK Collins, MSc ALA, Mrs YE Aitken MA DipLib ALA,
    Mrs AC Farr BA MA (part-time), Mrs PA Brewster BA ALA,
    (St James's) MK Gallico MA AIInfSc (Oncology Information Service),
    Mrs SP Bates BA DipLib (Oncology Information Service),
    Dr ME Carver MB ChB DipLib (Oncology Information Service - part
    time), Mrs EE Williams BSc (Oncology Information Service - part
    time), Mrs P Anson BA ALA, Miss JD Couchman BA
TYPE: Multidisciplinary
HOURS: Mon-Thurs 9-9 (9-5 in long vacation), Fri 9-5, Sat
    9-1 (9-12.30 in long vacation)
READERS: Staff and other users
STOCK POLICY: Duplicates of superseded editions of books discarded
LENDING: Books and journals. Photocopies supplied
COMPUTER DATA RETRIEVAL: DATASTAR online - charged computer time
                          only. CD-ROM from 1982
HOLDINGS: 49,000 books; 1,072 current journals; 68 videotapes (VHS)
CLASSIFICATION: NLM
NETWORK: YRAHCLIS
BRANCH: Saint James's University Hospital, Leeds

314
UNIVERSITY OF LEEDS, NUFFIELD CENTRE FOR HEALTH SERVICES STUDIES.
71-75 Clarendon Road, Leeds LS2 9PL
Tel: 0532 459034 x131
No other information available

315
UNIVERSITY OF LEEDS, ONCOLOGY INFORMATION SERVICE
University of Leeds, Leeds, LS2 9JT
Tel: 0532 335550   Fax: 0532 334381
STAFF: M Gallico MA ALA AIInfSc (Manager), Ms SP Bates BA DipLib,
        Dr ME Carver MB ChB DipLib (part time)
FOUNDED: 1974
TYPE: Medical
HOURS: Mon-Fri 9-5
READERS: Staff and other users
COMPUTER DATA RETRIEVAL: DATASTAR online - charged computer time
                only. CD-ROM from 1982
HOLDINGS: 11,000 journals
SPECIAL COLLECTION: Oncology
PUBLICATION: Oncology Information (monthly); AIDS information
        (monthly); Tumour Marker Update (bi-monthly);
    Pappillomavirus Report (bi-monthly)
NETWORK: Yorkshire Regional Cancer Organisation

316
UNIVERSITY OF LEEDS, SAINT JAMES'S MEDICAL LIBRARY
St James's University Hospital, Beckett Street, Leeds, West
Yorkshire, LS9 7TF
Tel: 0532 433144 x5638   Electronic mail: MDL6PB AT LEEDS.CMSI
STAFF: Mrs PA Brewster BA ALA
FOUNDED: 1972
TYPE: Medical
HOURS: Mon, Tues, Thurs 9-8, Wed, Fri 9-5, Sat 9-1 (Long Vacation
                Mon-Fri 9-5, sat 9-1)
READERS: Staff and other users
STOCK POLICY: Books, journals discarded after 15 years
LENDING: Books, journals, AV material. Photocopies provided
COMPUTER DATA RETRIEVAL: DATASTAR online - charged full   cost
                    CD-ROM from 1989
HOLDINGS: 7,120 books; 320 journals, 319 current titles;
            27 tape/slides, 27 videotapes (VHS)
CLASSIFICATION: NLM
NETWORK: YRAHCLIS

Leek

317
SAINT EDWARD'S HOSPITAL (MEDICAL) PSYCHIATRIC LIBRARY
Cheddleton, near Leek, Staffs ST13 7EB
Tel: 0538 360421
STAFF: Dr K Barrett (Honorary Librarian)
TYPE: Medical
HOURS: Mon-Fri 9-5. Key available at other times
READERS: Staff only
LENDING: Books only to staff
COMPUTER DATA RETRIEVAL: Access to terminal
HOLDINGS: c2,000 books; c20 current journals

Leicester

318
BRITISH PSYCHOLOGICAL SOCIETY
Saint Andrew's House, 48 Princess Road East, Leicester LE1
7DR

The British Psychological Society collection of periodicals
is deposited in the Psychological Library of the University
of London (Senate House) 071 636 4514 x42

319
LEICESTER GENERAL HOSPITAL MEDICAL LIBRARY
Gwendolen Road, Leicester LE5 4PW
Tel: 0533 490490 x4245
STAFF: Mrs J Stevenson ALA (part time)
TYPE: Multidisciplinary
HOURS: Mon-Fri 9-5
READERS: NHS staff only
STOCK POLICY: No definite policy
LENDING: Books only. Photocopies provided
COMPUTER DATA RETRIEVAL: Access to terminal - free.
        CD-ROM: on order
HOLDINGS: 3,000 books; 140 current journals
CLASSIFICATION: NLM

320
TOWERS MEDICAL LIBRARY
Towers Hospital, Humberstone, Leicester LE5 0TD
Tel: 0533 460460 x2642
STAFF: Mrs J Stevenson ALA (part-time)
TYPE: Medical, Nursing, Psychiatric
HOURS: Mon 10-2, Tues, Thu   9.15-1.15
READERS: Staff only
STOCK POLICY: No stock discarded
LENDING: Books only. Photocopies provided
COMPUTER DATA RETRIEVAL: Access to terminal.
HOLDINGS: 1,800 books; 40 journals, 36 current titles
SPECIAL COLLECTION: Psychiatric
CLASSIFICATION: NLM

321
UNIVERSITY OF LEICESTER, CLINICAL SCIENCES LIBRARY
Clinical Sciences Building, Leicester Royal Infirmary,
  PO Box 65, Leicester LE2 7LX
Tel: 0533 523102   Fax: 0533 523107
Electronic mail: RSU @ UK.AC.LEICESTER VAX
STAFF: Mrs JG Shaw BSc MPhil, R Summers BSc DipLib ALA
FOUNDED: 1978
TYPE: Multidisciplinary
HOURS: Mon-Fri 9-10, Sat 9-6, Sun 2-9
READERS: Staff and other users
STOCK POLICY: Books discarded after 10-20 years
LENDING: Books, slides only. Photocopies supplied
COMPUTER DATA RETRIEVAL: DATASTAR online - charged.
        CD-ROM from 1983
HOLDINGS: 14,200 books; 18,314 journals, 500 current titles;
        Tape/slides, 15,000 35mm slides, videotapes (VHS)
SPECIAL COLLECTION: Leicester Medical Society's collection
 of historical works (2,000 vols)
CLASSIFICATION: NLM
PUBLICATIONS: Library guides
NETWORKS: TRAHCLIS; UMSLG

Limerick

322
REGIONAL MEDICAL LIBRARY, POSTGRADUATE MEDICAL CENTRE,
Regional Hospital, Dooradoyle, Limerick, Republic of Ireland
Tel: 010 353 61 29288
STAFF: Ms M Dillon BA Mod DLIS (part-time), 4 other (part-time)
staff
TYPE: Medical, nursing
HOURS: Mon-Thurs 9-9, Fri 9-5
READERS: Staff, open to all medical personnel in the
Mid-West Region
LENDING: Books only
COMPUTER DATA RETRIEVAL: Access to terminal. Free
HOLDINGS: 2,200 books, 600 bound journals; 120 current
journals
CLASSIFICATION: DDC
NETWORK: Regional Medical Library for Mid-Western Health
Board Region
BRANCHES: Associated with Ennis General Hospital, Ennis, Co
Clare; General Hospital, Nenagh, Co Tipperary

Lincoln

323
LINCOLN MEDICAL LIBRARY
County Hospital, Greetwell Road, Lincoln LN2 5QY
Tel: 0522 512512 x2108
STAFF: Mrs LD Cooper ALA
FOUNDED: 1963
TYPE: Multidisciplinary
HOURS: Mon-Fri 9.30-5. Key available at other times
READERS: Staff, Lincolnshire DHA personnel, bona fide enquirers
STOCK POLICY: Books discarded after 10 years or when superseded by
new editions; Major journal titles offered on exchange
schemes
LENDING: Books, journals , health information leaflets.
Photocopies provided
COMPUTER DATA RETRIEVAL: Access to terminal.
HOLDINGS: 4,500 books; 155 journals, 150 current titles;
1,500 35mm slides
CLASSIFICATION: DDC
PUBLICATION: News bulletin
NETWORKS: TRAHCLIS; Lincs Library Service

Liverpool

324
BROADGREEN MEDICAL LIBRARY
Broadgreen Hospital, Thomas Drive, Liverpool L14 3LB
Tel: 051 228 4878 x3447
STAFF: Mrs JA Tyrer PGDipLib, Mrs P Smith
staff

TYPE: Multidisciplinary
HOURS: Mon-Fri 9.15-8.30, Sat 9.30-12
READERS: Staff and other users
STOCK POLICY: Out of date editions of books and journals
        over 4 years old discarded
LENDING: Books and journals
COMPUTER DATA RETRIEVAL: Access to terminal.
HOLDINGS: c 14,000 books; 65 current journals.
CLASSIFICATION: NLM
NETWORK: Mersey Region

325
FAZAKERLEY HOSPITAL, POSTGRADUATE MEDICAL LIBRARY
Lower Lane, Liverpool L9 7AL
Tel: 051 525 5980
STAFF: Mrs S Corfe (part time)
TYPE: Multidisciplinary
HOURS: 24 hours. Staffed Mon-Fri 9-3.30
READERS: Staff and other users
STOCK POLICY: Books discarded
LENDING: Reference only. Photocopies supplied
COMPUTER DATA RETRIEVAL: Access to terminal
HOLDINGS: 50 current journals; microfilms, 35mm slides, VHS
        videotapes

326
LIVERPOOL MEDICAL INSTITUTION
114 Mount Pleasant, Liverpool L3 5SR
Tel: 051 709 9125
STAFF: DM Crook BA ALA, Mrs M Samuels BA(Hons)
FOUNDED: 1779
TYPE: Medical
HOURS: Mon-Fri 9.30-6, Sat 9.30-12.30
READERS: Members and other users
STOCK POLICY: Books selectively discarded after 10 years
LENDING: Books and journals. Photocopies supplied
COMPUTER DATA RETRIEVAL: Access to terminal. CD-ROM from 1989
HOLDINGS: 150 current journals
CLASSIFICATION: Barnard
NETWORK: Contracted to serve Mersey RHA

327
LIVERPOOL SCHOOL OF TROPICAL MEDICINE
Pembroke Place, Liverpool L3 5QA
Tel: 051 708 9393
STAFF: Dr 'CM Deering BA PhD DipLib ALA
TYPE: Medical
HOURS: Mon-Fri 9-5
READERS: Staff, other users at discretion of Librarian
STOCK POLICY: No stock discarded
LENDING: Books ,journals and AV material
COMPUTER DATA RETRIEVAL: DATASTAR, BLAISE, DIALOG online. Charged
        computer time only
HOLDINGS: 10,000 books; 250 journals ; 100 tape/slides
CLASSIFICATION: Barnard

328
SEFTON SCHOOL OF HEALTH STUDIES, STAFF EDUCATION LIBRARY
Aintree Complex, Fazakerley Hospital, Longmoor Lane , Liverpool
    L9 7AL
Tel: 051 529 3609
STAFF: A Willan BA DipLib, Mrs P Owen, Mrs S Astley
TYPE: Nursing, psychiatric
HOURS: Mon-Fri 8.45-4.15
READERS: Nursing and teaching staff
STOCK POLICY: Out of date or damaged books discarded
LENDING: Books only. photocopies provided
HOLDINGS: c20,000 books; 60 current journals; 16mm cine films,
            tape/slides, videotapes (VHS)
CLASSIFICATION: Own
BRANCHES: Greaves Hall Hospital, Southport; Southport Royal
                    Infirmary, Southport

Livingston

329
ST JOHN'S HOSPITAL AT HOWDEN, POSTGRADUATE MEDICAL LIBRARY
Howden Road West, Livingston, West Lothian, EH54 6PP
Tel: 0506 419666 x2302
STAFF: Ms AR Walker BA
TYPE: Medical
HOURS: Open 24 hours
READERS: Staff, other users for reference only
STOCK POLICY: Journals discarded after 10 years; Out of date books
        discarded
LENDING: Books and journals. Photocopies provided
HOLDINGS: 1,000 books; 70 journals, 65 current titles;
            100 35mm slides, 70 tape/slides, 23 videotapes (VHS)
CLASSIFICATION: NLM
SPECIAL COLLECTIONS: Articles published by medical staff

Llanelli

330
LLANELLI GENERAL HOSPITAL, STAFF LIBRARY
Bryn Gwyn Mawr, Llanelli, Dyfed SA15 1NL
Tel: 0554 741222
STAFF: Mrs A Leeuwerke
FOUNDED: 1977
TYPE: Multidisciplinary
HOURS: Mon-Fri 8.30-4.30 (24 hours access for hospital
 doctors).
READERS: Staff and other users

    doctors).
    READERS: Staff and other users

    STOCK POLICY: Books selectively discarded after 10 years
    LENDING: Books and journals. Photocopies provided
    COMPUTER DATA RETRIEVAL: In-house terminal - free. CD-ROM from 1990
    HOLDINGS: 2,500 books; 90 journals, 85 current titles;
                        videotapes (VHS)
    CLASSIFICATION: NLM
    PUBLICATIONS: Accessions lists; library guide
    NETWORK: AWHILES

London

331
BACUP: BRITISH ASSOCIATION OF CANCER UNITED PATIENTS & THEIR
    FAMILIES AND FRIENDS
121-123 Charterhouse Street, London EC1M 6AA
Tel: 071 608 1785   Fax: 071 253 0123
STAFF: Ms D Husband MA DipLib ALA AIInfSc
FOUNDED: 1985
TYPE: Medical, patients
HOURS: Mon-Fri 9-5.30
READERS: Staff, other users via Cancer Information Service (071 608
                1661 -from outside London 0800 181199)
LENDING: Reference only. Photocopies supplied
COMPUTER DATA RETRIEVAL: DATASTAR, BLAISE online - free
HOLDINGS: 500 books; c30 current journals; 30 videotapes (VHS),
                press cuttings

332
BLOOMSBURY COLLEGE OF NURSE EDUCATION
Minerva House, North Crescent, Chenies St, London WC1E 7ER
Tel: 071 387 9300 x5124
STAFF: Ms J Williamson BA ALA
TYPE: Midwifery, nursing, paramedical
HOURS: Mon-Thu 8.30-6, Fri 8.30-5
READERS: Staff and students only
LENDING: Books and journals. Photocopies supplied
COMPUTER DATA RETRIEVAL: DATASTAR online - free. CD-ROM from 1989
HOLDINGS: 20,000 books; 200 journals, 165 current titles;
                80 tape/slides, videotapes (150 U-matic, 50 VHS)
CLASSIFICATION: NLM
PUBLICATION: Current awareness bulletin
NETWORK: NE Thames

333
BRENT AND HARROW SCHOOL OF NURSING
Central Middlesex Hospital, Park Royal, London NW10 7NS
Tel: 081 965 5733 x2512
STAFF: Mrs M Banasiewicz (part-time)
TYPE: Nursing
HOURS: Mon-Fri 8.30-5
READERS: Staff and students
STOCK POLICY: Books and journals discarded after 10 years
LENDING: Books only. Photocopies provided
HOLDINGS: 23 current journals
CLASSIFICATION: NLM (modified) - changing to DDC
NETWORK: NW Thames Region

334
BRITISH DENTAL ASSOCIATION, ROBERT & LILIAN LINDSAY LIBRARY
64 Wimpole Street, London W1M 8AL
Tel:071 935 0875
STAFF: Miss MA Clennett BA ALA MIInfSc, 2 other professional staff
TYPE: Dental
HOURS: Mon-Fri 9-5.30
READERS: Staff, other users for reference only except for dentists
          who are not members of BDA
STOCK POLICY: Non-dental obsolete texts, duplicate dental
  books and out of date journals discarded
LENDING: Books, AV material lent to members only, journals lent to
          members and other libraries. Photocopies provided
COMPUTER DATA RETRIEVAL: DATASTAR online. Charged full
  cost to non-members, flat rate for BDA members
HOLDINGS: 11,000 books, 2,000 pamphlets, 450 subject
  packages (collections of reprints on specific topics); c200
  current journals
CLASSIFICATION: Black (modified)
PUBLICATIONS: Catalogue of accessions and supplements;
  catalogue of rare book collection; Current journals

335
BRITISH INSTITUTE OF RADIOLOGY
36 Portland Place, London W1N 4AT
Tel: 071 580 4085   Fax: 071 255 3209
STAFF: Mrs G Ingham, Swedish graduate in Library Science
       (part-time)
FOUNDED: 1923
TYPE: Radiological
HOURS: Mon-Fri 9-5 (Tue until 7). Staffed Tue 11-7, Thu 11-5
READERS: Members and staff, RSM members and bona fide researchers
          for reference only

STOCK POLICY: General medical journals discarded after 2 years
LENDING: Books to Members only. Photocopies provided
HOLDINGS: 3,370 books; 140 journals, 108 current titles
CLASSIFICATION: Own
SPECIAL COLLECTION: Kathleen Clark Collection of the College of
    Radiographers; early radiologic literature

336
BRITISH LIBRARY SCIENCE REFERENCE AND INFORMATION SERVICE
25 Southampton Buildings, Chancery Lane, London WC2A 1AW
Tel: 071 323 7477   Telex: 266959 SCIREF G   Fax: 071 323 7930
STAFF: Director: MW Hill MA BSc MRIC CChem MIInfSc, 81 other
professional and managerial staff, 223 non-professional
staff
TYPE: Multidisciplinary
HOURS: Mon-Fri 9.30-9, Sat 10-1
READERS: Open to all readers for reference. Holdings at
postgraduate level
STOCK POLICY: Duplicate stock discarded
COMPUTER DATA RETRIEVAL: Computer search service. PRESTEL
available
HOLDINGS: 192,000 books; 30,500 current journals; 26
million patents
CLASSIFICATION: SRL classification system
PUBLICATIONS: Publications on Biotechnology and many other
topics. List of publications available on request
OTHER SERVICES: Photocopy, enquiry services, European
Biotechnology Information Project, Business Information
Service, Japanese Information Service in Science and
Technology and Commerce, Linguistic Aid
TELECOMMUNICATIONS: Facsimile, BT Gold and PRESTEL
available
HOLBORN READING ROOM, 25 Southampton Buildings, London WC2A
1AW Tel: 071 323 7477
Makes available the literature on the inventive sciences,
engineering, industrial technologies, patents and commerce.
Also includes food technology
COMPUTER DATA RETRIEVAL; Online Search service

337
ALDWYCH READING ROOM, 9 Kean Street, London WC2B 4AT
 Tel: 071 323 7288
Makes available the SRL's main collections of literature on
the life sciences and technologies, medicine,
biotechnology, agriculture, the earth sciences, astronomy
and pure mathematics. Many journals are on open access.
HOURS: Mon-Fri 9.30-5.30
CD-ROM SERVICE: MEDLINE (CSA), EXCERPTA MEDICA, LIFE SCIENCES
    COLLECTION, SCIENCE CITATION INDEX, etc

338
BRITISH MEDICAL ASSOCIATION LIBRARY
BMA House, Tavistock Square, London WC1H 9JP
Tel: 071 383 6060 (Enquiries), 071 383 6625 (loans)
Telex: 9312131899 NLG   Fax: 071 388 2544
Electronic mail: BT Gold 74:BMX030
STAFF: T McSean BA ALA, Mrs PA Bonnett BA ALA, WH Forrester BSc ALA
                AIIS, RM Jones BA MLS, Ms BS Carney MA ALA, T Norman
FOUNDED: 1887
TYPE: Medical
HOURS: Mon-Wed 9-6, Thu-Fri 9-8
READERS: Members of BMA, other users at librarian's discretion
STOCK POLICY: Books and journals discarded
LENDING: Books , journals, films, videos. Photocopies provided
COMPUTER DATA RETRIEVAL: DATASTAR,BLAISE online. Charged full
        cost. CD-ROM: CSA Medline from 1987, Compact Library-AIDS
HOLDINGS: 30,000 books; 3,000 journals, 1,200 current titles;
                100 microfilms, 900 16mm films, 140 videotapes (VHS)
CLASSIFICATION: NLM
SPECIAL COLLECTION: Hastings Collection (428 vols)
PUBLICATION: BMA library bulletin; Video catalogue; Journal
        catalogue

339
BRITISH SCHOOL OF OSTEOPATHY
1-4 Suffolk Street, London SW1Y 4HG
Tel: 071 930 9254
STAFF: W Podmore MA DipLib, P Moriarty, L Lynes
FOUNDED: 1980
TYPE: Medical
HOURS: Mon-Wed 9-7, Thu-Fri 9-5 (term time), Mon-Fri 9-5 (vacation)
READERS: Staff and other users
STOCK POLICY: Books discarded after a varying number of years
LENDING: Books, videos, tapes, slides, X-rays .Photocopies
        provided
COMPUTER DATA RETRIEVAL: BLAISE online. Charged computer time only
HOLDINGS: 10,000 books; 100 journals, 75 current titles;
                100 tape/slides, 60 videotapes (VHS)
 osteology models,
 X-rays, , audio cassettes
SPECIAL COLLECTION: Osteopathy (600 vols)
CLASSIFICATION: DDC
PUBLICATIONS: Recent accessions

340
BROOK GENERAL HOSPITAL POSTGRADUATE MEDICAL LIBRARY
Shooters Hill Road, Woolwich, London SE18 4LW
Tel: 081 856 5555 x3301
STAFF: Mrs R Bremer ALA, Mrs S Smith (part time)
FOUNDED: 1966
TYPE: Medical, paramedical
HOURS: Mon-Fri 9-5
READERS: Staff and other users
STOCK POLICY: Out of date books discarded. Journals no longer used
        offered to other libraries
LENDING: Books only. Photocopies provided
COMPUTER DATA RETRIEVAL: DATASTAR online - free
HOLDINGS: 1,760 books; 126 current journals. Tape/slides,
        videotapes (VHS)
CLASSIFICATION: NLM
PUBLICATION: Library bulletin
NETWORK: SE Thames Regional Library and Information Service

341
CENTRAL MIDDLESEX HOSPITAL
Acton Lane, London NW10 7NS
Tel: 081 965 5733 x250314
STAFF: Mrs BM Farrant BA DipLib ALA, Mrs S Cook, Mrs A Freuchan
        LDS RCSEng DipLib
FOUNDED: pre 1964
TYPE: Multidisciplinary
HOURS: Mon-Fri 9.15-5
READERS: Staff and other users
STOCK POLICY: Books selectively discarded after 10 years.
LENDING: Books only. Photocopies provided
COMPUTER DATA RETRIEVAL: HEADLINE, ACCESS online. Free
        CD-ROM from 1989
HOLDINGS: c3,000 books; 125 journals, 115 current titles
CLASSIFICATION: NLM
PUBLICATIONS: Monthly accessions list; Annual journals list
NETWORK: NW Thames Regional Library and Information Service

342
CENTRE FOR POLICY ON AGEING
25/31 Ironmonger Row, London EC1V 3QP
Tel: 071 253 1787   Fax: 071 490 4206
STAFF: Ms G Crosby BA(Hons) ALA, Ms H Monypenny BA DipLib
FOUNDED: c1975
TYPE: Social gerontology
READERS: Staff and other users
STOCK POLICY: Journals selectively discarded
LENDING: Reference only. Photocopies provided
COMPUTER DATA RETRIEVAL: In-house terminal
HOLDINGS: 200 journals
CLASSIFICATION: Own
PUBLICATIONS: New Literature on Old Age (bi-monthly); Selected
        bibliographies; Register of research

343
CHARING CROSS AND WESTMINSTER MEDICAL SCHOOL (Charing Cross site)
The Reynolds Building, Saint Dunstan's Road, London W6 8RP
Tel: 081 846 7152   Fax: 081 846 7222
Electronic mail: JANET: S.GODBOLT/N.WHITSED/LIBRARY @ UK.AC.LON.
                         CXWMS.UX
STAFF: Mrs LS Godbolt BA FLA, Mrs N Whitsed MSc ALA , HR Hague
   MA ALA, P Morrell BA ALA
  DipLib FRGS, 2 other (full-time), 5 (part-time) staff
TYPE: Multidisciplinary
HOURS: Mon-Thu 9-9, Fri 9-8, Sat 9-12
READERS: Staff, other bona fide enquirers
STOCK POLICY: Review items over 10 years old
LENDING: Books only. photocopies provided
COMPUTER DATA RETRIEVAL: DATASTAR, BLAISE online - standard
  charge. CD-ROM: Medline from 1975 - other databases available
HOLDINGS: 12,000 books; 400 journals 300 current titles; microfilms,
        tape/slides, 35mm slides, videotapes (U-matic,VHS),
        videodiscs
CLASSIFICATION: NLM
SPECIAL COLLECTION: Writings by Charing Cross staff (200 vols)
PUBLICATIONS: Library guide; accessions list; audio-visual
  holdings; journals list; subject guides; readers guides;
  other leaflets
BRANCHES: Charing Cross and Westminster Medical School:
  Westminster site (see next entry); West London Hospital;
ASSOCIATE LIBRARIES: West Middlesex University Hospital;
  Queen Mary's University Hospital, Roehampton;
  Kennedy Institute of Rheumatology, London W6
NETWORKS: NW Thames; University of London

344
CHARING CROSS AND WESTMINSTER MEDICAL SCHOOL (Westminster Site)
17 Horseferry Road, London SW1P 2AR
Tel: 071 746 8107   Fax: 071 828 7196
STAFF: WJ Robertson MA DipLib, R Wentz Dipl Bibl ,Ms A Thain BA ALA
TYPE: Multidisciplinary
HOURS: Always open. Staffed Mon-Fri 9-5.30
READERS: Staff and other users
STOCK POLICY: Pre-penultimate editions of books discarded
LENDING: Books and journals. Photocopies provided
COMPUTER DATA RETRIEVAL: DATASTAR online - standard charge.
                  CD-ROM from 1982
HOLDINGS: 4,500 books; 230 journals, 180 current titles
CLASSIFICATION: NLM
PUBLICATIONS: Monthly library bulletin; periodicals
  catalogue
NETWORK: NW Thames

345
CHARING CROSS SCHOOL OF NURSING
Riverside College of Nursing, Claybrook Road, Hammersmith,
    London W6 8LN
Tel: 081 846 1681
STAFF: Miss P Louison BA ALA
TYPE: Nursing
HOURS: Mon-Fri 8.30-4.30
READERS: Staff and nursing students
STOCK POLICY: Some books over 10 years old discarded
LENDING: Books only. photocopies provided
COMPUTER DATA RETRIEVAL: Access to terminal.
CLASSIFICATION: DDC 19th ed (modified)
NETWORK: NW Thames Regional Library and Information Service

346
CHARLES WEST SCHOOL OF NURSING,
Hospitals for Sick Children, 24 Great Ormond Street, London WC1N 3JH
Tel: 071 405 9200 x5843
STAFF: Mrs D Fisher BA ALA, Miss SJ Marsh BA DipLib
TYPE: Nursing
HOURS: Mon-Fri 8.30-5, Mon, Wed until 6
READERS: Nursing staff, other users by arrangement
STOCK POLICY: Books discarded after 10 years
LENDING: Books and journals. photocopies supplied
COMPUTER DATA RETRIEVAL: DATASTAR online
HOLDINGS: 17,000 books; 102 current journals; tape/slides,
        computer progroms, videotapes (VHS)
CLASSIFICATION: RCN
PUBLICATIONS: Library leaflet; Current Awareness Bulletin;
        Literature Search Guide
BRANCH: Queen Elizabeth Hospital for Children, School of
Nursing, London
NETWORK: NE Thames Regional Library Service

347
CHILD ACCIDENT PREVENTION TRUST RESOURCE CENTRE
28 Portland Place, London W1N 4DE
Tel: 071 636 2545   Fax: 071 323 5179
STAFF: A Sen MA MLitt PG Dip (Information Officer)
FOUNDED: 1979
TYPE: Multidisciplinary
HOURS: Mon-Fri 10-5
READERS: Staff, other users by appointment
STOCK POLICY: Books and journals discarded after variable intervals.
LENDING: Reference only. Photocopies provided
HOLDINGS: 95 journals; 35mm slides, tape/slides, 30 videotapes
CLASSIFICATION: Own
PUBLICATION: Accession list (monthly)

348
CIBA FOUNDATION
41 Portland Place, London W1N 4BN
Tel: 071 636 9456   Fax: 071 436 2840
STAFF: Dr CK Langley MA PhD, Ms L Geller, T Conyers, Ms H Russell
FOUNDED: 1947
TYPE: Multidisciplinary
HOURS: Mon-Fri 9-6, Sat-Sun 9-5.30. Staffed weekdays only
READERS: Staff, other users
STOCK POLICY: Journals discarded if no longer required, books after
        15 years.
LENDING: Reference only. Photocopies provided. Own titles for sale
COMPUTER DATA RETRIEVAL: DATASTAR online charged full cost
HOLDINGS: 8,000 books; 100 journals, 80 current titles
SPECIAL COLLECTIONS: Oppenheimer medical biographies (1,000 vols)

349
DEPARTMENT OF HEALTH AND SOCIAL SECURITY
Hannibal House, Elephant and Castle, London SE1 6TE
Tel: 071 972 2380/1/2   Fax: 071 972 2383
STAFF: JH Wormald BSc ALA (Head of Library & Information Services),
CH Horsey BSc DipLib ALA, DS Buchanan MA ALA, AB Cooper MLS ALA,
21 other professional staff.
FOUNDED: 1834
TYPE: Multidisciplinary
HOURS: Mon-Fri 9-5
READERS: Staff, accredited research workers by arrangement only
STOCK POLICY: Journals discarded after varying periods, books
        discarded after 10 years
LENDING: Books and journals. Photocopies provided
COMPUTER DATA RETRIEVAL: DATASTAR, BLAISE, DIALOG, PERGAMON,
        PROFILE, TEXTLINE (all online).
HOLDINGS: Over 200,000 books and bound journals; over 2,000
        current journals
SPECIAL COLLECTION: Early Poor Law pamphlets (51 vols
 containing approx. 700 pamphlets)
CLASSIFICATION: Bliss
PUBLICATIONS: Health Service abstracts; Social Service Abstracts;
 Health buildings library bulletin; Nursing Research Abstracts;
 Quality Assurance Abstracts (with King's Fund); Social Security
 library bulletin; Current literature on occupational pensions;
 Selected abstracts on occupational diseases; bibliographies on a
 range of subjects are produced as required
BRANCHES: Health Buildings Library, London; Medicines
 Library, London; Social Security Library, London; Russell Square
 Library, London; Richmond House library, London

350
DISABLED LIVING FOUNDATION
380-384 Harrow Road, London, W9 2HU
Tel: 071 289 6111
STAFF: Mrs P Lane ALA, Ms J Parkin BA
FOUNDED: 1972
TYPE: Nursing, psychiatric, all non-medical aspects of disability
HOURS: Mon-Fri 9.30-5
READERS: Staff, other users by appointment
STOCK POLICY: Journals discarded after 2 years, except essential
          runs, books discarded when superseded
LENDING: Reference only. Photocopies occasionally provided
COMPUTER DATA RETRIEVAL: In-house terminal
HOLDINGS: 7,000 books; 300 journals, 250 current titles;
                    3 videotapes (VHS)   •
CLASSIFICATION: Own
PUBLICATIONS: Resource papers, reading lists, journals list

351
FRIERN HOSPITAL
Friern Barnet Rd, New Southgate, London N11 3BP
081 368 1288 x2158
STAFF: Miss S Robertson BA , Mrs EF Browne
TYPE: Multidisciplinary
HOURS: Mon-Wed 9-4.30, Thu 9-6, Fri 9-4.30
READERS: Staff and other users
STOCK POLICY: Out of date editions of books discarded
LENDING: Books and journals. Photocopies provided
HOLDINGS: 4378 books; 117 journals 93 current titles
SPECIAL COLLECTION: Psychiatry and psychology (4,000 vols)
CLASSIFICATION: UDC
PUBLICATION: Current awareness bulletin on community care of
        mental illness.
NETWORK: NE Thames Regional Library and Information Service; PLCS

352
GREENWICH DISTRICT HOSPITAL
Vanbrugh Hill, London SE10 9HE
081 858 8141 x2158/9 ; 081 858 3947
STAFF: Mrs CE Russell BA(Hons) ALA
FOUNDED: 1971
TYPE: Multidisciplinary
HOURS: Mon-Fri 9-5
READERS: Staff and other users
STOCK POLICY: Stock discarded
LENDING: Books and journals. Photocopies provided
COMPUTER DATA RETRIEVAL: DATASTAR online - free. Access
 to PRESTEL via Woolwich Reference Library
HOLDINGS: 3,500 books; 150 journals, 85 current titles
CLASSIFICATION: NLM
NETWORK: LASER; SE Thames Regional Library and Information
 Service

353

HEALTH EDUCATION AUTHORITY, HEALTH PROMOTION INFORMATION CENTRE
Hamilton House, Mabledon Place, London WC1H 9TX
Tel: 071 383 3833   Fax: 071 387 0550
STAFF: Ms S Cook BA ALA (Manager),Ms F Martin BA DipLib ALA, R Amis
        BA(hons), Ms E Hermon BA(Hons), MS S Lyth BA(Hons) DipLib,
        Ms E Reed, Ms L Hoare BSc PGCE, Ms C Herman BA(Hons) (job
        share with Ms R Salter)
FOUNDED: 1974
TYPE: Health education/promotion
HOURS: Mon-Fri 9-5
READERS: Staff and other users
STOCK POLICY: Books and journals discarded at varying periods
LENDING: Books only. Photocopies provided for BLLD forms
COMPUTER DATA RETRIEVAL: DATASTAR online.
HOLDINGS: 12,000 books; 400 current journals; 500 sets 35mm slides,
        500 tape/slides, 2,000 videotapes (VHS), 4,000 teaching
        packs, 500 tapes, 500 posters, 1,000 leaflets, 300 models/
        games
CLASSIFICATION: UDC
SPECIAL COLLECTION: Health education dissertations (250)
PUBLICATIONS: Journal articles of interest to health educators
        (monthly), Recent additions to Library (bi-monthly),
        Recent additions to Resources (bi-monthly), Resource Lists

354

HIGHLANDS HOSPITAL POSTGRADUATE CENTRE
Highlands Hospital, World's End Lane, Winchmore Hill, London N21 1PN
081 366 6600 x6743
STAFF: Ms H Frankel (part-time)
TYPE: Multidisciplinary
HOURS: Mon-Fri 9-5. Key available out of hours. Staffed
 Mon-Fri 9.30-3.30 (except Thurs 9.30-3)
READERS: Staff and other users
STOCK POLICY: Books over 10 years old discarded with discretion
LENDING: Books , journals, skeletons. Photocopies provided
COMPUTER DATA RETRIEVAL: DATASTAR online. Free
HOLDINGS: 1,200 books; 65 current journals
CLASSIFICATION: NLM
NETWORK: NE Thames Regional Library and Information Service

355

HOMERTON HOSPITAL EDUCATION CENTRE, NEWCOMB LIBRARY
Homerton Row,   London E9 6SR
081 985 5555 x7751
STAFF: Miss IA Cantwell BA, Ms A Wood BA
FOUNDED: 1986 (Based on library at Hackney Hospital founded 1940s)
TYPE: Multidisciplinary

HOURS: Mon-Fri 7.15am-11pm. Staffed 9-6
READERS: Staff, other users by arrangement
STOCK POLICY: Books discarded after 10 years
LENDING: Books, journals, slides. Photocopies provided
COMPUTER DATA RETRIEVAL: DATASTAR online - charged full cost.
HOLDINGS: 6,500 books; 133 journals, 118 current titles;
                     tape/slides, videotapes (VHS)
CLASSIFICATION: NLM
PUBLICATIONS: Library services guide; new books
NETWORK: NE Thames Regional Library and Information Service

356
IMPERIAL CANCER RESEARCH FUND, LIBRARY & INFORMATION SERVICES
PO Box 123, 44/45 Lincoln's Inn Fields, London WC2A 3PX
Tel:071 269 3206   Telex: 265107   Fax: 071 405 1556
STAFF: Mrs M Davies BA(Hons) DipLib ALA MIInfSc (Head of Library
    & Information Services, Ms LS Farley BA ALA (part time),
    Mrs A Aldam BSc DipInfSc MIInfSc (part time), Ms J Lomas BA ALA
    MIInfSc, Mrs J Milligan MSc, W Russell-Edu, Miss L Shepherd BA,
        4 other full-time and 3 part time staff
TYPE: Medical, research
HOURS: Always open. Staffed Mon-Fri 9-5
READERS: Staff, other bona fide researchers for reference
 only during hours when library staff are present
LENDING: Books only. Photocopies provided
COMPUTER DATA RETRIEVAL: In-house terminal - free; CD-ROM from 1989
HOLDINGS: c10,000 books; c500 journals, c300 current titles
CLASSIFICATION: NLM
PUBLICATIONS: Library bulletin; periodicals holdings list; ICRF
        Scientific Report
BRANCH: Imperial Cancer Research Fund Laboratories, Clare
 Hall, South Mimms, Potter's Bar, Herts EN6 3LD

357
INSTITUTE FOR THE STUDY OF DRUG DEPENDENCE
1-4 Hatton Place, Hatton Garden, London EC1N 8ND
Tel: 071 430 1991   Fax: 071 404 4415
STAFF: P Defriez MA ALA MIInfSc (Head Librarian), J Witton BSc ALA
        DipLib (Head of Information Services),Ms K Carter BSc
        DipLib, Ms J Yeates BSc DipLib
 FOUNDED: 1968
TYPE: Multidisciplinary
HOURS: Mon-Fri 9.30-5.30
 READERS: Staff and other users
 STOCK POLICY: No stock discarded
 LENDING: Reference only. Photocopies provided
 COMPUTER DATA RETRIEVAL: In-house terminal
 HOLDINGS: 2,500 books; 350 journals, 150 current titles;
        45,000 document, 100 videotapes (VHS)
 PUBLICATIONS: Drug abuse current awareness bulletin; Drug
        abstracts monthly; Press digest

358
INSTITUTE OF CANCER RESEARCH: ROYAL CANCER HOSPITAL
Chester Beatty Laboratories, 237 Fulham Road, London SW3 6JB
Tel: 071 352 5946 (library only); 071 352 8133
STAFF: Ms GM Davies BA ALA, E Bull BSc DipLib, S Dobby ALA,
 J Randall BA ALA, 3 other (full-time) and 1 (part time) staff
TYPE: Multidisciplinary
HOURS: Always open. Staffed Mon-Fri 9-5.30
READERS: Staff, other users for reference only
STOCK POLICY: Duplicate journals over 20 years old
 discarded
COMPUTER DATA RETRIEVAL: In-house terminal - free
HOLDINGS: 8,000 books, 30,000 bound journals; 600 current
              journals. Microfiche
CLASSIFICATION: NLM
NETWORK: CLIC
BRANCH: Institute of Cancer Research, Clifton Avenue,
 Belmont, Sutton, Surrey SM2 5PX

359
INSTITUTE OF CHILD HEALTH
30 Guilford Street, London WC1N 1EH
Tel: 071 242 9789 x2424
STAFF: Miss ES Brooke ALA
FOUNDED: 1946
TYPE: Medical
HOURS: Mon-Fri 9-6 (Times may vary during Summer)
READERS: Medical staff, other users at discretion of Librarian
STOCK POLICY: Out of date stock discarded
LENDING: Reference only. No photocopy service, but will provide
          photocopies to other libraries occasionally
COMPUTER DATA RETRIEVAL: DATASTAR online. Only available to staff.
          CD-ROM from 1988
HOLDINGS: c5,500 books; 224 journals, 153 current titles
CLASSIFICATION: Barnard
NETWORK: University of London

360
INSTITUTE OF DENTAL SURGERY
Eastman Dental Hospital, Gray's Inn Road, London WC1X 8LD
Tel: 071 837 3646
STAFF: Ms B Cumbers BA ALA
FOUNDED: 1950
TYPE: Dental
HOURS: Mon, Thu 9-7, Tue Wed Fri 9-5.30
READERS: Staff and other users
STOCK POLICY: Books discarded irregularly
LENDING: Books and journals. Photocopies provided
COMPUTER DATA RETRIEVAL: DATASTAR online - charged computer time
          only. CD-ROM from 1983

HOLDINGS: 2,000 books; 200 journals, 91 current titles;
            25 tape/slides, 6 videotapes (VHS)
CLASSIFICATION: Own
PUBLICATIONS: Library guide; Staff publications list; Guides to
        literature searching; Irregular newsletter (Library
        Information for Eastman Staff and Students - LIES)
NETWORK: NE Thames Regional Library and Information Service;
        University of London

361
INSTITUTE OF MEDICAL LABORATORY SCIENCES
12 Queen Anne Street, London W1M 0AU
Tel: 071 636 8192   Fax: 071 436 4946
STAFF: JR Mercer AIMLS ARPS AIMI
FOUNDED: 1962
TYPE: Paramedical
HOURS: Mon-Fri 9-5 (by appointment)
READERS: Members of Institute and others interested in
Medical Laboratory Sciences
STOCK POLICY: Some journals discarded after 3 years
LENDING: Books and journals. Also lend IMLS Fellowship theses
 through and to other libraries (not to individuals)
HOLDINGS: 1050 books; 52 journals, 43 current
SPECIAL COLLECTION: Fellowship theses
CLASSIFICATION: Own
PUBLICATIONS: Catalogue of theses; list of current journals
        received
NETWORK: Outlier library, British Museum

362
INSTITUTE OF NEUROLOGY, ROCKEFELLER MEDICAL LIBRARY
The National Hospital, Queen Square, London WC1N 3BG
Tel; 071 837 6611 x4143/4144; 071 829 8709
Fax: 071 278 5069
STAFF: Ms MB Bailey ALA AIInfSc, Miss M Ford BA DipLib
FOUNDED: 1948
TYPE: Medical, biomedical
HOURS: Mon-Fri 9-6
READERS: Staff and other users
STOCK POLICY: Books and journals (except neurology texts) discarded
LENDING: Books only. Photocopies provided
COMPUTER DATA RETRIEVAL: In-house terminal - charged computer time
        only. CD-ROM
HOLDINGS: 16,000 books; 12,500 bound journals, 250 titles, 180
        current titles
SPECIAL COLLECTION: Historical neurology (1,000 vols)
CLASSIFICATION: UDC
BRANCHES: Maida Vale Hospital, London; affiliated to
National Hospital College of Speech Sciences

363
INSTITUTE OF PSYCHIATRY LIBRARY
De Crespigny Park, London SE5 8AF
Tel: 071 703 5411 x3204   Electronic mail: LIBRARY @ UK.AC.PSYCH.UX
STAFF: M Guha BA ALA, Ms C Martin BA ALA
TYPE: Psychiatric
HOURS: Mon-Thurs 9-8, Fri 9-5
READERS: Staff only
STOCK POLICY: No stock discarded
LENDING: Books and journals. Photocopies provided
COMPUTER DATA RETRIEVAL: DATASTAR, DIALOG online - premium charge
        to outside users. CD-ROM from 1984 - outside users charged
HOLDINGS: 30,000 books, 20,000 bound journals; 400 current titles
CLASSIFICATION: Bliss (modified)
NETWORK: PLCS

364
INSTITUTE OF PSYCHO-ANALYSIS
63 New Cavendish Street, London W1M 7RD
Tel: 071 580 4952
STAFF: AS Couch (Honorary Librarian-part time), Ms J Duncan
FOUNDED: 1926
TYPE: Psychoanalysis and related topics
HOURS: Mon-Fri 10-6
READERS: Staff, other users with special permission
STOCK POLICY: Books discarded
LENDING: Books and journals. Photocopies provided
HOLDINGS: 30,000 books; 26 journals, 20 current titles.
CLASSIFICATION: Own

365
INTERNATIONAL PLANNED PARENTHOOD FEDERATION
Regents College, Inner Circle, Regents Park, , London NW1 4NS
Tel: 071 486 0741   Telex: 919573 IPEPEE G   Fax: 071 487 7950
STAFF: Mrs R Ward ALA, Ms D Coleman ALA
FOUNDED: 1964
TYPE: Medical, welfare
HOURS: Mon-Fri 10-5
READERS: Staff and other users
STOCK POLICY: Books and journals discarded at variable intervals
LENDING: Books , AV material. Photocopies provided
COMPUTER DATA RETRIEVAL: CD-ROM from 1989
HOLDINGS: 6,000 books; 150 current journals; 5,000 microfilms,
        30 tape/slides, 2,000 35mm slides, 200 videotapes (VHS)
CLASSIFICATION: Own
PUBLICATION: Quarterly accessions list

366
ISLINGTON DISTRICT LIBRARY
Whittington Hospital, Highgate Hill, London N19 5NF
Tel: 071 272 3070 x4261   Fax: 071 263 4760
STAFF: Miss JM Stephen ALA, E Sidoli BA
FOUNDED: 1984
TYPE: Multidisciplinary
HOURS: Mon-Fri 9.30-9, Sat 9.30-1 (Staffed Mon-Fri 9.30-5)
READERS: Staff and other users
STOCK POLICY: Out of date books discarded
LENDING: Books only. Photocopies provided
COMPUTER DATA RETRIEVAL: DATASTAR online - free
HOLDINGS: 6,000 bound journals, 200 current titles
CLASSIFICATION: NLM
PUBLICATION: Accessions list
BRANCH: Royal Northern Hospital, Holloway Rd, London N7
NETWORK: NE Thames Regional Library Service

367
KENNEDY INSTITUTE OF RHEUMATOLOGY
6 Bute Gardens, London W6 7DW
Tel: 081 748 9966 x4007/4008   Fax: 081 748 5090
STAFF: Dr F Grainger BSci PhD DipIInfSci, TH Davies BA
FOUNDED: 1966
TYPE: Multidisciplinary
HOURS: Mon-Fri 9-5
READERS: Staff, other users on application
STOCK POLICY: Books over 10 years old discarded, journals discarded
     at variable intervals
LENDING: Books and journals to Institute staff only
COMPUTER DATA RETRIEVAL: DATASTAR online - outside users charged
     full cost. CD-ROM from 1989
HOLDINGS: 1,500 books; 100 current journals
CLASSIFICATION: LC

368
KING'S COLLEGE SCHOOL OF MEDICINE AND DENTISTRY (STRAND CAMPUS)
King's College London, Strand, London WC2R 2LS
Tel: 071 873 2139 Fax: 071 872 0207
STAFF: DG Law MA DipLib FLA, 80 other staff
FOUNDED: 1829
TYPE: Preclinical medicine
HOURS: Mon-Fri 9.30-9, (Vacation: 9.30-5)
READERS: Staff and other users
STOCK POLICY: Permanent retention
LENDING: Books only. Photocopies provided for BLLD forms
COMPUTER DATA RETRIEVAL: DATASTAR , DIALOG online - charged full
     cost. CD-ROM
HOLDINGS: 400,000 books; 400,000 journal volumes, c3,000 current
     titles
CLASSIFICATION: LC
BRANCHES: Denmark Hill (see next entry)
NETWORKS: University of London; SWALCAP

369
KING'S COLLEGE SCHOOL OF MEDICINE AND DENTISTRY (DENMARK HILL)
King's College Hospital, Bessemer Rd, London SE5 9PJ
Tel: 071 274 6222 x 4022   Fax: 071 326 3001
STAFF: Miss CG Hogg BA ALA, Mrs K Clark BLib ALA, Ms S Jardine
         BSc ALA, Ms J Ellin BA, 1 vacancy
TYPE: Multidisciplinary
HOURS: Mon-Fri 9-7. Staffed 9-6
READERS: Staff and students only
STOCK POLICY: Limited retention policy for smoe journal titles
LENDING: Books and journals. Self service photocopying

COMPUTER DATA RETRIEVAL: DATASTAR, BLAISE, DIALOG online - charged
         full cost. CD-ROM from 1983
HOLDINGS: 11,000 books; 400 journals, 260 current
CLASSIFICATION: Barnard
SPECIAL COLLECTION: King's publications, historical
PUBLICATIONS: Guide to library service; Dental current contents;
         pamphlets
BRANCH: Normanby College (combined School of Nursing,
 Midwifery and Physiotherapy), London
NETWORK: King's College London; LIBERTAS

370
KING'S FUND CENTRE
126 Albert Street, London NW1 7NF
071 267 6111   Fax: 071 267 6108
STAFF: Ms M Haines-Taylor BA MLS, Ms G Messenger MA ALA, C Renwick
         BLib, A Hutchinson BA, Mrs V Wildridge BA ALA
TYPE: Multidisciplinary, health administration
HOURS: Mon-Fri 9.30-5.30, Sat 9.30-5
READERS: Staff and other users
STOCK POLICY: Books discarded
LENDING: Reference only. Photocopies provided
COMPUTER DATA RETRIEVAL: DATASTAR, BLAISE, DIALOG online - charged
         computer time only
HOLDINGS: 26,000 books; 400 current journals; microfiche
CLASSIFICATION: Bliss
SPECIAL COLLECTION: 6,500 subject folders of journal articles
PUBLICATIONS: Accessions list; periodicals list

371
LEWISHAM HOSPITAL MEDICAL LIBRARY
Lewisham High Street, London SE13 6LH
Tel: 081 690 4311 x6454   Fax: 081 690 9829
STAFF: Miss J Brewer ALA, Miss J Coyte BA ALA (part-time),
         Ms J Jamieson
TYPE: Medical
HOURS: Mon-Fri 9-5
READERS: Staff and other users

STOCK POLICY: Out of date and damaged books withdrawn and
 replaced. Ephemeral journals discarded after 1 year
LENDING: Books and journals. photocopies provided
COMPUTER DATA RETRIEVAL: Access to terminal - free. PRESTEL
 available
HOLDINGS: 2,000 books, 3,000 bound journals; 130 current titles
CLASSIFICATION: DDC
NETWORK: SETRHA; Lewisham Public Libraries

372
LONDON COLLEGE OF FURNITURE
41 Commercial Rd, London E1 1LA
Tel: 071 247 1953 x254   Fax: 071 375 1903
STAFF: Ms A Rehahn BA MSc ALA MBIM, R Farr BA ALA, C Storey ALA,
       P Semple BA(Hons) DipLib, P Clarke BA(Hons) DipLib
FOUNDED: 1952
TYPE: Medical, paramedical, welfare
HOURS: Mon, Fri 9-5, Tue-Thu 9-7.15 (vacation 9-5)
READERS: Staff and other users
STOCK POLICY: Stock discarded
LENDING: Books and journals. Photocopies provided
COMPUTER DATA RETRIEVAL: BLAISE online - charged full cost
HOLDINGS: 39,000 books; 400 journals, 350 current titles;
              39 microfilms, 100 tape/slides, 30,000 35mm slides,
              900 videotapes (VHS)
CLASSIFICATION: DDC
SPECIAL COLLECTION: Design research for disability
PUBLICATION: Disability scene: a library reference list
BRANCH: Farrance Street, London E14
NETWORK: City of London Polytechnic Libraries

373
LONDON FOOT HOSPITAL AND COLLEGE OF PODIATRIC MEDICINE
33 Fitzroy Square, London W1P 6AY
Tel: 071 636 0602
STAFF: Mrs E South ALA (part time)
FOUNDED: 1913
TYPE: Paramedical
HOURS: Mon-Fri 8.30-5 (not staffed all the time)
READERS: Staff only
STOCK POLICY: Non-chiropody journals discarded after 5 years,
          non-chiropody books discarded after 10 years
LENDING: Books, videos, slides
COMPUTER DATA RETRIEVAL: In-house terminal. CD-ROM from 1990
HOLDINGS: 35 journals, 30 current titles; 3,000 35mm slides,
              25 videotapes (VHS)
CLASSIFICATION: NLM
NETWORK: NETRHA

374
LONDON HOSPITAL MEDICAL COLLEGE
Turner Street, Whitechapel, London E1 2AD
Tel: 071 377 7000   Telex: 893750   Fax: 071 377 7677
Electronic mail: (JANET) LIBRARY @ UK.AC.LON.LHMC.UX
STAFF: PS Hockney BSc DipLib ALA MIInfSci, Ms JM Thomas BSc DipLib
FOUNDED: Origins go back to 1785
TYPE: Multidisciplinary
HOURS: Mon-Fri 9-6
READERS: Staff and other users
STOCK POLICY: Books discarded after varying intervals
LENDING: Books only. Photocopies provided
COMPUTER DATA RETRIEVAL: DATASTAR online - charged. CD-ROM from
        1983
HOLDINGS: 35,000 books and bound journals; 600 journals, 350
        current journals
CLASSIFICATION: NLM
SPECIAL COLLECTION: Forensic medicine (100 vols); Alumni (200 vols)
PUBLICATIONS: Annual report; user guides
BRANCH: Mile End Hospital, London; Saint Clement's
Hospital, London
NETWORK: NE Thames Regional Library Service; University of London;
        City and East London Confederation

375
LONDON SCHOOL OF HYGIENE AND TROPICAL MEDICINE
Keppel Street, London WC1E 7HT
Tel: 071 636 8636 & 071 636 4154   Telex 8953437
Fax: 071 436 5389
STAFF: RB Furner BA ALA, JE Eyers BA DipLib MLS MIInfSc,
        Ms ME Gibson MLS ALA DHMSA, Ms JLL Thomson BA, 6 other
        full time and 2 part time staff
FOUNDED: 1899
TYPE: Medical, health administration
HOURS: Mon-Fri 9-7.30, Sat 9.30-12
READERS: Staff and other users
STOCK POLICY: Selective - fringe material only discarded
LENDING: Books only. Photocopies provided
COMPUTER DATA RETRIEVAL: DATASTAR online - charged full cost.
        CD-ROM from 1989
HOLDINGS: c30,000 books; c4,000 journals, 1,200 current titles;
                125 Tape/slides
CLASSIFICATION: Barnard
SPECIAL COLLECTIONS: Early works in public health and
  tropical medicine (800 vols); vaccination (400 vols)
PUBLICATIONS: Catalogue of the Ross Archives
NETWORKS: NE Thames Regional Library Service; University of London

376
MEDICAL RESEARCH COUNCIL , MEDICAL RESEARCH UNIT
26-29 Drury Lane, London WC2B 5RL
Tel: 071 836 8851
STAFF: Ms E Kishna (part time)
TYPE: Biophysics
HOURS: Mon-Fri 9.30-5.30
READERS: Staff and other users
LENDING: Books and journals. Photocopies provided
COMPUTER DATA RETRIEVAL: Access to terminal. Charged
HOLDINGS: 3,000 books; 200 journals, 150 current titles; fiche
CLASSIFICATION: LC
NETWORK: MRC

377
MEDICAL RESEARCH COUNCIL, NATIONAL INSTITUTE FOR MEDICAL RESEARCH
The Ridgeway, Mill Hill, London, NW7 1AA
Tel: 081 959 3666   Telex 922666   Fax: 081 906 4477
Electronic mail: (JANET) A-LIBRARY @ UK.AC.MRC.NIMT
STAFF: RJ Moore BA ALA MIInfSc MIBiol, JF Norman BSc DipLib ALA
        (Deputy Librarian), Miss R Wenham BSc DipLib
FOUNDED: 1920
TYPE: Basic biomedical sciences
HOURS: Always open. Staffed Mon-Fri 9-5
READERS: MRC staff, other users if clearly in need of facilities
STOCK POLICY: Some stock discarded
LENDING: Books and journals. Photocopies provided
COMPUTER DATA RETRIEVAL: DIALOG online - only for MRC staff.
          CD-ROM from 1983 - only for MRC staff
HOLDINGS: c20,000 books; c900 journals, c500 current titles
CLASSIFICATION: Barnard
PUBLICATION: Influenza bibliography
NETWORK: Medical Research Council; MISER

378
MINISTRY OF AGRICULTURE, FISHERIES AND FOOD LIBRARY
Room 807, Nobel House, 13 Smith Square, London SW1P 3JR
Tel: 071 238 6571
STAFF: P Ryan BA, Mrs S Griffiths BA
  FOUNDED: Opened 1939 as Ministry of Food Library
TYPE: Food and nutrition
HOURS: Mon-Fri 9-5
READERS: Staff only
STOCK POLICY: Books and journals discarded after 5-10 years
LENDING: Books and journals. Photocopies provided
COMPUTER DATA RETRIEVAL: Online databases: DATASTAR, BLAISE,
          DIALOG, ESA - free. PRESTEL available
HOLDINGS: 30,000 books; 700 journals, 620 current titles
CLASSIFICATION: UDC
PUBLICATION: Accessions list
NETWORK: Ministry of Agriculture, Fisheries and Food

379
NATIONAL CHILDREN'S BUREAU, LIBRARY & INFORMATION SERVICE
8 Wakley Street, London EC1V 7QE
Tel: 071 278 9441   Fax: 071 278 9512
STAFF: Ms N Hilliard BA ALA (Head), I Murray BA ALA (Librarian),
 Ms L Payne BA MLib (Information Officer)
FOUNDED: 1970
TYPE: Multidisciplinary (Children)
HOURS: Mon-Fri 10-5
READERS: Staff and other users
STOCK POLICY: No stock discarded
LENDING: Reference only. Photocopies provided
COMPUTER DATA RETRIEVAL: In-house terminal
HOLDINGS: 160 journals; Organizations database (2,000 entries)
CLASSIFICATION: Bliss
PUBLICATIONS: Children & Parliament; Highlights

380
NATIONAL HEART & LUNG INSTITUTE
Dovehouse Street, London SW3 6LY
Tel: 071 352 8121 x3098   Fax: 071 376 3442
STAFF: Miss LF Dorrington ALA MIInfSc, Mrs C Pullin BA DipLib,
 M Hunt BSc DipInfSc
TYPE: Medical, nursing
HOURS: Mon-Fri 9-7
READERS: Staff, other users by arrangement
LENDING: Books only
COMPUTER DATA RETRIEVAL: In-house terminal - free
HOLDINGS: 5,000 books; 250 current journals; AV material
SPECIAL COLLECTIONS: Brompton; Robert Young; Peacock;
 history of medicine and diseases of the chest and heart
CLASSIFICATION: NLM
PUBLICATION: Library guide; Current journal holdings
NETWORK: University of London; NW Thames Regional Library and
          Information Service
BRANCHES: Mulberry Heart Library, London Chest Hospital,
                     Bonner Road, London

381
NATIONAL HOSPITALS COLLEGE OF SPEECH SCIENCES & NURSING STUDIES
   UNIT, JOINT LIBRARY
Chandler House, 2 Wakefield Street, London WC1N 1PG
Tel: 071 837 0113
STAFF: Mrs PL Munro BA ALA (NHCSS), Miss A Brown BSc MSc (NSU)
            (part time)
FOUNDED: NHCSS - 1974; NSU - 1984
TYPE: Multidisciplinary
HOURS: Term: Mon-Tue 9-6.30,Wed-Fri 9-5. Vacation: Mon-Fri 9-5
READERS: Staff and students, other users for reference only

STOCK POLICY: Some out of date books discarded.
LENDING: Books only. Photocopies supplied
COMPUTER DATA RETRIEVAL: Access to DATASTAR - charged computer
time only. CD-ROM from 1982
HOLDINGS: 5,000 books; 111 journals, 63 current titles
CLASSIFICATION: DDC
SPECIAL COLLECTIONS: Test Library
PUBLICATION: Accessions list
NETWORK: Affiliated to Institute of Neurology; NE Thames

382
NEWHAM HEALTH DISTRICT LIBRARY
Newham Hospital, Glen Road, Plaistow, London E13 8SL
Tel: 071 476 1400
STAFF: Mrs AL Head ALA
FOUNDED: 1974
TYPE: Multidisciplinary
HOURS: Mon-Fri 8.30-4.30
READERS: Staff and other users
LENDING: Books only. Photocopies supplied
COMPUTER DATA RETRIEVAL: Access to DATASTAR - charged full cost
HOLDINGS: 5,000 books; 140 journals, 105 current titles
CLASSIFICATION: NLM
BRANCH: St Andrew's Hospital, Devons Rd, London E3
NETWORK: NE Thames Regional Library and Information Service

383
NORTH EAST THAMES REGIONAL LIBRARY SERVICE
David Ferriman Library, North Middlesex Hospital, Sterling Way,
London N18 1QX
Tel: 081 884 3391   Fax: 081 884 2773
STAFF: JF Hewlett MSc ALA
TYPE: Multidisciplinary, health care librarianship
COMPUTER DATA RETRIEVAL: Access to terminal.
PUBLICATIONS: Directory of libraries; union list of serials
NETWORK: NE Thames Regional Library and Information Service

384
NORTH LONDON POSTGRADUATE MEDICAL CENTRE
Saint Ann's Hospital, Block 6, Saint Ann's Road, Tottenham,
London N15 3TH
Tel: 081 800 0121
STAFF: DD Whitlock BSc FRSC CChem
TYPE: Multidisciplinary
HOURS: Always open. Staffed 9-4.30
READERS: Medical staff
LENDING: Reference only
HOLDINGS: 500 books; 60 journals
CLASSIFICATION: NLM
SPECIAL COLLECTION: Orthopaedics

385
NORTH MIDDLESEX HOSPITAL, DAVID FERRIMAN LIBRARY
Sterling Way, London N18 1QX
Tel: 081 807 3071 x3006/2714
STAFF: Ms LR Madelin ALA (District Librarian), N Orr BA DipLib
FOUNDED: 1989 in its present form
TYPE: Multidisciplinary
HOURS: Mon 8-6, Tue 9-8, Wed 8-6, Thu 9-8, Fri 9-6, Sat 9-12
READERS: Staff, other users for reference on application to
         Librarian
LENDING: Books only. Photocopies provided
COMPUTER DATA RETRIEVAL: DATASTAR online
HOLDINGS: 132 journals, 130 current titles
CLASSIFICATION: NLM and RCN (being converted to NLM)
NETWORKS: NETRLS; close links with Middlesex Polytechnic Library
          and Harringey Public Libraries

386
NORTH WEST THAMES REGIONAL LIBRARY AND INFORMATION SERVICE
c/o Westminster Branch Library, Charing Cross and
 Westminster Medical School, 17 Horseferry Road, London
 SW1P 2AR
071 630 1574 (Direct line); 071 828 9811 x2660
STAFF: Ms FM Picken ALA, 1 other (part-time) staff
TYPE: Health administration, librarianship
HOURS: Exclusively postal use of stock. Staffed irregular
 hours, telephone answering machine
READERS: Staff only
LENDING: Books and journals
COMPUTER DATA RETRIEVAL: Access to terminal. Charged
 computer time only
HOLDINGS: 60 books, 100 bound journals; 50 current
 journals. 35 mm slides
SPECIAL COLLECTION: Librarianship
CLASSIFICATION: NLMC
PUBLICATIONS: Guide on guides; union list of serials; guide
 on library bulletin
NETWORK: NW Thames Regional Library and Information Service

387
OFFICE OF POPULATION CENSUSES AND SURVEYS
Saint Catherine's House, 10 Kingsway, London WC2B 6JP
Tel: 071 242 0262 x2236   Fax: 071 242 0262 x2167
STAFF: Mrs CA Cole MA ALA, , D McComb BA ALA, Ms V Hills BA ALA
TYPE: Statistics, government
HOURS: Mon-Fri 9.30-4

READERS: Staff and other users
LENDING: Books and journals. Photocopies supplied
COMPUTER DATA RETRIEVAL: In-house terminal.
HOLDINGS: 50,000 books; 400 journals, 350 current titles;
                    300 microfilms
CLASSIFICATION: Bliss 2nd ed
PUBLICATIONS: Accessions list; bibliographies;bulletins

388
POISONS UNIT (LEWISHAM AND NORTH SOUTHWARK H.A.)
New Cross Hospital, Avonley Road, London SE14 5ER
Tel: 071 639 9852   Fax: 071 639 2101
STAFF: Ms H Checketts BA DipEd DipLib
FOUNDED: 1970
TYPE: Medical, toxicological, pharmacological
HOURS: Mon-Fri 8.30-4.30
READERS: Staff and other users
STOCK POLICY: Stock discarded
LENDING: Books and journals. Photocopies provided
COMPUTER DATA RETRIEVAL: DATASTAR online - other libraries charged
                    full cost. CD-ROM from 1982
HOLDINGS: 721 books; 61 current journals
CLASSIFICATION: NLM
NETWORK: SE Thames ; MISGR

389
PRINCESS ALEXANDRA AND NEWHAM COLLEGE OF NURSING AND MIDWIFERY
Philpot Street, London E1 2EA
Tel: 071 377 7423/7424
STAFF: Ms LJ Parr BA DipLib MA ALA, Ms A Raffan BA
FOUNDED: c1895
TYPE: Nursing, midwifery
HOURS: Mon, Wed, Fri 8.30-5.30, Tues 8.30-8
READERS: Staff and students
STOCK POLICY: Some books discarded after 10 years
LENDING: Books only. Photocopies provided
COMPUTER DATA RETRIEVAL: DATASTAR online - charged
HOLDINGS: 10,000 books; 60 current journals; 54 videotapes (VHS)
CLASSIFICATION: RCN
BRANCH: St Andrew's Hospital, Newham; London Hospital (Mile End)
NETWORK: NE Thames Regional Library Service

390
PUBLIC HEALTH LABORATORY SERVICE, CENTRAL LIBRARY
Central Public Health Laboratory , 61 Colindale Avenue,
 London NW9 5HT
Tel:081 200 4400 x4616   Telex 8953942 (DEFEND G)
Fax: 081 200 7875   Electronic mail: BT Gold 79: PHL018
STAFF: Mrs SA Bloomfield BSc DipLib ALA, Mrs HT Westmancoat BLib
   (part time), Miss JC Cann BSc DipLib, DJ Keech MSc DipLib ALA,
     Miss AJ Trigg BA
FOUNDED: 1946
TYPE: Microbiology, infectious diseases
HOURS: Mon-Fri 9-5.30
READERS: Staff, bona fide enquirers by arrangement
STOCK POLICY: Superseded editions of books discarded
LENDING: Books and journals. Photocopies provided
COMPUTER DATA RETRIEVAL: DATASTAR, DIALOG online - free to PHLS
          staff - others charged
HOLDINGS: 9,000 books; 400 journals, 350 current titles
CLASSIFICATION: Barnard (modified)
PUBLICATIONS: PHLS Library Bulletin; PHLS HIV Bulletin
BRANCH: PHLS Centre for Applied Microbiology and Research,
 Porton Down, Wiltshire

391
QUEEN CHARLOTTE'S MATERNITY HOSPITAL, SCHOOL OF MIDWIFERY
Goldhawk Road, London W6 0XG
Tel: 081 748 4666
No furthur information available

392
QUEEN ELIZABETH HOSPITAL FOR CHILDREN, SELWYN SELWYN-CLARKE LIBRARY
Hackney Road, London E2 8PS
Tel: 071 739 8422 x1
STAFF: C Duncun MA DipLib
FOUNDED: 1969
TYPE: Medical (paediatrics), paramedical
HOURS: Mon-Fri 9-5
READERS: Staff, medical students
LENDING: Books, journals, tape/slides. Photocopies provided
HOLDINGS: 638 books; 94 current journals; 51 tape/slide sets
CLASSIFICATION: NLM

393
QUEEN ELIZABETH MILITARY HOSPITAL, MEDICAL LIBRARY TRAINING SCHOOL
Stadium Road, Woolwich, London SE18 4QH

Tel: 081 856 5533 x2421   Fax: 081 856 5533 x2317
STAFF: Ms L Kerr MA DipLib ALA
FOUNDED: 1978
TYPE: Multidisciplinary
HOURS: Mon-Fri 8-9. Staffed Mon-Fri 8.30-4
READERS: Members of Army Medical Service, others by appointment
STOCK POLICY: Old editions of books discarded
LENDING: Books, AV material. Photocopies provided
COMPUTER DATA RETRIEVAL: DATASTAR, DIALOG online. CD-ROM from 1983
HOLDINGS: 6,000 books; 100 current journals; 100 tape/slides,
                65 35mm slides, 500 videotapes (VHS)
CLASSIFICATION: NLM
NETWORK: Ministry of Defence Medical Library Service

394
QUEEN MARY'S UNIVERSITY HOSPITAL, DISTRICT LIBRARY
Roehampton Lane, London SW15 5PN
Tel: 081 789 6611 x2093   Fax: 081 780 1089
Electronic mail: Datamail - Helen A Alper
STAFF: Mrs H Alper AIL ALA
FOUNDED: 1987
TYPE: Multidisciplinary
HOURS: Mon-Fri 9-5. Key available out of hours
READERS: Staff and other users
STOCK POLICY: Books discarded after 10 years if out of date,
        Journals discarded after discussion within Region
LENDING: Books and journals. Photocopies provided
COMPUTER DATA RETRIEVAL: DATASTAR online - free. CD-ROM from 1988
HOLDINGS: 2,000 books; 190 journals, 175 current titles
CLASSIFICATION: NLM
PUBLICATION: Guide to library services
NETWORK: SW Thames RLIS

395
ROYAL ARMY MEDICAL COLLEGE
Millbank, London SW1P 4RJ
Tel: 071 873 6340   Fax: 071 873 6348
STAFF: Mrs CM Goddard BA ALA (Head of MOD Medical Library Services),
 College Librarian post vacant, 1 part time clerical assistant
TYPE: Medical
HOURS: Mon-Fri 9-5
READERS: Members of the Army Medical Services, other users
 by appointment
STOCK POLICY: Out of date books and journals discarded
LENDING: Books only. Photocopies provided
COMPUTER DATA RETRIEVAL: DATASTAR, DIALOG, OCLC online - free.
                CD-ROM from 1989
HOLDINGS: 10,000 books; 200 current journals
CLASSIFICATION: NLM
NETWORK: Ministry of Defence Medical Library Service
BRANCHES: In military hospitals at home and overseas

396
ROYAL COLLEGE OF GENERAL PRACTITIONERS, INFORMATION RESOURCES
   CENTRE
14 Princes Gate, London SW7 1PU
Tel: 071 581 3232   Fax: 071 225 3047
STAFF: Miss M Hammond DipSocCertCrim, Mrs C Stockbridge-Bland BA
   MA ALA, L Malcolm BSc DipLib, D Bates BA(Hons), Ms M McFarland
   MA(Hons) DipLib, Mrs S Gear ALA, Ms A Mason BA(Hons) ALA
FOUNDED: 1958
TYPE: Medical
HOURS: Mon-Fri 9-5.30
READERS: Staff and members of RCGP
STOCK POLICY: General journals discarded after 5 years, books
              discarded when no longer of use
LENDING: College publications only. Photocopies provided
COMPUTER DATA RETRIEVAL: DATASTAR, BLAISE, DIALOG PROFILE online -
              standard charge.
HOLDINGS: 3,500 books; 234 journals, 192 current titles;
           80 practice annual reports, 250 practice premises plans, 300
           practice information leaflets, 100 specimens of patient
           record cards
SPECIAL COLLECTION: General practice (3,000 vols)
CLASSIFICATION: Barnard
PUBLICATION: New reading for general practitioners
NETWORK: NW Thames

397
ROYAL COLLEGE OF MIDWIVES, ARNOLD WALKER-FLORENCE MITCHELL LIBRARY
11 Queen Anne Street, London W1M 9FD
Tel: 071 580 6523   Fax: 071 436 3951
STAFF: Mrs J Ayres BA DipLib, J Ions, 2 other staff
FOUNDED: Informal collection since 1881
TYPE: Midwifery, nursing
HOURS: Mon-Fri 9-5
READERS: Staff and other users
STOCK POLICY: Permanent retention
LENDING: Books, bibliographies. Photocopies provided
COMPUTER DATA RETRIEVAL: In-house terminal. CD-ROM from 1990
HOLDINGS: 5,000+ books; 80 journals, 67 current titles
CLASSIFICATION: Own
PUBLICATION: Current awareness service (quarterly); Midwifery
                     index

398
ROYAL COLLEGE OF NURSING
20 Cavendish Square, London W1M OAB
Tel: 071 409 3333   Fax: 071 408 0190
STAFF: A Shepherd BA ALA DMS MBIM, Ms J Lord BA(Hons) ALA,
    Miss H Thomas MA DipLib ALA, Mrs A Watson MSc BSc, 1 vacancy,
    6 other staff
TYPE: Multidisciplinary
HOURS: Term : Mon-Fri 8.30-7 ;Vacation: Mon-Thu 8.30-6, Fri 8.30-5
READERS: Members and other users
STOCK POLICY: Non nursing books discarded
LENDING: Books only. Photocopies provided
COMPUTER DATA RETRIEVAL: DATASTAR, DIALOG online - charging by
        arrangement. CD-ROM
HOLDINGS: 45,000 books; 400+ journals, 300 current titles
SPECIAL COLLECTIONS: Steinberg collection of nursing research
 (525 vols); historical collection
CLASSIFICATION: RCN
PUBLICATIONS: Nursing bibliography (monthly) ; catalogue of
 Steinberg collection of nursing research
BRANCHES: RCN Birmingham Centre for Nursing Education, 162 Hagley
 Road, Edgbaston, Birmingham B16 9NY; RCN, Northern Ireland Board,
 17 Windsor Ave, Belfast BT8 6EE

399
ROYAL COLLEGE OF OBSTETRICIANS AND GYNAECOLOGISTS, MARKLAND LIBRARY
27 Sussex Place, Regent's Park, London NW1 4RG
Tel: 071 262 5425 or 071 402 2317   Fax: 071 723 0575
STAFF: Miss PC Want ALA, Ms G Edwards BA ALA
TYPE: Medical
HOURS: Mon-Fri 10-5
READERS: Fellows and Members of the College, other users must be
            introduced by a Fellow
STOCK POLICY: No stock discarded
LENDING: Reference only. Photocopies only supplied as back -up to
         usual sources
COMPUTER DATA RETRIEVAL: BLAISE online - special terms apply
HOLDINGS: c4,000 books; 370 journals, 180 current titles
 journals
SPECIAL COLLECTION: Historical (2,000 vols)
CLASSIFICATION: Barnard
PUBLICATION: Short-title catalogue of books printed before
 1851 in the library of the RCOG, 2nd ed 1968

400
ROYAL COLLEGE OF PHYSICIANS OF LONDON
11 Saint Andrew's Place, London NW1 4LE
Tel: 071 935 1174   Fax: 071 487 5218
STAFF: G Davenport BA ALA (Librarian), Miss JA Allum BA ALA,
  (Archivist), Miss TM Parker BA DAA (Archivist)
FOUNDED: 1518
TYPE: History of medicine, medical biography
HOURS: Mon-Fri 9.30-5.30
READERS: Staff and all bona fide research workers
STOCK POLICY: Out of date reference books discarded,
  clinical journals discarded after 3 years, other medical
  colleges and academics discarded after 10 years
LENDING: Books and journals. Photocopies provided
COMPUTER DATA RETRIEVAL: In-house terminal
HOLDINGS: 50,000 books and bound journals; 100 current
  journals; 3,000 35mm slides, prints (engravings, etc) photographs,
    48 microfilms, videotapes (1 U-matic, 70 VHS)
CLASSIFICATION: UDC
SPECIAL COLLECTION: Evan Bedford Library of Cardiology (1,300 vols),
        Library of Marquis of Dorchester [1606-80] (c3,400 vols)
PUBLICATIONS: Brief introduction to the library; Evan Bedford
        Library of Cardiology: catalogue (1977); AH Driver. A
        Catalogue of the engraved portraits ... (1952); W Munk. The
        roll of the Royal College of Physicians of London. 3 vols
        (1878); continued as Lives of the Fellows ... vols 4-8
        (1955-89)

401
ROYAL COLLEGE OF PSYCHIATRISTS
17 Belgrave Square, London SW1 8PG
Tel: 071 235 2351   Fax: 071 245 1231

STAFF: Dr GE Berrios (Honorary Librarian), Mrs S Floate DipLib
  (Librarian) , Mrs M Harcourt-Williams (Archivist) (part time)
TYPE: Psychiatric
HOURS: Mon-Fri 9.30-4.30
READERS: Staff and Members of the College. Bona fide
  research workers only by appointment
STOCK POLICY: Out of date books discarded. Some journals
  discarded after 5 years
LENDING: Books and photocopies to members of College only
COMPUTER DATA RETRIEVAL: In-house terminal
HOLDINGS: 5,000 books; 55 journals, 50 current titles
SPECIAL COLLECTION: Antiquarian psychiatric (500 vols)
CLASSIFICATION: Own
PUBLICATIONS: Books suitable for a psychiatric library; Reading
                lists for psychiatric trainees

402
ROYAL COLLEGE OF SURGEONS OF ENGLAND
35-43 Lincoln's Inn Fields, London WC2A 3PN
Tel: 071 405 3474   Telex: 936573 RCSEN G   Fax: 071 831 9438
STAFF: IF Lyle ALA, FK Sherwood BSc DipLib ALA MIInfSc,
 Mrs CM Craig BA DipLib
FOUNDED: 1800
TYPE: Multidisciplinary
HOURS: Mon-Fri 10-6, closed throughout August
READERS: Diplomates of the College, other users by letter of
     introduction from a Fellow, or at the Librarian's discretion
STOCK POLICY: Permanent retention
LENDING: Books, journals, videotapes to other libraries only.
               Photocopies supplied
COMPUTER DATA RETRIEVAL: DATASTAR online - charged
HOLDINGS: 50,000 books; 3,000 journals, 650 current titles;
                  30 microfilms, 30 tape/slides, 1,000 35mm
                  slides, 40 videotapes (VHS)
SPECIAL COLLECTIONS: Hunter-Baillie collection autograph letters
   and manuscripts (1,500 items); John Hunter, his contemporaries
   and pupils - printed books, manuscripts and autograph letters
   (1,100 items); Lord Lister - printed books, autograph letters and
   manuscripts (250 items); Richard Owen - printed books, autograph
     letters and manuscripts (750 items); Arthur Keith - printed
     books, autograph letters and manuscripts (300 items); engraved
     portraits (3,000 items); book-plates (2,000 items); medals
   (150 items);Julian Brunner collection (surgery of the hand) (400
   vols); Menzies Campbell collection of early dental literature
     (300 items)
CLASSIFICATION: Barnard
PUBLICATIONS: List of current periodical holdings; English books
                  before 1701

403
ROYAL COLLEGE OF VETERINARY SURGEONS' WELLCOME LIBRARY
32 Belgrave Square, London SW1X 8QP
Tel: 071 235 6568   Fax: 071 245 6100
STAFF: Miss B Horder BA ALA
FOUNDED: 1940s
TYPE: Veterinary
HOURS: Mon-Fri 10-5
READERS: Staff, other users on introduction by member or librarian
STOCK POLICY: Books and journals discarded at varying intervals
LENDING: Books and journals. Photocopies provided
COMPUTER DATA RETRIEVAL: DIALOG, ESA-DIALTECH, BRS online - charged
               flat rate. CD-ROM from 1989
HOLDINGS: c26,000 books; 250 current journals
SPECIAL COLLECTION: Historical collection on veterinary
   science (2,500 vols)
CLASSIFICATION: Barnard for main collection, UDC for historical
                  collection
NETWORK: Special source library for British Library

404
ROYAL FREE HOSPITAL SCHOOL OF MEDICINE
Medical Library, Royal Free Hospital, Rowland Hill Street,London
 NW3 2PF
Tel: 071 794 0500 x3203 (Enquiries),x3201 (Librarian),
                        x4996/7 Assistant Librarians
STAFF: Miss AE Fletcher BA ALA, Miss P Summers ALA, JJ Cox MA DipLib
        ALA, 4 other (full-time) and 1 (part-time) staff
TYPE: Medical
HOURS: Mon-Fri 9-10, Sat 9-5 (custodian Mon-Fri 7-10, Sat 1-5)
READERS: Staff and students,University of London (reference only),
            other users by letter of introduction
STOCK POLICY: Out of date textbooks discarded
COMPUTER DATA RETRIEVAL: DATASTAR, DIALOG online - charged full
            cost. CD-ROM from1966
HOLDINGS: c20,000 books; 520 journals, 340 current titles;
            60 tape/slides, 37 videotapes (VHS)
CLASSIFICATION: NLM
PUBLICATIONS: Newsletter; library guides; accessions lists;
            guides to various services; CD-ROM; Online services;
            reference sources; Index Medicus
NETWORK: NE Thames

405
ROYAL FREE HOSPITAL SCHOOL OF NURSING
Royal Free Hospital, Pond Street, Hampstead, London NW3 2QG
Tel: 071 794 0500 x3737
STAFF: Ms J Ellis BA ALA, 1 other (full-time) staff
FOUNDED: 1974
TYPE: Nursing
HOURS: Mon 8.40-6, Tues-Fri 8.40-4.30
READERS: Nursing staff, tutors and students only
STOCK POLICY: Books over 10 years old discarded
LENDING: Books only. Photocopies provided
HOLDINGS: 10,000 books; 65 journals, 53 current titles;
            20 Videotapes (VHS)
CLASSIFICATION: NLM
NETWORK: NE Thames Regional Library and Information Service

406
ROYAL NATIONAL INSTITUTE FOR THE BLIND, REFERENCE LIBRARY
224 Great Portland Street, London W1N 6AA
Tel: 071 388 1266
STAFF: CP Yates MA ALA, A McLeod BSc ALA, T Stansbury BLib ALA
FOUNDED: 1959
TYPE: Welfare
HOURS: Mon-Fri 9.30-5
READERS: Staff and other users
STOCK POLICY: No stock discarded
LENDING: Books and journals. Photocopies provided

HOLDINGS: 4,400 books; 300 journals, 175 current titles
CLASSIFICATION: Own
PUBLICATIONS: Select accessions list, other bibliographies and
        information leaflets
NETWORK: BLDSC back up library

407
ROYAL NATIONAL INSTITUTE FOR THE DEAF
105 Gower Street, London WC1E 6AH
Tel: 071 387 8033
STAFF: Miss ME Plackett BA ALA, Deputy Librarian vacancy ,
        Ms C-A Orbell BA ALA
FOUNDED: 1911
TYPE: Multidisciplinary
HOURS: Mon-Fri 9.30-5 (Thurs 9.30-6.30 during term)
READERS: Staff and other users
STOCK POLICY: Stock rarely discarded
LENDING: Books only. Photocopies provided
COMPUTER DATA RETRIEVAL: In-house terminal
HOLDINGS: 8,000 books; 500 journals, 300 current titles;
                55 microfilms, 150 Videotapes (U-matic)
CLASSIFICATION: Own
PUBLICATIONS: Current awareness service;

408
ROYAL PHARMACEUTICAL SOCIETY OF GREAT BRITAIN
1 Lambeth High Street, London SE1 7JN
Tel: 071 735 9141   Fax: 071 735 7629
STAFF: Miss PM North BPharm FRPharmS MIInfSci (Head of Library &
        Technical Information Service), Miss MF Mackenzie DHMSA ALA
        (Librarian), 2 other full time staff
FOUNDED: 1841
TYPE: Pharmaceutical
HOURS: Mon-Fri 9-5
READERS: Fellows and Members, other bona fide persons by arrangement
STOCK POLICY: Permanent retention
LENDING: Books only to Fellows and Members. Photocopies provided
COMPUTER DATA RETRIEVAL: DATASTAR, DIALOG online.
HOLDINGS: 65,000 books; 500 current journals
SPECIAL COLLECTIONS: Herbals; pharmacopoeias (2,000 vols)
CLASSIFICATION: UDC
BRANCH: ROYAL Pharmaceutical Society of Great Britain (Scottish
Branch), Edinburgh

409

ROYAL POSTGRADUATE MEDICAL SCHOOL
Hammersmith Hospital, Du Cane Road, London W12 0HS
Tel: 081 740 3246   Fax: 081 740 3203
STAFF: Miss LA Curtis BA DipLib ALA, Miss EA Davis BSc ALA, Ms JMC
    Stone BA ALA, PC Stokes BA ALA, JR Matthews BA ALA
FOUNDED: 1935
TYPE: Medical
HOURS: Mon-Fri 9-9 (9-6 during August), Sat 9.30-12.30.
                              (August Mon-Fri 9-6)
READERS: Staff and other users
STOCK POLICY: Books discarded after 10-60 years
LENDING: Books only. Photocopies provided
COMPUTER DATA RETRIEVAL: DIALOG online - outsiders pay full cost,
              own users pay computer time only. CD-ROM from 1966
HOLDINGS: 8,000 books; 875 current journals
CLASSIFICATION: NLM
BRANCH: Institute of Obstetrics and Gynaecology (see next entry)
NETWORK: University of London

410

ROYAL POSTGRADUATE MEDICAL SCHOOL, INSTITUTE OF OBSTETRICS AND
GYNAECOLOGY
Queen Charlotte's & Chelsea Hospital, Goldhawk Road, London W6 0XG
Tel: 081 748 4666 x5314   Fax: 081 741 1838
STAFF: Mrs G Going ALA
TYPE: Medical, obstetric
HOURS: Mon-Fri 9-5
READERS: Staff, other users by arrangement with librarian
STOCK POLICY: No stock discarded
LENDING: Books only. Photocopies provided
COMPUTER DATA RETRIEVAL: BLAISE online - charged full cost
          CD-ROM from 1966
HOLDINGS: 2,150 books; 2,500 bound journals, 64 current titles
CLASSIFICATION: Own
NETWORK: NW Thames Region library & Information Service

411

ROYAL SOCIETY OF MEDICINE
1 Wimpole Street, London W1M 8AE
071 408 2119 Telex 298902 ROYMED G   Fax: 071 408 0062
STAFF: DWC Stewart BA ALA, JE Ayres MA DipLib ALA, Ms L Griffiths BA
    MLS ALA, JM Harris BA DipLib ALA, 8 other professional staff
FOUNDED: 1805
TYPE: Medical
HOURS: Mon-Fri 9-9.30, Sat 10-5.
READERS: Members of the Society, other users on introduction by
                        Member
LENDING: Books, journals, some AV material. Photocopies provided
COMPUTER DATA RETRIEVAL: DATASTAR, BLAISE, DIALOG online - charged

computer time only. CD-ROM from 1989
HOLDINGS: 120,000 books; 8,000+ journals, 2,030 current titles;
             800 . microfilms,   tape/slides,   videodisc,   <500   35mm
             slides,   videotapes (<10 U-matic, <10 VHS)
CLASSIFICATION: UDC
SPECIAL COLLECTION: Comfort Collection on Gerontology (500 vols)
PUBLICATIONS: Current periodicals list
NETWORK: BLDSC back-up library

412
ROYAL VETERINARY COLLEGE (University of London)
Camden Library, Royal College Street, London NW1 OTU
Tel: 071 387 2898   Fax: 071 388 2342
STAFF:Ms L Warden BA ALA, Miss F Houston ALA, Ms J Kingsley BA(Hons)
FOUNDED: 1791
TYPE: Medical, Veterinary
HOURS: Mon-Fri 10-4.50. Some evening opening
READERS: Staff, other users for reference only
LENDING: Books, journals, pamphlets lent internally. Photocopies
                       provided
COMPUTER DATA RETRIEVAL: BLAISE online - charged. CD-ROM from 1989.
                       PRESTEL available
HOLDINGS: c15,000 books; 652 journals, 430 current titles
CLASSIFICATION: · Barnard
SPECIAL COLLECTION: Historical (c3,000 vols)
PUBLICATIONS: Library guide; postcards from historical collection
BRANCH: Hawkshead Library, Hawkshead House, Hawkshead Lane, North
                       Mymms, Hatfield, Herts AL9 7TA
                       Tel: 0707 55486   Fax: 0707 52090
NETWORK: University of London

413
SAINT BARTHOLOMEW'S HOSPITAL MEDICAL COLLEGE
West Smithfield, London EC1A 7BE
Tel: 071 601 8888 x7837
STAFF: Miss JS Morris BSc DipLib, Miss J Hayles BA ALA, A Besson
 PhD DipLib ALA, Miss C Cheney BA ALA
TYPE: Multidisciplinary
HOURS: Mon-Fri 9-9 (not staffed 6-9)
READERS: Staffand students only.
STOCK POLICY: Out of date books discarded
LENDING: Books and journals. photocopies provided
COMPUTER DATA RETRIEVAL: DATASTAR, DIALOG online - charged full
             cost. CD-ROM from 1966
HOLDINGS: 20,000 books;c40,000 bound journals, 300 current titles
CLASSIFICATION: NLM
PUBLICATIONS: Library guide
BRANCHES: Charterhouse Branch Library, London

414
SAINT BARTHOLOMEW'S COLLEGE OF NURSING AND MIDWIFERY
Saint Bartholomew's Hospital, West Smithfield, London
  EC1A 7BE
Tel: 071 601 8653
STAFF: P Moorbath MSc ALA DipLib PGCE
FOUNDED: 1962
TYPE: Nursing
HOURS: Mon-Fri 8.30-5. (Tue 8-6)
READERS: Staff, all nurses in the District
STOCK POLICY: Out of date books discarded
LENDING: Books only. photocopies provided
HOLDINGS: 12,000 books; 80 current journals; 50 sets 35mm slides,
                    videotapes (180 Betamax, 75 VHS)
CLASSIFICATION: RCN (slightly revised)
SPECIAL COLLECTION: Radiography (150 vols)
NETWORK: NE Thames Regional Library and Information Service

415
SAINT CHARLES HOSPITAL MEDICAL LIBRARY
Saint Charles Hospital, Exmoor Street, London W10 6DZ
Tel: 081 968 2323
STAFF: MR Taylor BA(Hons) DipLib ALA (part time)
TYPE: Medical, psychiatric
HOURS: Always open. Staffed Mon-Fri 9-5
READERS: Medical staff
STOCK POLICY: Books discarded after c10 years
LENDING: Books only. Photocopies supplied
HOLDINGS: 893 books; c750 journals, 60 current titles
CLASSIFICATION: NLM
NETWORK: NW Thames Regional Library and Information Service

416
SAINT CHRISTOPHER'S HOSPICE, HALLEY STEWART LIBRARY
51-59 Lawrie Park Road, Sydenham, London SE26 6DZ
Tel: 081 778 9252
STAFF: Mrs D Brady
FOUNDED: 1978
TYPE: Multidisciplinary
HOURS: Mon-Fri 9-5
READERS: Staff, other users for reference only
STOCK POLICY: Discarded at Librarian's discretion
COMPUTER DATA RETRIEVAL: Access to terminal
HOLDINGS: c1,600 books; 35 journals, 30 current titles;
        1,000 35mm slides, videotapes (20 U-matic, 80 VHS)
CLASSIFICATION: Own
SPECIAL COLLECTION: Terminal Care & Bereavement (1,000+ vols)
PUBLICATIONS: Bibliographies, library guide
NETWORK: SE Thames RLIS

417

SAINT GEORGE'S HOSPITAL MEDICAL SCHOOL

Hunter Wing, Cranmer Terrace, London SW17 0RE

Tel: 081 672 1255 x4855   Telex 945291 SAGEMS G   Fax: 081 767 4696

Electronic mail: LIBRARY @ UK.AC.LON.SGHMS.UX

STAFF: Mrs S Gove BSc DipLib FZS, Ms M Logan-Bruce BA, Miss S
 Gilbert BA MSc, Mrs N Thevakarrunai ALA, Mrs J Yeoh BA DipLib

FOUNDED: 1833

TYPE: Multidisciplinary

HOURS: Mon-Fri 9-9, Sat 9.30-12.30

READERS: Staff, students and other users

STOCK POLICY: Duplicate journals and older editions of books
                          discarded

LENDING: Books, AV material. Photocopies supplied

COMPUTER DATA RETRIEVAL: DATASTAR online - charged computer time
                          and reference cost. CD-ROM from 1988

HOLDINGS: c25,000 books; c1,000 journals, 550 current titles;
                    c150 tape/slides, c1,000 videotapes (VHS), audiotapes

SPECIAL COLLECTIONS: Books about Saint George's or by Saint
 George's staff; history of medicine (3,000 vols)

CLASSIFICATION: NLM

PUBLICATIONS: Library guide; accessions list; newsletter; AV list;
                          Quick references

NETWORK: SW Thames Regional Library and Information Service

BRANCH: Atkinson Morley's Hospital, Wimbledon; Bolingbroke
 Hospital, London; Springfield Hospital, Tooting

418

SAINT MARY'S HOSPITAL MEDICAL SCHOOL

Norfolk Place, Paddington, London W2 1PG

Tel: 071 723 1252 x5192

STAFF: ND Palmer BA ALA, Miss SE Smith BA MLS ALA, Miss RC Shipton
 BA ALA

TYPE: Medical

HOURS: Mon-Fri 9-9,(Mon-Fri 9-7 vacation)

READERS: Staff, other users at discretion of Librarian for
 reference only

STOCK POLICY: Superseded editions of books (except those of
 historical interest) discarded

LENDING: Books only. Photocopies provided

COMPUTER DATA RETRIEVAL: DATASTAR online - charged full cost.
                          CD-ROM from 1983

HOLDINGS: 5,000 books; 27,000 bound journals, 307 current titles;
                          60 tape/slides, 14 videotapes (VHS)

SPECIAL COLLECTION: Publications by past and present staff
 of Saint Mary's Hospital

CLASSIFICATION: Own

BRANCH: Saint Mary's is a constituent part of Imperial College of
                          Science, Technology and Medicine

NETWORK: NW Thames

419
SAINT MARY'S SCHOOL OF NURSING
Mint Wing, Saint Mary's Hospital, Praed Street, London W2 1NY
Tel: 071 725 1307
STAFF: JW Barrington BA DipGenLing DipLib ALA
TYPE: Nursing, midwifery
HOURS: Mon-Thurs 8.30-6, Fri 8.30-5. Staffed 9.30 till close
READERS: Staff, other users at discretion of Librarian
STOCK POLICY: Most books and journals over 10 years old discarded
LENDING: Books only. Photocopies provided (Inter Library Loans
                only)
COMPUTER DATA RETRIEVAL: In-house terminal.
HOLDINGS: 9,300 books; 132 journals, 125 current titles
CLASSIFICATION: DDC (modified)
BRANCH: St Charles Hospital, Exmoor St, London W10
NETWORK: NW Thames Regional Nursing Libraries

420
SAINT THOMAS' HOSPITAL. DISTRICT LIBRARY (WEST LAMBETH
  HEALTH AUTHORITY)
Lambeth Palace Road, London SE1 7EH
01 928 9292 x2507
STAFF: Miss D Finlayson BA ALA (District Librarian),
              Mrs R Nicholson ALA,
TYPE: Health administration, patients and staff
HOURS: Mon-Fri 8.45-5, Sat 10-1145
READERS: Staff, other users within reason
STOCK POLICY: Out of date books discarded, most journals
  discarded after 2 years
LENDING: Books and journals (music cassettes & talking books to
            patients). Photocopies provided
HOLDINGS: 17,000 books and unbound journals (1,500 on
  health administration); 50 current journals
SPECIAL COLLECTION: Health Service Administration
CLASSIFICATION: DDC
PUBLICATIONS: Recent additions to library; journal holdings
NETWORK: SE Thames Regional Library and Information Service
BRANCHES: South Western Hospital Multidisciplinary & Patients
            and Staff Libraries, London; Tooting Bec Hospital
                Multidisciplinary & Patients and Staff Libraries, London

421
SAINT THOMAS' HOSPITAL, NIGHTINGALE SCHOOL OF NURSING,
  LEARNING RESOURCES CENTRE
2 Lambeth Palace Road, London SE1 7EP
Tel: 071 928 9292 x2699   Fax: 071 401 3651
STAFF: Ms B Janzer BSc MLS, Ms M Salehi-Jones BA DipLib (part-time)
TYPE: Medical, Nursing
HOURS: Mon-Thurs 9-5, Fri 9-4.45
READERS: Nursing staff and other users
STOCK POLICY: Books and journals discarded at varying intervals

LENDING: Books only
COMPUTER DATA RETRIEVAL: DATASTAR online - free. CD-ROM
HOLDINGS: 8,000 books; 76 journals, 68 current titles.
     255 Tape/slides, 35mm slides, 460 videotapes (VHS)
CLASSIFICATION: NLM
NETWORK: SE Thames Regional Library and Information Service

422
SCHOOL OF PHARMACY UNIVERSITY OF LONDON
29-39 Brunswick Square, London WC1N 1AX
Tel: 071 837 7651   Fax: 071 278 0622
STAFF: Mrs L Lisgarten BA MIInfSc ALA, Miss K Henderson BA ,
Miss E Howell BA, 3 other (part-time) staff
TYPE: Medical, pharmacy
HOURS: Mon-Fri 9-8 (Mon-Fri 9-5 in long vacation)
READERS: Staff and other users
LENDING: Books only
COMPUTER DATA RETRIEVAL: DIALOG online - charged computer time
           only. CD-ROM from 1987
HOLDINGS: 15,000 books, 11,000 bound journals; 220 current
journals. Microfilms
SPECIAL COLLECTIONS: Pharmacy; pharmacology; toxicology
CLASSIFICATION: UDC
PUBLICATIONS: Library guide; quarterly accessions list
NETWORK: University of London

423
SOUTH BANK POLYTECHNIC
Borough Road, London SE1 0AA
Tel: 071 928 8989 x2987   Fax: 071 261 1865
Electronic mail: BT Gold 74: LE1 043
STAFF: J Akeroyd MPhil BSc DipLibInfSc ALA MIInfSc (Head of Library
and Learning Resources), Ms RE Clarke BA DipLib ALA SRN NDNCert
HVCert (responsible for nursing and health administration),
24 other professional staff, 30 other staff (some part-time)
TYPE: Multidisciplinary
HOURS: Mon-Fri 9-9 (Vacations 9-5)
READERS: Staff and students, limited access to external users
STOCK POLICY: Books and journals discarded when no longer
required for teaching or research
LENDING: Books only, AV material overnight. Photocopies provided
COMPUTER DATA RETRIEVAL: DATASTAR, BLAISE, DIALOG Online - charged
        full cost to outside users. CD-ROM from 1987
HOLDINGS: c10,00 health books; 107 health journals, 65 current
health titles; microfilms, tape/slides, 35mm slides,
videotapes (U-matic, VHS)
CLASSIFICATION: DDC
PUBLICATIONS: Library guide; periodicals list by subject;
guide to searching the literature of nursing; community
health and social services
NETWORK: SEAL; SE Thames ; NISG
BRANCH: South Bank Polytechnic, Wandsworth Road, London

424
SOUTH WESTERN HOSPITAL MULTIDISCIPLINARY LIBRARY
Landor Road, Stockwell, London SW9 9NU
Tel: 071 733 7755
STAFF: Ms M Salehi-Jones BA DipLib
TYPE: Multidisciplinary
HOURS: Key always available. Staffed Mon-Fri 2-5
READERS: Staff only
STOCK POLICY: Books discarded.
LENDING: Books only. Photocopies provided
HOLDINGS: 2,500 books; 25 journals, 20 current titles
  journals
CLASSIFICATION: NLM
SPECIAL COLLECTION: Geriatrics
NETWORK: SE Thames Regional Library and Information Service

425
SPASTICS SOCIETY, CENTRAL LIBRARY & INFORMATION UNIT
12 Park Crescent, London W1N 4EQ
Tel: 071 636 5020   Fax: 071 436 2601
STAFF: Ms H Gray ALA (Head), Ms J Kenyon BA (Assistant Librarian),
    Ms R Marks (Assistant Information Officer)
FOUNDED: 1952
TYPE: Multidisciplinary
HOURS: Mon-Fri 9.15-5.15
READERS: Staff and other users
STOCK POLICY: Books and journals discarded at Librarian's discretion
LENDING: Books, videos only. Photocopies provided
COMPUTER DATA RETRIEVAL: In-house terminal
HOLDINGS: 70 current journals
CLASSIFICATION: Own
SPECIAL COLLECTIONS: Cerebral palsy
PUBLICATION: Bookshop price list
NETWORKS: informal links with other London disability charity
        libraries

426
TAVISTOCK CLINIC JOINT LIBRARY
Tavistock Centre, Belsize Lane, London NW3 5BA
Tel: 071 435 7111   Fax: 071 431 5382
STAFF: Mrs ML Walker ALA, Ms A Haselton BA DipLib ALA,
  Ms H Oliver BA DipLib
FOUNDED: 1947
TYPE: Multidisciplinary
HOURS: Mon-Fri 8-10. Staffed Mon-Fri 9.30-5.30
READERS: Staff, other users - limited access at Librarian's
              discretion
STOCK POLICY: No stock discarded
LENDING: Books, journals and AV material. Photocopies provided
COMPUTER DATA RETRIEVAL: DATASTAR, BLAISE, DIALOG online - standard
                  charge

HOLDINGS: 26,000 books; 765 journals; 342 current titles;
                           100 audiotapes, 100 videotapes (VHS)
CLASSIFICATION: Bliss 2nd ed
NETWORK: NE Thames; BLDSC back-up library

427
THOMAS GUY AND LEWISHAM SCHOOL OF NURSING
Shepherd House, Guys Hospital, St Thomas St, London SE1 9RT
Tel: 071 955 5000 x3191
STAFF: AF Doherty ALA
TYPE: Multidisciplinary
HOURS: Mon-Fri 9-5, (Thu 9-7)
READERS: Nursing and midwifery staff trained and untrained.
STOCK POLICY: Books and journals discarded at varying intervals
LENDING: Books only. Photocopies provided
COMPUTER DATA RETRIEVAL: DATASTAR online - free
HOLDINGS: 5,000 books; 50 current journals.
CLASSIFICATION: NLM
BRANCH: Lewisham School of Nursing
NETWORK: SE Thames Regional Library and Information Service

428
TOBACCO ADVISORY COUNCIL
7th Floor, Glen House, Stag Place, London SW1E 5AG
Tel: 071 828 2041 telex: 8953754
Mrs P Elcome
TYPE: Medical, welfare
READERS: Staff only
LENDING: Reference only
COMPUTER DATA RETRIEVAL: In-house terminal
HOLDINGS: Books, journals, microfilms, videotapes (U-matic, VHS)

429
TOOTING BEC HOSPITAL, MULTIDISCIPLINARY LIBRARY,
Education Centre , Tooting Bec Road, London SW17 8BL
Tel: 081 672 9933 x2273
STAFF: Ms M Wensley BA ALA, 1 other (part-time) staff
   FOUNDED: 1980
TYPE: Multidisciplinary
HOURS: Mon-Fri 8.30-4.30
READERS: Staff and other users
STOCK POLICY: Selected journal titles discarded after 15 years,
                  pharmacology books discarded after 10 years
LENDING: Books and journals. Photocopies provided
COMPUTER DATA RETRIEVAL: Access to terminal.
HOLDINGS: 3,000 books; 60 journals, 42 current titles
CLASSIFICATION: NLM
PUBLICATIONS: Monthly current awareness bulletin
NETWORK: SE Thames ; West Lambeth Health Authority

430
UNITED MEDICAL AND DENTAL SCHOOLS OF GUY'S AND SAINT THOMAS'
HOSPITALS
Guys Campus : Wills Library & FS Warner Dental Library
London Bridge, London SE1 9RT   Tel: 071 955 4348 Fax: 071 357 7563
Electronic mail: P.GALE @ UK.AC.LON.UMDS.UXG; A.GUNN @ UK.AC.LON.
          UMDS.UXG; A.BASTER DLIBRARY @ UK.AC.LON.UMDS.UXG
St Thomas's Campus, Lambeth Palace Road, London, SE1 7EH
Tel: 071 928 9292 x2367
STAFF: Miss P Gale MA, Miss Y Hibbott MA MLS ALA AIL, Mrs A Gunn MSc
    MIInfSc ALA, A Baster MA, D Hodgson BA DipLib, Miss J Colclough BA
    DipLib
TYPE: Medical, dental
HOURS: Medical: Mon-Fri 9-9, Wills library Sat 9-1
READERS: Staff and students, some other users
STOCK POLICY: Superseded editions of books and dead sets of
    journals discarded
LENDING: Books only. Photocopies provided for BLDSC forms
COMPUTER DATA RETRIEVAL: DATASTAR, DIALOG online - charged full
        cost. CD-ROM: Medline, from 1982, Oxford Txtbook of Medicine
HOLDINGS: 60,000 books; c800 journals, 700 current titles; 45
        tape/slides (dental), videotapes (5 Betamax, 45 VHS)
CLASSIFICATION: NLM
SPECIAL COLLECTION: Books by Guy's men, history of medicine
    (2,500 vols)
PUBLICATION: Library guide, new books list, periodicals list
NETWORK: University of London

431
UNITED MEDICAL AND DENTAL SCHOOLS OF GUY'S AND ST THOMAS'S
HOSPITALS, COMMUNITY MEDICINE LIBRARY
St Thomas's Campus, London SE1 7EH
Tel: 071 928 9292 x3152   Fax: 071 928 1468

Miss H Lodge BLib
TYPE: Community medicine
HOURS: Mon-Fri 9-5
READERS: Staff, other users by appointment
STOCK POLICY: Books discarded when no longer required
LENDING: Books only. Photocopies provided
COMPUTER DATA RETRIEVAL: DATASTAR online - charged computer time
HOLDINGS: 4,000 books; 780 journals, 60 current titles
CLASSIFICATION: DDC
SPECIAL COLLECTION: Registrar General annual reports from 1840
PUBLICATIONS: Accession lists
NETWORK: SE Thames RLIS

432
UNITED MEDICAL AND DENTAL SCHOOLS OF GUY'S AND ST THOMAS'S
HOSPITALS, INSTITUTE OF DERMATOLOGY
St John's Dermatology Centre, St Thomas's Hospital, Lambeth Palace
Road, London SE1 7EH
Tel: 071 928 9292 x1313
STAFF: Miss PM Tharratt
TYPE: Medical (Dermatology and allied subjects)
HOURS: Mon-Fri 9.30-5.30
READERS: Staff, other users with suitable identification
STOCK POLICY: Some books and journals discarded
LENDING: Books and duplicate journals. Photocopies provided
COMPUTER DATA RETRIEVAL: Access to terminal
HOLDINGS: 2,300 books; 187 journals, 117 current titles
CLASSIFICATION: Barnard (probably changing to NLM)
NETWORK: SE Thames RLIS

433
UNITED MEDICAL AND DENTAL SCHOOLS OF GUY'S AND ST THOMAS'S
HOSPITALS, PAEDIATRIC RESEARCH UNIT LIBRARY
Prince Philip Research Laboratories, 8th Floor, Guy's Tower,
London Bridge, SE1 9RT
Tel: 071 955 4135; 071 955 x5000
Fax: 071 955 4644 Electronic mail: A000005231000.PRULIB
STAFF: Mrs BA Merchant BSc MIInfSc ALA , 2 other part time staff
FOUNDED: 1963
TYPE: Medical genetics
HOURS: Mon-Fri 9-5
READERS: Staff and other users
STOCK POLICY: Superseded books discarded
LENDING: Books and journals. Photocopies provided
COMPUTER DATA RETRIEVAL: DATASTAR online. Free only to
 staff in Paediatric Research Unit
HOLDINGS: 4,000 books; 145 journals, 80 current titles;
                86,000 reprints
CLASSIFICATION: Books: Barnard (adapted)
PUBLICATIONS: Library guide; accessions list; periodicals
 holdings list
NETWORK: SE Thames Regional Library and Information Service;
          University of London

434

UNIVERSITY COLLEGE AND MIDDLESEX SCHOOL OF MEDICINE, BOLDERO
LIBRARY
Riding House Street, London W1P 7PN
071 380 9454   Fax: 071 436 0184
Electronic mail: JANET - LIBRARY @ UK.AC.UCL.SM.UXM
STAFF: Mrs J Cropper BSc DipLib (Boldero Librarian and Medical
          Libraries Coordinator), JA Dawson BSc DipInfSc
FOUNDED: 1835 (as Middlesex Hospital Medical School)
TYPE: Medical
HOURS: Mon-Thu 9.30-9, Fri 9.30-6
READERS: Staff and students, other users with identification for
          reference
LENDING: Books and journals. Self service photocopier
COMPUTER DATA RETRIEVAL: DATASTAR online - charged full cost.
          CD-ROM: from 1983
HOLDINGS: 4,000 books; 250 journals, 200 current titles; 70
          tape/slides, 30 videotapes (VHS)
CLASSIFICATION: NLM
SPECIAL COLLECTION: Books by Middlesex authors (250 vols)
PUBLICATION: Library newsletter (internal use only)
NETWORK: University of London

435

UNIVERSITY COLLEGE AND MIDDLESEX SCHOOL OF MEDICINE, CLINICAL
SCIENCES LIBRARY
University Street, London WC1E 6JJ
Tel: 071 387 9300 x5154
STAFF: GR Peacock BA DipLib, Miss J Gauld BA ALA
FOUNDED: 1906 (as University College Hospital Medical School)
TYPE: Medical, dental
HOURS: Mon, Wed, Fri 9-7, Tue, Thu 9-9, Sat 9.30-12.30
READERS: Staff and UCL students
STOCK POLICY: Out of date editions of books discarded
LENDING: Books only. Photocopies provided
COMPUTER DATA RETRIEVAL: DATASTAR online - charged full cost.
          CD-ROM from 1983
HOLDINGS: 15,000 books; 500 journals, 350 current titles; 30
          videotapes (VHS)
CLASSIFICATION: NLM
SPECIAL COLLECTION: Sir Robert Carswell (pathological
 drawings) (2,000 drawings)
PUBLICATION: Library guide
BRANCH: Royal Ear Hospital, London
NETWORKS: NE Thames RLS; University of London

436

UNIVERSITY COLLEGE AND MIDDLESEX SCHOOL OF MEDICINE, INSTITUTE OF
LARYNGOLOGY AND OTOLOGY
330-332 Gray's Inn Road, London WC1X 8EE
Tel: 071 837 8855 x4145
STAFF: PC Zwarts
TYPE: Medical (otology, rhinology, laryngology, audiology)

HOURS: Mon, Fri 9.30-5.30, Tues, Wed, Thurs 9.30-7
READERS: Staff only
LENDING: Books only. Photocopies provided
HOLDINGS: 2,200 books;3,300 bound journals,50 current titles
CLASSIFICATION: Barnard

437
UNIVERSITY COLLEGE AND MIDDLESEX SCHOOL OF MEDICINE, INSTITUTE OF
        OPHTHALMOLOGY
Judd Street, London WC1H 9QS
Tel: 071 387 9621 x238/239
The Institute will be moving from Judd St in Summer 1991. All
intending visitors should telephone prior to a visit as much of the
stock will be inaccessible.

STAFF: Mrs CS Lawrence MA DipLib ALA MIInfSc, Miss C Williams BA,
        Miss R Harris BA (part time)
FOUNDED: 1948
TYPE: Medical, postgraduate ophthalmology & visual science
HOURS: Mon, Wed, Thurs 9-5.30, Tues 9-7, Fri 9-4.30
READERS: Staff, other users for reference only by arrangement
STOCK POLICY: Out of date works on peripheral subjects
 discarded, peripheral journals discarded
LENDING: Books and journals. Photocopies provided
COMPUTER DATA RETRIEVAL: Access to terminal. Charged full cost
HOLDINGS: c9,000 books; 200 current journals
SPECIAL COLLECTION: Historical ophthalmology and visual
 science
CLASSIFICATION: Own
BRANCH: Moorfields Eye Hospital (Nursing/Residents library)
NETWORK: British Postgraduate Medical Federation ; NE Thames
        Regional Library Service

438
UNIVERSITY COLLEGE AND MIDDLESEX SCHOOL OF MEDICINE, INSTITUTE OF
ORTHOPAEDICS
Royal National Orthopaedic Hospital, 45-51 Bolsover Street,
 London W1P 8AQ
Tel: 071 387 5070   Fax: 081 954 8560
STAFF: PF Smith MA DPhil ALA, DK Chatarji BSc MA MPhil DipLibSci,
 Mrs D Henderson (part time)
FOUNDED: 1946
TYPE: Orthopaedic
HOURS: Mon-Fri 9.30-5.30 (Stanmore Mon-Fri 9-5)
READERS: Staff, other users at Librarian's discretion
STOCK POLICY: No stock discarded
LENDING: Books and journals. Photocopies provided
COMPUTER DATA RETRIEVAL: DATASTAR, BLAISE online (at Stanmore
        branch) - Charged full cost. CD-ROM from 1989
HOLDINGS: 5,000 books; 278 journals, 165 current titles
SPECIAL COLLECTION: Orthopaedics: historical collection (c440 vols)
CLASSIFICATION: NLM
BRANCH: Sir Herbert Seddon Teaching Centre, Royal National
 Orthopaedic Hospital, Stanmore, Middlesex HA7 4LP (081 954 2300)
NETWORK: University of London

439
UNIVERSITY COLLEGE AND MIDDLESEX SCHOOL OF MEDICINE, INSTITUTE OF
UROLOGY
172 Shaftesbury Avenue, London WC2H 8JE
Tel: 071 240 9115
STAFF: Mrs D Leach BA DipLib
TYPE: Medical
HOURS: Mon-Fri 9.30-1.30
READERS: Staff of Institute, staff of hospitals in group
LENDING: Books and journals
COMPUTER DATA RETRIEVAL: Access to terminal. Free
HOLDINGS: 650 books; 2,000 bound journals, 40 current titles
SPECIAL COLLECTION: Urology and nephrology
CLASSIFICATION: Barnard

440
UNIVERSITY COLLEGE AND MIDDLESEX SCHOOL OF MEDICINE, THANE MEDICAL
SCIENCES LIBRARY
Gower Street, London WC1E 6BT
Tel: 071 387 7050 x2632
STAFF: Miss DM Mercer MSc DipLib ALA
TYPE: Medical (preclinical)
HOURS: Mon-Fri 9.30-9 (9.30-7 Xmas, Easter vacations,9.30-5 Summer)
READERS: Staff and other users (9.30-5.30 except vacations)
LENDING: Books only. self service photocopier
COMPUTER DATA RETRIEVAL: DATASTAR online - charged computer time
              only. CD-ROM
HOLDINGS: 20,000 books; 600 journals, 400 current titles
CLASSIFICATION: Garside

441
WELLCOME INSTITUTE FOR THE HISTORY OF MEDICINE
183 Euston Rd, London NW1 2BQ
**FROM March 1990, for approximately 2 years, the Library will be in
 temporary accomodation at 200 Euston Rd, London, NW1 2BQ
 Tel: 071 387 4499**
STAFF: EJ Freeman BA ALA, RM Price MA ALA, HJM Symons MA ALA,
    Ms KJC Hooper MA, Ms J Lake BA ALA, PL Davey BA ALA, Miss HB
    Sutton BA DipLib, RJ Palmer BA PhD ALA, NMWT Allan MA PhD ALA,
   D Wujastyk BSc MA DPhil, WM Schupbach MA, Ms' GP Nuding MA PhD,
   Miss PM Hully BA FLA
FOUNDED: c1890, opened to the public 1949
TYPE: History of medicine and science
HOURS: Mon, Wed, Fri 9.45-5.15, Tue, Thu 9.45-7.30
READERS: Staff and other users
STOCK POLICY: No stock discarded
LENDING: Reference only. Photocopies supplied
COMPUTER DATA RETRIEVAL: In-house terminal
HOLDINGS: mss, printed books; c6,000 journals, c400 current titles;
          650 microfilms, 43 moving image films

CLASSIFICATION: Barnard and NLM
SPECIAL COLLECTIONS: Oriental (over 11,000 mss, c3,000 printed
        books); American (150 mss, c14,000 printed books)
PUBLICATIONS: Medical history (quarterly journal); Current Work in
        the History of Medicine (bibliographical quarterly);
        Library and exhibition catalogues, etc

442
WEST LONDON INSTITUTE OF HIGHER EDUCATION
Borough Rd, Isleworth, Middlesex TW7 5DU
Tel: 081 891 0121
STAFF: Ms P Wharram BA MLS (Director of Library Services)
FOUNDED: 1977 from Borough Rd College (1808), Maria Grey College
                (1878) and part of Chiswick Polytechnic (1850)
TYPE: Multidisciplinary
HOURS: Mon-Thu 9-9, Fri 9-5, Sat 9-12
READERS: Staff and students, other users for reference only
STOCK POLICY: Books and journals discarded when appropriate
LENDING: Books, journals occasionally. Photocopies provided
COMPUTER DATA RETRIEVAL: DATASTAR, BLAISE, DIALOG, WILSONLINE,
        COMPASS 2000, QUESTEL, PERGAMON INFO - all online - free at
        present. CD-ROM from 1988
HOLDINGS: 101 current journals relevant to health & paramedical
        subjects
CLASSIFICATION: DDC
SPECIAL COLLECTION: Sports medicine
BRANCHES: Two equal sites

443
WESTMINSTER CITY LIBRARIES MEDICAL LIBRARY
Marylebone Library, Marylebone Road, London NW1 5PS
Tel: 071 798 1039
STAFF: Mrs S Stallion ALA, Miss VA Perkins BA ALA
TYPE: Multidisciplinary
HOURS: Mon 10-7, Tue-Fri 9.30-7, Sat 9.30-5
READERS: Open to any member of the public
STOCK POLICY: Closed runs of journals discarded, books discarded
                at varying intervals
LENDING: Books only. Photocopies provided
COMPUTER DATA RETRIEVAL: Access to DIALOG - charged full cost.
HOLDINGS: 36,000 books; 120 current journals
CLASSIFICATION: DDC
PUBLICATION: Quarterly accessions list
NETWORK: LASER

444
WHIPPS CROSS HOSPITAL MEDICAL EDUCATION CENTRE
Leytonstone, London E11 1NR
Tel: 081 539 5522 or 081 539 3026 Electronic mail: DATAMAIL WHIPPSX
STAFF: Ms DM Hall BA ALA (District Librarian), Mrs G Palmer (part
time)
TYPE: Medical, dental
HOURS: Mon-Fri 8.30-7. Staffed Mon 9-1.30, Tues and Thurs 9-4.30
READERS: Staff, other users on application
STOCK POLICY: Books and journals discarded at varying intervals
LENDING: Reference only. Photocopies supplied
COMPUTER DATA RETRIEVAL: DATASTAR online - free
HOLDINGS: 1,500 books; 100 journals, 80 current titles
CLASSIFICATION: NLM
NETWORK: NE Thames

445
WOLFSON SCHOOL OF NURSING
30 Vincent Square, London SW1P 2NW
Tel: 071 828 9811 x464
No furthur information available

Londonderry

446
MULTIDISCIPLINARY EDUCATION CENTRE
Altnagelvin Hospital, Londonderry BT47 1JB
Tel: 0504 45171
STAFF: FA O'Deorain BSc(Hons) DipLib ALA, 1 other (full-time) and 2
(part-time) staff
TYPE: Multidisciplinary
HOURS: Mon, Thurs 9-9.30, Tues, Wed, Fri 9-5.30
READERS: Staff and other users
STOCK POLICY: Out of date books discarded
LENDING: Books and journals
COMPUTER DATA RETRIEVAL: In-house terminal. Free
HOLDINGS: 8,000 books and bound journals; 130 current
journals. 16 mm cine films, tape/slides, 35 mm slides,
videotapes (VHS)
CLASSIFICATION: LC
PUBLICATIONS: Accessions lists; bibliographies
NETWORK: NIHSSL

Loughborough

447
FISONS plc-PHARMACEUTICAL DIVISION
Research and Development Laboratories, Bakewell Road,
Loughborough, Leics LE11 0RH
Tel: 0509 611011   Fax: 0509 611222
STAFF: Ms P Teggart BSc(Hons) DipAgEng DipLib ALA, Ms A Wray BA MA

Loughborough, Leics LE11 0RH
Tel: 0509 611011   Fax: 0509 611222
STAFF: Ms P Teggart BSc(Hons) DipAgEng DipLib ALA, Ms A Wray BA MA
TYPE: Pharmaceutical
HOURS: Staffed 8.30-5.30
READERS: Staff, other users by prior arrangement only
STOCK POLICY: Journals discarded after 20 years, books discarded
             after 10 years
LENDING: Books internally only, journals to overnight users.
          Photocopies provided
COMPUTER DATA RETRIEVAL: DATASTAR online - free. CD-ROM from 1988
HOLDINGS: 4,000 books; 400 journals, 350 current titles
CLASSIFICATION: Own

448
3M HEALTH CARE LIMITED
1 Morley Street, Loughborough, Leics LE11 1EP
Tel: 0509 611611   Telex 34587 HEALTH G   Fax: 0509 237288
STAFF: M Sanderson BA ALA, H Martin BSc BA ALA
TYPE: Pharmaceutical, Health care products
HOURS: Mon-Fri 9-5.
READERS: Staff only
STOCK POLICY: Journals discarded after varying periods, books
              discarded after 11 years
LENDING: Books, journals and microfiche. Photocopies provided
COMPUTER DATA RETRIEVAL: Online databases: DATASTAR, BLAISE, DIALOG,
              ORBIT, INFOLINE
PUBLICATIONS: Library guides; Current awareness bulletin; Library
              bulletin

Luton

449
LUTON AND DUNSTABLE HOSPITAL MEDICAL CENTRE
Luton and Dunstable Hospital, Luton, Beds LU4 0DZ
Tel: 0582 491122 x2170
STAFF: Librarian post vacant, Assistant post vacant
FOUNDED: 1967
TYPE: Multidisciplinary
HOURS: Always open. Staffed Mon-Fri 8.30-5
READERS: Staff and other users
STOCK POLICY: Out of date books discarded
LENDING: Books, journals, human bones. Photocopies provided
COMPUTER DATA RETRIEVAL: DATASTAR online - external users charged
             flat rate. CD-ROM from 1982
HOLDINGS: 1800 books; 2,000 bound journals, 122 current titles;
             collection of human bones
CLASSIFICATION: NLM
PUBLICATIONS: Library guide; journal holdings list
BRANCH: General patients library, Luton & Dunstable Hospital
NETWORK: NW Thames Regional Library and Information Service

Macclesfield

450
EAST CHESHIRE ASSOCIATION FOR MEDICAL EDUCATION
Postgraduate Medical Centre, Macclesfield District General
Hospital, Prestbury Rd, Macclesfield, SK10 3BL
Tel:0625 21000
STAFF: Mrs M Perry ALA (part time)
TYPE: Multidisciplinary
HOURS: Mon-Fri 9-5
READERS: Staff, other users on written application
LENDING: Books and journals. Photocopies supplied
HOLDINGS: 2,650 books; 50 bound journals; 59 current titles
CLASSIFICATION: DDC
NETWORK: Mersey Region

451
ICI PHARMACEUTICALS, MERESIDE LIBRARY
Mereside, Alderley Park, Macclesfield, Cheshire SK10 4TG
Tel: 0625 515149   Fax: 0625 586278
STAFF: Mrs GD Swash MA ALA
FOUNDED: 1957
TYPE: Multidisciplinary
HOURS: Staffed Mon-Fri 9-5.
READERS: Company staff only
STOCK POLICY: Books and journals discarded
LENDING: Books and journals
COMPUTER DATA RETRIEVAL: In-house terminal - free. PRESTEL
 available. CD-ROM from 1989
HOLDINGS: 10,000 books;2,000 journals, 1,500 current titles.
CLASSIFICATION: UDC
BRANCH: Commercial Library, Alderley House Works Library,
 Macclesfield

Maidenhead

452
WYETH LABORATORIES
Huntercombe Lane South, Taplow, Maidenhead, Berks SL6 0PH
Tel: 0628 604377   Telex: 847640   Fax: 0628 666368
No further information available

Maidstone

453
THE EUROPEAN SCHOOL OF OSTEOPATHY
104 Tonbridge Road, Maidstone, Kent ME13 8SL
Tel: 0622 671558
STAFF: Mrs LH Brice BA DipLib ALA
FOUNDED: c1982
TYPE: Osteopathy, complementary medicine, medical (as
 relevant)

HOURS: Mon- Fri 9-5.30
READERS: Staff and other users
STOCK POLICY: Journals discarded after 2 years, Books
          rarely discarded
LENDING: Books only. Photocopies provided
COMPUTER DATA RETRIEVAL: Access to terminal. Charged
HOLDINGS: 2,000 books; c20 journals; 1,000 35mm slides,
                videotapes (20 Betamax, 40 VHS)
CLASSIFICATION: Own
SPECIAL COLLECTION: Osteopathy/manipulation (200 vols)
NETWORK: SE Thames

454
MAIDSTONE HOSPITAL, OAKWOOD LIBRARY
Hermitage Lane, Maidstone, Kent, ME16 9QQ
Tel: 0622 29000 x647
STAFF: Mrs G Procter ALA, Mrs I Gallagher ALA , Mrs P Davey
          BSc DipLib ALA (part time)
FOUNDED: 1974
TYPE: Multidisciplinary
HOURS: Mon-Thurs 9-5, Fri 9-4.30.
READERS: Staff, other users for reference only
STOCK POLICY: Out of date books discarded. Journals over 10
 years old discarded if available elsewhere in SETRHA
LENDING: Books, limited AV only. Photocopies provided
COMPUTER DATA RETRIEVAL: DATASTAR online free
HOLDINGS: 9,000 books; 176 journals, 165 current titles
                titles; 36 tape/slides
CLASSIFICATION: DDC
PUBLICATIONS: Library guide; Spotlight (newsletter)
NETWORK: SE Thames Regional Library and Information Service
BRANCHES: Maidstone Health Authority Headquarters, Maidstone;
 Preston Hall Hospital PGC,Maidstone, ME20 7NJ; Kent County
 Ophthalmic and Aural Hospital , Maidstone; Maidstone Hospital
 Postgraduate Medical Education Centre

Manchester
455
BOOTH HALL CHILDREN'S HOSPITAL, MEDICAL LIBRARY
Charlestown Road, Blackley, Manchester M9 2AA
Tel: 061 795 7000
STAFF:Dr B Wolman MD FRCP DCH (Honorary Librarian)
TYPE: Medical, paediatric
HOURS: Mon-Fri 9-5 (Unstaffed). Key available after hours
READERS: Medical staff and other users
STOCK POLICY: No stock discarded
LENDING: Reference only. Photocopies provided
HOLDINGS: 1,500 books; 560 bound journals, 40 current titles
CLASSIFICATION: Own

456
CHRISTIE HOSPITAL AND HOLT RADIUM INSTITUTE
Wilmslow Road, Withington, Manchester M20 9BX
Tel: 061 445 8123 x308   Fax: 061 434 7728
STAFF: Mrs M Hinde BA ALA, Assistant Librarian post vacant
TYPE: Medical, nursing , physics
HOURS: Mon-Thurs 9-5.30, Fri 9-5
READERS: Graduates of hospital and nursing staff. Other
  users by appointment or at discretion of librarian
STOCK POLICY: Books and journals discarded when space
            demands
LENDING: Books, journals and slides.   Photocopies
          provided
COMPUTER DATA RETRIEVAL: DATASTAR online - charged full
          cost
HOLDINGS: 5,000 books; c250 journals, 230 current titles;
            c500 35mm slides
CLASSIFICATION: Barnard
PUBLICATION: Library newsletter (monthly)

457
MANCHESTER ROYAL INFIRMARY, JEFFERSON MEDICAL LIBRARY
Oxford Road, Manchester M13 9WL
Tel: 061 276 1234 x4344
STAFF: Mrs SK Reddy MA BLSc DipLib ALA (part time), Mrs R
        Banerjee (part time)
FOUNDED: 1971
TYPE: Medical
HOURS: Mon-Fri 10-5. (5-12 with security system)
READERS: Medical staff and other users
STOCK POLICY: Some books discarded after 10 years,
              some journals discarded after 5 years
LENDING: Books and journals
HOLDINGS: 1,200 books; 80 current journals; video-
              tapes (VHS)
CLASSIFICATION: NLM
SPECIAL COLLECTION: Jefferson (Neurology) (30 vols)
BRANCH: Archives Library

458
JOHN RYLANDS UNIVERSITY LIBRARY OF MANCHESTER
The University, Oxford Road, Manchester M13 9PP
Tel: 061 275 3729/3751 Telex 668932 MCHRUL G   Fax: 061 273 7488
  Electronic mail: YMULB @ UK.AC.UMIST
STAFF: Dr MA Pegg PhD (Director/University Librarian), Mrs VA
  Ferguson BA DipLib FLA (Assistant Librarian: Medicine):
  Rylands Information Centre: Mrs PA Rangeley BA (Head), Dr DM
    Leitch BSc PhD (Science Librarian), Dr AF Neville MSc PhD
    (Information Officer), Dr N Kimber BSc PhD DipLib (Biological
    Sciences), Miss P Cumming ALA (Manchester Medical Collection)
FOUNDED: 1835 (Manchester Medical Society Library)
TYPE: Multidisciplinary
HOURS: Mon-Fri 9-9.30, Sat 9-1 (Term, Easter vacation,

except Holy Week), Mon-Fri 9.30-5.30, Sat 9.30-1 (Christmas
vacation, Holy Week, Summer vacation). Full services not
all available after 5.00
READERS: Staff, students and members of the Manchester
Medical Society and UMIST members. Other users by
arrangement
STOCK POLICY: Duplicate books, journals and some ephemeral
material discarded
LENDING: Books and journals
COMPUTER DATA RETRIEVAL: Online databases: DATASTAR, BLAISE, STN,
DIALOG, ESA, WILSONLINE, PROFILE, ECHO, TELESYSTEME QUESTEL.
Charged full cost. CD-ROM
HOLDINGS: 135,000 books; 180,000 bound journals; 1,000
current journals. Tape/slides, 35 mm slides, videotapes
(VHS)
SPECIAL COLLECTIONS: Manchester Collection - history of
medicine in the Manchester area (1,000 vols) and archives;
medical books 1480-1800 (6,000 vols) (Deansgate Building);
medical books 1800-1940 (25,000 vols); Marie Stopes collection
(600 vols) (Main Library)
CLASSIFICATION: Own
PUBLICATION: Catalogue of medical books in Manchester
University Library 1480-1700 by EM Parkinson; Bulletin of the
John Rylands University Library of Manchester 1900- (3 pa);
Library News in Medicine (Newsletter for the Medical Faculty);
North West Health services Librarians Association Union List of
Periodicals
BRANCHES: Medical Faculty Library, Stopford Building,
Manchester M13 9PT; Deansgate Building, Deansgate, Manchester M3
3EM

459
NORTH MANCHESTER POSTGRADUATE MEDICAL CENTRE
North Manchester General Hospital, Manchester M8 6RH
Tel: 061 795 4567
STAFF: Mrs PC Mallinson, Mrs S Coffey (part-time)
FOUNDED: 1973
TYPE: Multidisciplinary
HOURS: Mon-Thurs 9-8, Fri 9-5
READERS: Staff and other users
STOCK POLICY: Journals discarded after 19 years, books discarded
after 20 years
LENDING: Books and journals. Photocopies provided
COMPUTER DATA RETRIEVAL: DATASTAR online - charged computer time
only
HOLDINGS: 3,000 books; 143 journals, 124 current titles;
6 tape/slides,10 35mm slides, videotapes (2 U-matic, 25 VHS)

CLASSIFICATION: DDC
SPECIAL COLLECTIONS: British Journal of Surgery & Maudsley
Monographs (both from vol 1)
PUBLICATION: Library bulletin
BRANCH: Moncall Hospital
NETWORK: NORWHSLA

460
NORTH WESTERN REGIONAL HEALTH AUTHORITY, MANAGEMENT LIBRARY
Gateway House, Piccadilly South, Manchester M60 7LP
Tel: 061 237 2138   Fax: 061 236 1134
STAFF: Ms SCR Padden BA(Hons) ALA, Mrs K Turtle BA ALA
TYPE: Health administration
HOURS: Mon-Fri 8-4.30
READERS: Staff, other users for reference only
STOCK POLICY: Books and journals discarded at varying intervals
LENDING: Books and journals
COMPUTER DATA RETRIEVAL: DATASTAR online - other libraries/users
                charged full cost
HOLDINGS: c5,000 books; c50 current journals
CLASSIFICATION: Bliss
PUBLICATIONS: Quarterly recent additions bulletin; Monthly current
                awareness; bibliographies
NETWORK: NORWHSLA; NHS Management Librarians Group

461
PRESTWICH HOSPITAL PROFESSIONAL LIBRARY
Bury New Road, Prestwich, Manchester M75 7BL
Tel: 061 773 9121 x104
STAFF: J Coulshed BA DipLib
TYPE: Multidisciplinary
HOURS: Mon-Fri 9-5
READERS: Staff and other users at discretion of librarian
LENDING: Books and journals. Photocopies provided
COMPUTER DATA RETRIEVAL: DATASTAR online - free
HOLDINGS: 4,000 books; 70 journals, 55 current titles;
                tape/slide, 35mm slide, videotape (VHS)
CLASSIFICATION: RCP
PUBLICATIONS: Whats In Current Awareness Bulletin; Forensic CAB;
                Community CAB
NETWORK: PLCS; NORWHSLA

462
PRESTWICH HOSPITAL SCHOOL OF NURSING
Bury New Road, Prestwich, Manchester M25 7BL
Tel: 061 789 7373 x2347
No furthur information available

463
ROYAL MANCHESTER CHILDREN'S HOSPITAL, MEDICAL LIBRARY
Hospital Road, Pendlebury, Manchester M27 1HA
Tel: 061 794 4696
STAFF: Mrs JE Kelly BA ALA (part-time)
FOUNDED: 1978
TYPE: Medical, paediatric
HOURS: Mon-Fri 9-4.30.
READERS: Staff only
STOCK POLICY: Journals (except paediatric) discarded after 5 years,
              books discarded after 10 years
LENDING: Books and journals. Photocopies provided
COMPUTER DATA RETRIEVAL: DATASTAR online - charged computer time
                          only
HOLDINGS: 568 books; 70 journals, 62 current titles
CLASSIFICATION: NLM
PUBLICATIONS: Library bulletin
NETWORK: NORWHSLA

464
SAINT MARY'S HOSPITAL MEDICAL LIBRARY
Research Floor, Saint Mary's Hospital, Whitworth Park,
 Manchester M13 0JH
Tel: 061 276 1234
STAFF: Mrs W Lamb (part-time)
TYPE: Multidisciplinary
HOURS: Mon-Fri 9.30-7. Staffed 22½ hours per week
READERS: Staff only
STOCK POLICY: Books discarded when information out of date
COMPUTER DATA RETRIEVAL: In-house terminal
HOLDINGS: 900 books; 1,630 bound journals, 77 current titles;
                     tape/slides
CLASSIFICATION: Own
PUBLICATION: List of Staff publications
NETWORK: NORWHSLA

465
SOUTH WEST MANCHESTER COLLEGE OF NURSING
Mauldeth House, Mauldeth Road West, Manchester M21 2RL
Tel: 061 881 7233 x286
STAFF: Miss T Roberts BA(Hons), Miss H Bridges
TYPE: Nursing
HOURS: Mon-Thurs 8.30-5, Fri 8.30-4
READERS: Nurses only
STOCK POLICY: Books reviewed after 5 years
LENDING: Books only. Photocopies provided
COMPUTER DATA RETRIEVAL: Access to terminal. Charged full
 cost
HOLDINGS: c8,000 books; 33 current journals. 16mm cine
 films, tape/slides, 35mm slides, videotapes (VHS)
CLASSIFICATION: DDC
NETWORK: North West Nursing Librarians Group
BRANCH: Wythenshawe Post Basic Department, Manchester M23 9LT

466
TRAFFORD SCHOOL OF NURSING
Trafford General Hospital, Moorside Rd, Davyhulme, Manchester
          M31 3SL
Tel: 061 748 4022 x512
STAFF: B Durham BA(Hons) ALA
TYPE: Nursing
HOURS: Mon-Thu 8.30-4.30, Fri 8.30-4
READERS: Nursing staff, other users for reference only
STOCK POLICY: Books discarded at varying intervals
LENDING: Books only. Photocopies provided
COMPUTER DATA RETRIEVAL: DATASTAR online - charged full cost
HOLDINGS: 2,500 books; 39 journals,18 current titles;
                    50 tape/slides, 100 videotapes (VHS)
CLASSIFICATION: DDC
PUBLICATIONS: Current awareness bulletin
NETWORK: NORWHSLA
BRANCH: Saint Anne's Hospital (Continuing Education
 Department), Bowden

467
WITHINGTON HOSPITAL MEDICAL LIBRARY
Nell Lane, West Didsbury, Manchester M20 8LR
Tel: 061 447 3878/9
STAFF: Miss E Jordan BA ALA, Miss DL Jones BA
TYPE: Multidisciplinary
HOURS: Mon, Tue, Thu 9-8.30, wed, Fri 9-5.45
READERS: Staff, GP's and Community Medicine personnel
STOCK POLICY: Books discarded at varying intervals
LENDING: Books and journals
COMPUTER DATA RETRIEVAL: DATASTAR online - charged full cost
HOLDINGS: c7,000 books; 250 current journals; 50 tape/slides
SPECIAL COLLECTION: Geriatrics (400 vols)
CLASSIFICATION: DDC
PUBLICATIONS: Monthly current awareness list
NETWORK: NORWHSLA

468
WYTHENSHAWE POSTGRADUATE CENTRE MEDICAL LIBRARY
Wythenshawe Hospital, Southmoor Road, Manchester M23 9LT
Tel: 061 946 2348
STAFF: Mrs JA White (part-time)
FOUNDED: 1970
TYPE: Medical
HOURS: Mon-Thu 9-5, Fri 9-4
READERS: Staff and other users
STOCK POLICY: Books and journals discarded selectively
LENDING: Books, journals and AV material. Photocopies provided
COMPUTER DATA RETRIEVAL: DATASTAR online - charged computer time
                                only
HOLDINGS: 3,500 books; 130 journals, 120 current titles;

35mm slides, videotapes (VHS)
CLASSIFICATION: NLM
NETWORK: NORWHSLA

Mansfield

469
INTAKE TRUST MEDICAL LIBRARY
Mansfield and District General Hospital, West Hill Drive,
 Mansfield, Notts NG18 1PH
Tel: 0623 22515
STAFF: Mrs I Stubbs (part-time)
TYPE: Medical
HOURS: Mon-Fri 8-8. Staffed 8.30-4
READERS: Staff and GP's in area
STOCK POLICY: Very out of date editions of books discarded
LENDING: Journals lent and photocopies provided through ILL
COMPUTER DATA RETRIEVAL: Access to terminal
HOLDINGS: 5,000 books; 200 journals, 125 current titles
 journals
CLASSIFICATION: Own
BRANCH: King's Mill Hospital, Sutton in Ashfield
NETWORK: TRAHCLIS

470
MANSFIELD AND WORKSOP SCHOOL OF NURSING
Ashfield Avenue, Mansfield, Notts NG18 2AE
Tel: 0623 22515 x533
No furthur information available

Margate

471
THANET DISTRICT GENERAL HOSPITAL, POSTGRADUATE MEDICAL LIBRARY
St Peter's Road, Margate, Kent, CT9 4AN
Tel: 0843 225544 x2536
Librarian vacancy.
TYPE: Multidisciplinary
HOURS: Mon-Fri 9-5
READERS: Staff and other users
STOCK POLICY: Journals discarded after 20 years
LENDING: Books, videos. Photocopies provided
COMPUTER DATA RETRIEVAL: DATASTAR online
HOLDINGS: 60 current journals; 20 videotapes (VHS)
NETWORK: SE Thames RLIS

Merthyr Tydfil

472
PRINCE CHARLES HOSPITAL
Merthyr Tydfil, Mid-Glamorgan, CF47 9DT
Tel: 0685 721721 x8251
STAFF: Mrs LH Foster BA(Hons)
FOUNDED: 1978
TYPE: Multidisciplinary
HOURS: Mon-Fri 9-5.
READERS: Staff, other users on application
LENDING: Books and journals. Photocopies supplied
COMPUTER DATA RETRIEVAL: Access to terminal. Free
HOLDINGS: 5,700 books; 128 journals, 98 current titles
CLASSIFICATION: DDC
PUBLICATIONS: Journal holdings

Middlesbrough

473
SOUTH TEES MEDICAL LIBRARY
Education Centre, South Cleveland Hospital, , Martin Road,
Middlesborough Cleveland, TS4 3BW
Tel: 0642 850850 x20695
STAFF: Mrs J Bethel ALA
TYPE: Multidisciplinary
HOURS: Mon-Fri 9-8, Sat 9-12
READERS: Staff only
STOCK POLICY: Journals discarded after 12 years, only current
             and previous editions of books kept.
LENDING: Books and journals. Photocopies supplied
COMPUTER DATA RETRIEVAL: DATASTAR online - free
HOLDINGS: 7,000 books; 238 journals, 225 current titles;
             tape/slides
CLASSIFICATION: DDC
PUBLICATIONS: Guide to the library; periodicals list
NETWORK: Northern Regional Association of Health Service
             Librarians

Midhurst

474
KING EDWARD VII HOSPITAL , MEDICAL LIBRARY
Midhurst, West Sussex GU29 0BL
Tel: 0730 812431   Fax: 0730 816333
STAFF: JN Harris FLA (part-time)
TYPE: Medical, paramedical
HOURS: Always open. Staffed Tue and Fri 9-4
READERS: Staff, other users by introduction
STOCK POLICY: Out of date editions of books discarded
COMPUTER DATA RETRIEVAL: Access to terminal.
HOLDINGS: 500 books; 80 journals 50 current titles
CLASSIFICATION: UDC
PUBLICATIONS: Periodicals list

Milton Keynes

475
HEALTH MATTERS
795 Avebury Boulevard, Central Milton Keynes, MK9 3NW
Tel: 0908 677200
STAFF: Mrs MG Muller BA DipLib ALA
FOUNDED: 1987
TYPE: Multidisciplinary
HOURS: Tue 10-5, Wed 10-1, Thu 2-7, Fri 10-5
READERS: Staff and other users
STOCK POLICY: Books and journals discarded at Librarian's discretion
LENDING: Leaflets, reference lists, contacts with self-help groups.
            Photocopies provided
COMPUTER DATA RETRIEVAL: DATASTAR online - free
HOLDINGS: 570 books
CLASSIFICATION: Own
PUBLICATIONS: Simplified language versions of medical information

476
HOECHST (UK) LIMITED
Walton Manor, Walton, Milton Keynes MK7 7AJ
Tel: 0908 665050 x206   Telex: 826033   Fax: 0908 665564
STAFF: Mrs JM Henley BSc MLib ALA MIInfSc (Consultant Librarian)
TYPE: Pharmacy
HOURS: Mon-Fri 9-5.30 - not always staffed
READERS: Staff, other users by prior arrangement
STOCK POLICY: Books and journals discarded
LENDING: Books only. Photocopies provided
COMPUTER DATA RETRIEVAL: DATASTAR, BLAISE, DIALOG, ESA, SDC,
                        INFOLINE, PROFILE online
HOLDINGS: 2,000 books; 200 journals, 150 current titles
CLASSIFICATION: UDC
PUBLICATIONS: Guide to services; journals listing

477
MILTON KEYNES HOSPITAL, POSTGRADUATE EDUCATION CENTRE
Standing Way, Eaglestone, Milton Keynes, MK6 5AZ
Tel: 0908 660033 x2175   Fax: 0908 660539
STAFF: Ms G Needham BA DipLib ALA
FOUNDED: 1984
TYPE: Multidisciplinary
HOURS: Mon-Fri 9-5 . Ansaphone at other times
READERS: Staff and other users
STOCK POLICY: Books discarded after 5-10 years, journals discarded
        after 10 years
LENDING: Books only. Photocopies provided
COMPUTER DATA RETRIEVAL: DATASTAR, BLAISE, DIALOG online - free
HOLDINGS: 5,000 books; 150 journals, 130 current titles
CLASSIFICATION: NLM
PUBLICATIONS: Weekly contents page bulletin; Press cuttings bulletin
NETWORK: Oxford Regional LIS

478
NORTHUMBRIA COLLEGE OF NURSING, NURSE EDUCATION LIBRARY
Northgate Hospital, Morpeth, Northumberland, NE61 3BP
Tel: 0670 512281 x314
STAFF: Mrs CM Smith MA DipLib ALA (part time)
TYPE: Nursing, psychiatric
HOURS: Mon-Fri 9-5 (Staffed 6 hours per week)
READERS: Access permitted via Librarian
STOCK POLICY: Books discarded after 10 years
HOLDINGS: 1,500 books; 30 journals, 24 current titles; 35mm slides
CLASSIFICATION: DDC 19
PUBLICATION: Current contents of nursing and allied journals
NETWORK: NRAHSL

479
NORTHUMBRIA COLLEGE OF NURSING, NURSE EDUCATION LIBRARY
St George's Hospital, Morpeth, Northumberland, NE61 2NU
Tel: 0670 512121 x3650
STAFF: Mrs CM Smith MA DipLib ALA (part time)
TYPE: Nursing, psychiatric
HOURS: Mon-Fri 9-5 (Staffed 6 hours per week)
READERS: Access permitted via Librarian
LENDING: Books, videos, tape/slides. Photocopies provided
HOLDINGS: 1,000 books; 10 journals, 6 current titles; videotapes,
              tape/slides
CLASSIFICATION: DDC 19
PUBLICATION: Current contents
NETWORK: NRAHSL

480
SAINT GEORGE'S HOSPITAL POSTGRADUATE MEDICAL LIBRARY
Morpeth, Northumberland, NE61 2NU
Tel: 0670 512121 x3365

N Miller BA(Hons) DipLib (part time)
FOUNDED: 1987
TYPE: Psychiatric
HOURS: Mon-Fri 8.45-5 (Staffed Mon & Wed 8.45-12.30)
READERS: Staff and other users
LENDING: Books very occasionally. Photocopies provided
COMPUTER DATA RETRIEVAL: Access to DATASTAR, BLAISE, DIALOG,
        PERGAMON - free
HOLDINGS: 46 journals, 27 current titles
CLASSIFICATION: DDC
NETWORKS: Northern Region ; Northumberland County Library

Newbury

481
INSTITUTE FOR ANIMAL HEALTH
Compton Laboratory, Compton, Newbury, Berks, RG16 0NN
Tel: 0635 578411   Telex: 265871 quote ref: ARS 006

Fax: 0635 578844   Electronic mail: JANET IRADLIB @UK.AC.AFRC.IRAD
STAFF: Mrs R Zoro BSc ALA MIInfSc
FOUNDED: late 1930s
TYPE: Animal health and diseases (farm animals)
HOURS: Mon-Thu 8.30-5, Fri 8.30-4.30
READERS: Staff, other users by appointment
STOCK POLICY: Books discarded after 20 years
LENDING: Books and journals within AFRC libraries; Reprints of
         publications to other enquirers
COMPUTER DATA RETRIEVAL: DATASTAR, DIALOG online - online searches
         carried out for other AFRC sites - no charge
HOLDINGS: 1,500 books; c250 journals, 120 current titles
CLASSIFICATION: UDC
BRANCHES: 3 other sites
NETWORK: AFRC

Newcastle upon Tyne

482
FREEMAN HOSPITAL TEACHING CENTRE LIBRARY
Freeman Hospital, Freeman Road, High Heaton, Newcastle upon
 Tyne NE7 7DN
Tel: 091 2843111
STAFF: Mrs V Murray BA ALA DMS, Mrs J Dyson ALA (part-time)
TYPE: Multidisciplinary
HOURS: Mon-Fri 9-5 (Thu until 9), Sat 9-1
READERS: Staff and other users
STOCK POLICY: books and journals discarded
LENDING: Books and journals. Photocopies provided
COMPUTER DATA RETRIEVAL: CD-ROM from 1990
HOLDINGS: 10,500 books; 160 journals, 140 current titles
CLASSIFICATION: DDC
SPECIAL COLLECTION: Cardiology
PUBLICATIONS: User's guide; Current journal holdings; Library
                Bulletin; Library skills workbook
NETWORK: Northern Regional Association of Health Service
            Librarians; Northern Regional Library System

483
NEWCASTLE GENERAL HOSPITAL POSTGRADUATE MEDICAL CENTRE
Newcastle upon Tyne NE4 6BE
Tel: 091 273 8811 x22545
STAFF: AE Middleton BA ALA (part-time), 2 other (part-time) staff
TYPE: Multidisciplinary
HOURS: Mon-Fri 9.30-5.
READERS: Staff and other users in NHS/Newcastle HA
STOCK POLICY: Superseded editions of books discarded, some
                journals discarded after 3/10 years
LENDING: Books only. Photocopies provided
COMPUTER DATA RETRIEVAL: In-house terminal. CD-ROM from 1990
HOLDINGS: 5,000 books; 150 journals, 135 current titles
SPECIAL COLLECTION: Medical history (120 vols)
CLASSIFICATION: DDC
PUBLICATIONS: Accessions list; Journals list
NETWORK: Northern Regional Association of Health Service Librarians

484
NEWCASTLE UPON TYNE POLYTECHNIC LIBRARY
Ellison Place, Newcastle upon Tyne NE1 8ST
Tel: 091 232 6002 x4131   Telex: 53519 NEWPOL G   Fax: 091 261 6911
Electronic mail: Telecom Gold 74:LEI 030
STAFF: I Winkworth BA DipLib MPhil ALA Library staff responsible
    for health collection: H Hedley BA ALA, JG Walton BSc FETC MA ALA
FOUNDED: 1969
TYPE: Multidisciplinary
HOURS: Mon-Fri 9-9 (Mon-Fri 9-5 during vacation), Sat 9-5.30
READERS: Staff and employees of Northern Regional Health
 Authority
STOCK POLICY: Books discarded after varying periods
LENDING: Books only. Photocopies provided
COMPUTER DATA RETRIEVAL: DATASTAR, BLAISE, DIALOG online - free.
             CD-ROM: MEDLINE, SOCIOFILE, PSYCLIT, CINAHL
             PRESTEL available
HOLDINGS: 449,000 books; c2,900 current journals; microfilms,
             tape/slides, videotapes (U-MATIC,VHS)
CLASSIFICATION: DDC
PUBLICATIONS: Health information service (current awareness)
NETWORK: Northern Regional Association of Health Service
 Librarians

485
NORTHERN REGIONAL HEALTH AUTHORITY
Benfield Road, Walkergate, Newcastle upon Tyne NE6 4PY
Tel: 091 224 6222   Fax: 091 276 5717
STAFF: JM Sellers BA ALA, Miss VJ Burgess BA
FOUNDED: 1979
TYPE: Health administration
HOURS: Mon-Fri 9-5
READERS: Staff, other users by appointment
STOCK POLICY: Journals discarded after 2 years, books discarded
                    after varying periods
LENDING: Books and journals. Photocopies provided
COMPUTER DATA RETRIEVAL: DATASTAR online - free
HOLDINGS: c 6,000 books; 120 current journals ; c250 35mm slides
CLASSIFICATION: UDC
NETWORK: Northern Regional Association of Health Service
 Librarians

UNIVERSITY OF NEWCASTLE UPON TYNE, MEDICAL AND DENTAL
LIBRARY
The Medical School, Framlington Place, Newcastle upon Tyne
NE2 4HH
Tel: 091 222 6000   Electronic mail: O'DONOVAN @ UK.AC.NEWCASTLE
STAFF: Mrs K O'Donovan BA ALA MIInfSci (Medical and Dental
  Librarian), Mrs H Farn MA ALA, Mrs L Appiah BA ALA,
   Mrs D Gleadhill BA MA ALA, 6 other (full-time), 4 part time staff
FOUNDED: Medical School founded 1834, moved to present location
                in 1984
TYPE: Dental, medical
HOURS: Mon-Fri 9-9, Sat 9-4.30 (vacations Mon-Fri 9-5, Sat 9-1)
READERS: University and NRHA staff
STOCK POLICY: Books discarded after varying periods
LENDING: Books and pre-current journals. Photocopies provided
COMPUTER DATA RETRIEVAL: DATASTAR, BLAISE online - charged full
            cost. CD-ROM from 1976
HOLDINGS: 12,000 books, 40,000 bound journals; 500 current
  journals; tape/slides, videotapes (U-matic, VHS)
SPECIAL COLLECTION: History of medicine: Pybus collection
  of 15th-20th century medical books, letters and engravings
CLASSIFICATION: DDC
NETWORK: Northern Regional Association of Health Service
  Librarians; Northern Region Library Service

Newport

487
GWENT POSTGRADUATE MEDICAL CENTRE, MEDICAL LIBRARY
The Friars, Friars Road, Newport, Gwent, NP9 4EZ
Tel: 0633 252244 x4661/2
STAFF: GDC Titley BA(Hons) ALA
TYPE: Medical, psychiatric
HOURS: Mon 9-5, Tues 9-7, Wed 9-6, Thurs 9-7,Fri 9-4.30
           Staffed Mon 9-5, Tue 11-7, Wed 11-6, Thu 11-7, Fri 9-4.30
READERS: Staff, other users by prior application
STOCK POLICY: Books discarded at varying intervala
LENDING: Books, journals and videos. Photocopies provided
COMPUTER DATA RETRIEVAL: DATASTAR online
HOLDINGS: c4,000 books; 150 journals, 130 current titles;
                35 videotapes (VHS)
CLASSIFICATION: DDC 19
NETWORK: AWHILES
BRANCHES: St Cadoc's Hospital, Newport, Gwent; Llanfrechfa
  Grange Hospital, Cwmbran, Gwent

Newtownabbey

488
UNIVERSITY OF ULSTER
Shore Road, Newtownabbey, Co Antrim, Northern Ireland, BT37 0QB
Tel: 0232 365131   Telex: 747493   Fax: 0232 852926
STAFF: BG Baggett BSc MIInfSc, Ms P Holloway (Sub-Librarian, Social
   and Health Sciences), Ms P Campton (Sub-Librarian, Social and
   Health Sciences at Coleraine), over 30 other professional staff
FOUNDED: 1970
TYPE: Multidisciplinary
HOURS: Mon-Thu 9am-10pm, Fri 9-4.30, Sat 10-1 (Term time). No
    evening or Saturday opening in vacations
READERS: Staff and other users
STOCK POLICY: Books and journals discarded after a variable period
LENDING: Books and AV material. Photocopies provided
COMPUTER DATA RETRIEVAL: DIALOG, ORBIT online -free. PRESTEL
HOLDINGS: 600,000 books; 5,000 current journals; microfilms, 100
    tape/slides, 40,000 35mm slides, videotapes (500 Betamax,
    1,000 VHS)
CLASSIFICATION: DDC & LC
PUBLICATIONS: Library guides
BRANCHES: Other University campuses at Coleraine, Londonderry and
    Belfast

North Shields

489
NORTH TYNESIDE POSTGRADUATE MEDICAL CENTRE
Preston Hospital, North Shields, Tyne and Wear NE29 0LR
Tel: 091 259 6660 x3609
STAFF: Mrs L Snowdon BA ALA (part-time)
FOUNDED: 1984
TYPE: Medical
HOURS: Always open. Staffed Tues, Wed, Thurs 9.30-2.30
READERS: Staff only
STOCK POLICY: Journals discarded after 5 years
LENDING: Books only. Photocopies provided
COMPUTER DATA RETRIEVAL: DATASTAR online - standard charge.
     CD-ROM from 1987
HOLDINGS: 2,000 books; 70 current journals
CLASSIFICATION: DDC
NETWORK: Northern Regional Association of Health Care Librarians

Northallerton

490
FRIARAGE HOSPITAL STUDY CENTRE, DISTRICT LIBRARY
Northallerton, North Yorkshire DL6 1JG
Tel: 0609 779911 x2526   Fax: 0609 775749
STAFF: Mrs C Porter BSc MA ALA MIInfSc (Study Centre Manager),
     Mrs MA Snowden BA DipLib (part time)

FOUNDED: 1968
TYPE: Multidisciplinary
HOURS: 8-11pm. Staffed Mon-Fri 8.30-5.30
READERS: Staff and other users
STOCK POLICY: Superseded editions discarded
LENDING: Books, journals and AV material. Photocopies provided
COMPUTER DATA RETRIEVAL: DATASTAR online - other libraries
charged full cost. PRESTEL available
HOLDINGS: 5,300 books; 165 journals, 155 current titles;
35 tape/slides, 200 35 mm slides, 150 videotapes (VHS)
CLASSIFICATION: DDC
PUBLICATION: Guide to the library; Journals list
NETWORK: Northern Regional Association of Health Service
Librarians; YRAHCLIS

Northampton

491
CRIPPS POSTGRADUATE MEDICAL CENTRE
General Hospital, Billing Road, Northampton NN1 5BD
Tel: 0604 235929
STAFF: Nrs AP Skinner BSc ALA (part time), Mrs M Waite (part time),
Mrs A Forty (part time), Mrs A adams (part time)
FOUNDED: 1968
TYPE: Multidisciplinary
HOURS: Always open. Staffed Mon-Fri 9-5.
READERS: Staff, other users when staffed
STOCK POLICY: Journals discarded after 20 years
LENDING: Books, journals overnight only. Photocopies provided
COMPUTER DATA RETRIEVAL: DATASTAR online - free. PRESTEL available
HOLDINGS: 5,200 books; 130 current journals
CLASSIFICATION: NLM
NETWORK: Oxford Region Library and Information Service

492
NORTHAMPTON HEALTH AUTHORITY, DISTRICT LIBRARY SERVICE
Highfield, Cliftonville Rd, Northampton NN1 5DN
Tel: 0604 235911/12   Fax: 0604 235900
STAFF: Miss J Holdsworth BA ALA
FOUNDED: 1978
TYPE: Health administration
HOURS: Mon-Thurs 9-5, Fri 9-4
READERS: Staff and other users
STOCK POLICY: Books and journals discarded after 10 years
LENDING: Books only. Photocopies provided
COMPUTER DATA RETRIEVAL: DATASTAR online - free
HOLDINGS: 6,231 books; 82 current journals
SPECIAL COLLECTION: Health care management and planning
CLASSIFICATION: DDC
PUBLICATIONS: Bi-monthly subject list; Daily press cuttings
bulletin; Bi-monthly current contents bulletin
NETWORK: Oxford Region Library and Information Service

493
SAINT ANDREW'S HOSPITAL
Billing Road, Northampton NN1 5DG
Tel: 0604 29696   Fax: 0604 232325
Tel: Mrs A Ruch (part time), Mrs G Jenkins (part time),
        Mrs M Latkins (part time)
TYPE: Multidisciplinary
HOURS: Mon-Fri 9-5
READERS: Staff only
STOCK POLICY: Books discarded after 5 years
LENDING: Books only. photocopies provided
COMPUTER DATA RETRIEVAL: DATASTAR online - free
HOLDINGS: c6,000 books; 110 current journals; c10 videotapes (VHS)
CLASSIFICATION: NLM
NETWORK: Oxford Region; PLCS

494
SAINT CRISPIN HOSPITAL, MENTAL HEALTH UNIT LIBRARY
Duston, Northampton NN5 6UN
Tel: 0604 52323
STAFF: Mrs D Stephen BA ALA
TYPE: Medical, psychiatric
HOURS: Mon-Thurs 9.30-1.30
READERS: Staff and other users
STOCK POLICY: Journals discarded after 20 years
LENDING: Books and journals. photocopies provided
COMPUTER DATA RETRIEVAL: DATASTAR online free
HOLDINGS: 3,200 books; 60 journals, 48 current titles;
                     microfilms, tape/slides, 40 Videotapes (VHS)
CLASSIFICATION: Barnard
PUBLICATIONS: Current awareness bulletin
NETWORK: Oxford Region Library and Information Service

Northwood

495
LES CANNON MEMORIAL LIBRARY, HAREFIELD AND NORTHWOOD
 POSTGRADUATE MEDICAL CENTRE
Mount Vernon Hospital, Northwood, Middlesex HA6 2RN
Tel: 09274 21031   Fax: 0923 835803
STAFF: RM Osborn BA AKC DipLib
FOUNDED: 1973
TYPE: Multidisciplinary
HOURS: Mon-Fri 9-5.
READERS: Staff, other users on application
STOCK POLICY: Books discarded at veying intervals
LENDING: Books and journals. Photocopies provided
COMPUTER DATA RETRIEVAL: DATASTAR online - charged. CD-ROM from 1983
HOLDINGS: 1,700 books; 4,000 bound journals, 200 current titles
SPECIAL COLLECTIONS: Cancer research; plastic and

maxillofacial surgery
CLASSIFICATION: Barnard
BRANCH: Harefield Hospital
NETWORK: NW Thames Regional Library and Information Service

Norwich

496
NORFOLK AND NORWICH HOSPITAL, SIR THOMAS BROWNE LIBRARY
Brunswick Road, Norwich, NR1 3SR
Tel: 0603 628377 x3572
STAFF: Mrs JL Malcolm BA DipLib ALA, Mrs A Collins BA(Hons) ALA
   (part time), Mrs BJ Cole BA(Hons) ALA (part time), Mrs S Skene
   BA(Hons) ALA (part time)
FOUNDED: 1973
TYPE: Multidisciplinary
HOURS: Mon-Thu 9-8, Fri 9-5.30, Sat 9-1
READERS: Staff and other users
STOCK POLICY: Books discarded after 10 years
LENDING: Books, journals, tape/slides. Photocopies provided
COMPUTER DATA RETRIEVAL: DATASTAR online - free
HOLDINGS: 6,000 books; 214 current journals
CLASSIFICATION: NLM
BRANCH: West Norfolk Hospital
NETWORK: Norfolk And Norwich Information Exchange Scheme

Nottingham

497
THE BOOTS COMPANY plc
Industrial Division, Pennyfoot Street, Nottingham NG2 3AA
Tel: 0602 492496   Telex: 377811   Fax: 0602 492614
STAFF: TM Smyth ALA, PD Owen ALA MIL, Miss JM Leverton ALA, Miss EW
Wragg ALA, 9 other full-time staff
FOUNDED: 1946
TYPE: Multidisciplinary
HOURS: Mon-Fri 9-4.
READERS: Staff, other users by prior application
STOCK POLICY: Books and journals discarded at varying intervals
LENDING: Books and journals (subject to Company demands).
                     Photocopies provided
COMPUTER DATA RETRIEVAL: In-house terminal.
HOLDINGS: 25,000+ books; 3,000+ journals, 2,000+ current titles
CLASSIFICATION: UDC
PUBLICATIONS: Recent additions list; daily contents lists:
   biology, chemistry, medicine, pharmacology, general
   science; weekly contents list: computers and office
   technology; cosmetics/toiletries and packaging; health and
   safety; healthcare and food science; serials holdings list
   (irregular); list of current serials (irregular)
BRANCHES: The Boots Company Limited Chemical Sciences
   Library; Consumer Products Development Library;
   Pharmaceutical Formulation; Toxicology/Pathology Library

498
CITY HOSPITAL POSTGRADUATE MEDICAL EDUCATION CENTRE MEDICAL
  LIBRARY
Hucknall Road, Nottingham NG5 1PB
Tel: 0602 691169
STAFF: Mrs JH Ryan BA DipLib ALA
FOUNDED: 1970, extended 1981
TYPE: Multidisciplinary
HOURS; Mon-Fri 8.30-5
READERS: Staff and other users
STOCK POLICY: Out of date books discarded
LENDING: Books and journals. Photocopies provided
COMPUTER DATA RETRIEVAL: DATASTAR online - charged 50% of cost
HOLDINGS: 2,000 books; 135 journals, 115 current titles;
                        35 videotapes (VHS)
CLASSIFICATION: Own

499
MAPPERLEY HOSPITAL, MEDICAL LIBRARY
Porchester Road, Mapperley, Nottingham NG3 6AA
Tel: 0602 691300
STAFF: BC Spencer BA ALA, Mrs G Lewis ALA (part time),
            Ms C Fisher (part-time)
FOUNDED:
TYPE: Nursing, psychiatric
HOURS: Access always available. Staffed 19 hours per week
READERS: Psychiatric and ancillary staff (not nurses)
LENDING: Books and journals
COMPUTER DATA RETRIEVAL: Access to terminal. Charged
 computer time only
HOLDINGS: 2,500 books, 400 bound journals; 34 current
 journals
SPECIAL COLLECTIONS: Psychiatric; nursing (165 vols)
CLASSIFICATION: Own (psychiatric), NLM (nursing)
PUBLICATION: Current awareness bulletin

500
UNIVERSITY OF NOTTINGHAM MEDICAL LIBRARY
Queen's Medical Centre, Nottingham NG7 2UH
Tel: 0602 709445   Telex 37346   Fax: 0602 709449
STAFF: AJ Coggins BA ALA, Miss JM Mawby BSc DipEd
   ALA, Miss J Noblett MA ALA, AF Barker BA, Mrs W Stanton BA DipLib
   ALA, Mrs EG Fletcher BA, 9 other full time and 7 part time staff
TYPE: Multidisciplinary
HOURS: Mon-Fri 9-9.45, Sat 9-4.45. Staffed Mon-Fri 9-7, Sat

9-12.30
READERS: Staff and other users
STOCK POLICY: Books and journals discarded at varying intervals
LENDING: Books only. photocopies supplied
COMPUTER DATA RETRIEVAL: DATASTAR, BLAISE, DIALOG online - charged:
                internal - 50% of non-staff costs, external - full
                costs. CD-ROM: Medline from 1982. PRESTEL available
HOLDINGS: 86,000 books; 1200 journals, 730 current titles plus 365
                reports & series titles; microfilms, tape/slides,
                35mm slides, videotapes (U-matic, VHS)
SPECIAL COLLECTIONS: Nursing & Midwifery (15,000 vols); Nottingham
                Medico-chirurgical Society Library (1,600 vols)
CLASSIFICATION: NLM
PUBLICATIONS: Periodicals list; guide to the medical
 library; accessions bulletin; reports & series list
NETWORKS: SLS (SWALCAP) Ltd; NISG; TRAHCLIS

Nuneaton

501
COVENTRY AND WARWICKSHIRE SCHOOL OF NURSING
Nunscroft Nurse Education Centre, 139 Earles Rd, Nuneaton, CV11 5HP
Tel: 0203 384201 x674
STAFF: Mrs M Wilson ALA (part time)
TYPE: Nursing
HOURS: Mon-Fri 9-5 (Staffed Mon, Wed 11-3)
READERS: Staff and students
LENDING: Reference only. Photocopies provided
COMPUTER DATA RETRIEVAL: Access to terminal
CLASSIFICATION: RCN modified
NETWORK: West Midlands Regional Health libraries

502
GEORGE ELIOT CENTRE LIBRARY
George Eliot Hospital, College Street, Nuneaton CV10 7DJ
Tel: 0203 384201 x325/310
STAFF: Mrs D Clay ALA
TYPE: Multidisciplinary
HOURS: Mon-Fri 9-5.30. Key available at other times
READERS: Staff, other users with Librarian's permission
STOCK POLICY: Books discarded at varying intervals
LENDING: Books only. Photocopies provided
COMPUTER DATA RETRIEVAL: DATASTAR online - free.
HOLDINGS: 1,550 books; 150 current journals; 44 tape/slides,
                36 videotapes (VHS)
CLASSIFICATION: DDC (modified)
PUBLICATIONS: Library guide; accessions lists; journal holdings
NETWORK: CADIG; West Midlands Regional Health Libraries

503
FRANK LORD POSTGRADUATE MEDICAL CENTRE
Royal Oldham Hospital, Rochdale Rd, Oldham, Lancs, OL1 2JH
Tel: 061 624 0420 x4061
STAFF:Mrs M Kenway (Administrator/Librarian)
FOUNDED: 1969
TYPE: Medical
HOURS: Mon-Fri 9-5 (evening and weekend access)
READERS: Staff, other users for reference
STOCK POLICY: Journals discarded after 20 years, books discarded at
              discretion of Librarian
LENDING: Books and journals. Photocopies provided
HOLDINGS: 1,390 books; 104 journals, 88 current titles; 35mm slides,
          tapes, 15 videotapes (VHS)
CLASSIFICATION: Own
PUBLICATIONS: Recent additions, missing lists

504
WEST PENNINE COLLEGE OF HEALTH STUDIES
Westhulme Hospital, Oldham,
061 624 0420 x4525
STAFF: Mrs B Brierley
FOUNDED: 1970
TYPE: Multidisciplinary
HOURS: Mon-Fri 8.30-4.30
READERS: Staff and other users
STOCK POLICY: Clinical books over 10 years old and journals
 (except Nursing Times and Nursing Mirror) over 5 years old
 discarded
LENDING: Books and journals
HOLDINGS: 3,681 books; 15 current journals
PUBLICATION: Current awareness file
NETWORK: North West Nursing Librarians Group

505
ORMSKIRK AND DISTRICT POSTGRADUATE MEDICAL EDUCATION CENTRE
Ormskirk and District General Hospital, Wigan Road,
 Ormskirk, Lancashire L39 2AZ
Tel: 0695 577111
STAFF: Dr G Flood (Honorary Librarian),Ms SE Annis BA ALA (part
                    time)
FOUNDED: 1982
TYPE: Medical

HOURS: Staffed Mon-Fri 9.30-4.30. 24 hour access
READERS: Staff only
STOCK POLICY: Out of date books discarded
LENDING: Books, AV material. Photocopies provided
COMPUTER DATA RETRIEVAL: Access to terminal.
HOLDINGS: 2,000 books; 66 journals, 60 current titles;
6 packs 35mm slides, 10+ videotapes (VHS)
CLASSIFICATION: DDC
SPECIAL COLLECTION: Local history (35 vols)
NETWORK: NORWHSLA

Orpington

506
ORPINGTON HOSPITAL MEDICAL LIBRARY
Sevenoaks Rd, Orpington, Kent, BR6 9JU
Tel: 0689 27050 x2411
STAFF: Mrs MA Goulding BSc (part time)
TYPE: Medical
HOURS: tue, Thu, Fri 9.30-3.30
READERS: Staff, other users by request
STOCK POLICY: Books discarded after 20 years
LENDING: Books only. Photocopies provided
COMPUTER DATA RETRIEVAL: DATASTAR online - free
HOLDINGS: 46 journals, 20 current titles
CLASSIFICATION: NLM
NETWORK: SETRLIS

507
WEST KENT POSTGRADUATE MEDICAL CENTRE
Farnborough Hospital, Farnborough Common, Orpington, Kent, BR6 8ND
Tel: 0689 62423
STAFF: B Madge ALA, Mrs MA Goulding BSc (part time)
FOUNDED: 1973
TYPE: Medical, paramedical
HOURS: Staffed Mon-Fri 9-5. Key available at other times
READERS: Staff and other users
STOCK POLICY: Books discarded after 10 years or when new edition
available
LENDING: Books, journals and AV material. Photocopies provided
COMPUTER DATA RETRIEVAL: DATASTAR online - free. CD-ROM from 1990.
PRESTEL available
HOLDINGS: 2,565 books; 175 journals, 154 current titles;
32 tape/slides, 46 sets 35mm slides, 120 videotapes
(VHS), 30 audiocassettes
CLASSIFICATION: NLM
BRANCHES: Bromley Hospital, Orpington Hospital
NETWORK: SE Thames Regional Library and Information Service

508
FRANCIS COSTELLO LIBRARY, INSTITUTE OF ORTHOPAEDICS
Robert Jones and Agnes Hunt Orthopaedic Hospital, Oswestry,
 Shropshire SY10 7AG
Tel: 0691 655311 x3388
STAFF: Miss MF Carter BA DipLib ALA
FOUNDED: 1971
TYPE: Multidisciplinary
HOURS: Always open. Staffed Mon-Thurs 8.45-5, Fri 8.45-4
READERS: Staff only
LENDING: Books, AV material . Photocopies provided
COMPUTER DATA RETRIEVAL: DATASTAR online - charged full cost
HOLDINGS: 2,300 books; 150 journals, 115 current titles;
                120 tape/slides, 30 sets 35mm slides, videotapes
                (30 U-matic, 105 VHS)
CLASSIFICATION: NLM
SPECIAL COLLECTION: Orthopaedics
PUBLICATIONS: Library guides; bi-monthly library bulletin;
BRANCHES: School of Nursing, Oswestry; School of Physiotherapy,
                Oswestry
NETWORK: West Midlands Regional Health Libraries; Shropshire
                Library & Information services for Health; Orthopaedic
                Librarians Group

Otley

509
WHARFEDALE GENERAL HOSPITAL POSTGRADUATE MEDICAL CENTRE
Wharfedale General Hospital, Newall Carr Road, Otley, West
 Yorkshire LS21 2LY
Tel: 0943 465522
STAFF: Mrs M Ashford ALA (part time)
FOUNDED: 1968
TYPE: Medical
HOURS: Mon-Fri 9-7 (Staffed until 1)
READERS: Staff and local GP's
STOCK POLICY: Certain less important free journals discarded after
                1 year. Editions before penultimate discarded
LENDING: Books, journals and AV material. Photocopies provided
COMPUTER DATA RETRIEVAL: Access to terminal and CD-ROM
HOLDINGS: 1,412 books; 147 journals, 56 current titles;
                        c2,000 35mm slides, 16 videotapes (VHS)
CLASSIFICATION: NLM
PUBLICATION: Recent accessions list; Library guide; Postgraduate
                Centre Meetings Bulletin

510
CAIRNS LIBRARY
John Radcliffe Hospital, Headington, Oxford OX3 9DU
Tel: 0865 817818   Fax: 0865 742070
Electronic mail: FORREST @ UK.AC.OXFORD.VAX
STAFF: Mrs M Forrest ALA, Mrs C Lefebvre BA MSc, Ms A Maddison BA
         DipInfSc, Miss A Lusher BA MSc, Mrs D Smith BSc(Econ)
         DipLib, 4 other full time staff
FOUNDED: 1979
TYPE: Multidisciplinary
HOURS: Always open. Staffed Mon, Fri 9-5, Tues, Wed, Thurs 9-6
READERS: Staff and other users (restricted use)
STOCK POLICY: Books discarded after c10 years or when new edition
              is available.
LENDING: Books, journals and AV material. Photocopies provided
COMPUTER DATA RETRIEVAL: DATASTAR, BLAISE, DIALOG, ESA-IRS online -
              all other users charged full cost.CD-ROM from 1989
HOLDINGS: 9,807 books; 644 journals, 474 current titles;
140 tape/slides, videotapes (16 U-matic, 1 VHS)
CLASSIFICATION: NLM
PUBLICATION: Library guide
BRANCH: Cairns library, Radcliffe Infirmary, Oxford
NETWORK: Oxford Region Library and Information Service; University
              of Oxford

511
CAIRNS LIBRARY
Radcliffe Infirmary, Woodstock Road, Oxford OX2 6HE
Tel: 0865 249891 x4478
STAFF: R Snowball BA PhD DipLibInfStud ALA, 1 other (part-time)
                      staff
TYPE: Multidisciplinary
HOURS: Always open. Staffed Mon- Fri 9-5
READERS: Staff and other users (restricted use)
STOCK POLICY: Books discarded after c10 years or when new edition
              available.
LENDING: Books and journals. photocopies provided
COMPUTER DATA RETRIEVAL: DATASTAR, BLAISE, DIALOG, ESA-IRS online -
              other libraries/users charged full cost
HOLDINGS: 2,500 books; 120 journals, 80 current titles
CLASSIFICATION: NLM
NETWORK: Oxford Region Library and Information Service; University
              of Oxford

512
DORSET HOUSE SCHOOL OF OCCUPATIONAL THERAPY, CASSON LIBRARY
58 London Road, Headington, Oxford OX3 7PE
Tel: 0865 62831
STAFF: Mrs S Croft DipCOT (part-time), Mrs P Blake (part-time)
TYPE: Multidisciplinary
HOURS: Staffed Mon-Fri9-3
READERS: Staff and other users
STOCK POLICY: Out of date books offered to students/staff.
 Out of date journals offered to local libraries (then
 disposed)
LENDING: Books (preferably during school holidays)
COMPUTER DATA RETRIEVAL: Access to terminal
HOLDINGS: 5,500 books. Tape/slides, videotapes (VHS)
SPECIAL COLLECTION: Occupational therapy/rehabilitation
CLASSIFICATION: DDC
NETWORK: Oxford Region Library and Information Service

513
KILNER LIBRARY OF PLASTIC SURGERY
Plastic Surgery Dept, Radcliffe Infirmary, Oxford, OX2 6HE
Tel: 0865 249891
STAFF: Mr AM Godfrey FRCSEd (Honorary Librarian)
HOLDINGS: 25 current journals

514
LITTLEMORE HOSPITAL MEDICAL LIBRARY
Littlemore Hospital, Littlemore, Oxford OX4 4XN
Tel: 0865 778911 x325
STAFF: Mrs AE Gray BA (part time)
TYPE: Psychiatric
HOURS: Key available to readers at all times. Staffed
 Tues, Thurs 9-12.30
READERS: Staff and other users
LENDING: Books only. photocopies provided
COMPUTER DATA RETRIEVAL: Access to DATASTAR.
HOLDINGS: 7,0books; 70 journals, 50 current titles
SPECIAL COLLECTION: Psychiatry
CLASSIFICATION: NLM
NETWORK: Oxford Region Library and Information Service; PLCS

515
NUFFIELD DEPARTMENT OF ORTHOPAEDIC SURGERY, GIRDLESTONE MEMORIAL
LIBRARY
Nuffield Orthopaedic Centre, Headington, Oxford OX3 7LD
Tel: 0865 64811 x285   Fax: 0865 742348
STAFF: Mrs LC Allen (part-time), Mrs E Hollis (part-time)
TYPE: Orthopaedic, nursing, rehabilitation
HOURS: Mon-Fri 9-4.45
READERS: Staff and other users
STOCK POLICY: Books and journals discarded at varying intervals

LENDING: Books and journals. photocopies supplied
COMPUTER DATA RETRIEVAL: DATASTAR online - free. CD-ROM from 1983
HOLDINGS: 2,000 books; 99 journals, 65 current titles
CLASSIFICATION: NLM
SPECIAL COLLECTION: History of orthopaedics (20 vols)
PUBLICATIONS: Handbook; journal list; accessions list
BRANCHES: Oxford Rehabilitation Research Unit, Oxford;
 Oxford Orthopaedic Engineering Centre, Oxford
NETWORK: Oxford Region Library and Information Unit

516
OXFORD REGION LIBRARY AND INFORMATION SERVICE
Cairns Library, John Radcliffe Hospital, Headington, Oxford OX3 9DE
Tel: 0865 817531
STAFF: Dr P Leggate MA DPhil FIInfSci, JR Van Loo BA ALA DMS MIInfSc
HOURS: Mon-Fri 9-5
PUBLICATIONS: Directory of libraries; Union list of periodicals

517
OXFORD REGIONAL HEALTH AUTHORITY
Old Road, Headington, Oxford OX3 7LF
Tel: 0865 64861   Fax: 0865 68330
STAFF: Mrs DE Leonard ALA (part time)
TYPE: Multidisciplinary
HOURS: Mon-Fri 9-5.20
READERS: Staff and other users
STOCK POLICY: Out of date and superseded editions of books
 discarded. Journals over 5 years old discarded
LENDING: Books only
COMPUTER DATA RETRIEVAL: In-house terminal. Free
HOLDINGS: 21,000 books and bound journals; 150 current
 journals. Commercial microfiche systems
CLASSIFICATION: Bliss (modified), UDC, SfB
PUBLICATIONS: Monthly bulletin; library guide; periodicals
 list
NETWORK: Oxford Region Library and Information Service

518
UNIVERSITY OF OXFORD, DEPARTMENT OF HUMAN ANATOMY
South Parks Road, Oxford OX1 3QX
Tel: 0865 272157   Fax: 0865 272420
Electronic mail: CDS @ VAX.OXFORD.AC.RL
STAFF: Miss J Ballinger (part time)
FOUNDED: c1860
TYPE: Multidisciplinary
HOURS: Always open. Staffed Mon-Fri 9-12.30, 2-5
READERS: Staff, other users on a limited scale
STOCK POLICY: Books and journals discarded at varying intervals
LENDING: Books and journals to own users only
COMPUTER DATA RETRIEVAL: VAX/MEDLINE online - all users charged
                full cost
HOLDINGS: 4,800 books and bound journals; 47 current journals

519
UNIVERSITY OF OXFORD, RADCLIFFE SCIENCE LIBRARY
Parks Road, Oxford OX1 3QP
Tel: 0865 72800   Fax: 0865 272821
STAFF: Dr DF Shaw CBE MA DPhil FInstP (Keeper of Scientific Books),
 PJR Warren BA ALA (Deputy Keeper of Scientific Books),
 55 other staff
FOUNDED: 1749
TYPE: Multidisciplinary
HOURS: Mon-Fri 9-10, Sat 9-1 (Mon-Fri 9-5 or 7, Sat 9-1 during
                                              vacation)
READERS: Staff and other users
LENDING: Books and journals only on inter-library loan
 through BLLD
COMPUTER DATA RETRIEVAL: DIALOG, etc, online - charged full cost
                         CD-ROM from 1987
HOLDINGS: 300,000 books; 30,000 journals, 11,000 current titles;
                         Microfiche.
SPECIAL COLLECTIONS: Portraits; various historical MS
 collections relating to Dr John Radcliffe (1653-1714) and
 other Radcliffe Librarians
CLASSIFICATION: Own
PUBLICATIONS: Oxford University Union List of Scientific
 Serials 1983 (microfiche) (revised annually -latest
 revision issued December 1989); A review of Oxford
 University science libraries, 1977; Oxford University
 science libraries - a guide, 1981; various pamphlets on the
 history of medicine in Oxford
NETWORK: Dependant library of Bodleian Library

520
WARNEFORD HOSPITAL LIBRARY
Old Road, Headington, Oxford OX3 7JX
Tel: 0865 245651 x4412
Tel: Mrs AE Gray BA ALA, 1 other staff
TYPE: Psychiatric
HOURS: Mon-Fri 9-5. Key available to readers at all other
 times
READERS: Staff and other users
LENDING: Books only. Photocopies provided
COMPUTER DATA RETRIEVAL: DATASTAR online - outside users charged
                full cost
HOLDINGS: 1,500 books; 25 journals, 15 current titles
CLASSIFICATION: NLM
NETWORK: Oxford Region Library and Information Service;
 PLCS

Paisley

521
ROYAL ALEXANDRA HOSPITAL
Corsebar, Paisley PA2 9PN
Tel: 041 887 9111 x4127

STAFF: Miss J Polson ALA, Mrs J Kerr, Miss E Paton BA (part time)
FOUNDED: 1986
TYPE: Multidisciplinary
HOURS: Always open. Staffed Mon-Fri 8.30-4.30
READERS: Staff, other users on application
STOCK POLICY: Out of date books discarded
LENDING: Books only. Photocopies supplied
COMPUTER DATA RETRIEVAL: In-house terminal. CD-ROM from 1976
HOLDINGS: 12,000 books; 200 current journals;
CLASSIFICATION: DDC
NETWORK: Scottish region

Papworth Everard

522
PAPWORTH HOSPITAL
Papworth Everard, Cambs, CB3 8RE
Tel: 0480 830541
STAFF: Mrs L Edmonds BA ALA (part time)
TYPE: Medical
HOURS: Mon-Fri 9-2
READERS: Staff and other users
STOCK POLICY: Books discarded
LENDING: Books and journals to staff only. Photocopies provided
COMPUTER DATA RETRIEVAL: Access to DATASTAR online
HOLDINGS: 64 journals, 58 current titles
CLASSIFICATION: NLM
PUBLICATIONS: Library guide; List of current journals
NETWORK: East Anglian Health Care Libraries

Penarth

523
LLANDOUGH HOSPITAL MEDICAL LIBRARY
Penarth, South Glamorgan CF6 1XX
Tel:0222 708601 x5497
STAFF: Ms R Soper BA DipLib ALA , Ms BM Vose BSc, Ms JA Bishop BA
TYPE: Multidisciplinary
HOURS: Mon-Fri 9.30-5
READERS: Staff, other users at Librarian's discretion
STOCK POLICY: Non-unique titles discarded
LENDING: Books and journals. photocopies supplied
COMPUTER DATA RETRIEVAL: DATASTAR online - free
HOLDINGS: 1,500 books; 65 journals, 60 current titles
CLASSIFICATION: DDC
BRANCH: This library is a branch of the University of Wales College
                        of Medicine main library
NETWORK: AWHILES

Perth

524
PERTH COLLEGE OF NURSING AND MIDWIFERY
125 Glasgow Road, Perth PH2 0LU
Tel: 0738 25284
STAFF: Mrs CB McGregor ALA
TYPE: Nursing, midwifery
HOURS: Mon-Thu 8-8, Fri 8-7.30. Staffed Mon-Fri 8.30-5
READERS: Staff, other users for reference only
STOCK POLICY: Out of date material discarded
LENDING: Books, videotapes only.Photocopies supplied
HOLDINGS: 5,500 books; 45 current journals; 38 tape/slides,
                        46 sets 35mm slides, 150 videotapes (VHS)
CLASSIFICATION: DDC
PUBLICATIONS: Library guide; Recent accessions lists
BRANCH: Midwifery library

525
PERTH ROYAL INFIRMARY
Perth PH1 1NX
Tel: 0738 23311
No further information available

Peterborough

526
PETERBOROUGH DEPARTMENT OF NURSE EDUCATION
Peterborough District Hospital, Thorpe Road, Peterborough, PE3 6DA
Tel: 0733 67451
STAFF: Mrs P Billyard
FOUNDED: 1980
TYPE: Nursing
HOURS: Mon, Wed, Fri 8.30-5, tue, thu 8.30-7
READERS: Nurse tutors and nurses in training
STOCK POLICY: Books discarded after 10 years
LENDING: Books and journals
HOLDINGS: 5,019 books; 34 current journals
CLASSIFICATION: RCN
NETWORK: East Anglian Region

527
PETERBOROUGH POSTGRADUATE MEDICAL CENTRE, LAXTON LIBRARY,
Peterborough District Hospital, Thorpe Road, Peterborough, PE3 6DA
Tel: 0733 67451
STAFF: Mrs MA Rushford ALA (District Medical Librarian)
FOUNDED: 1973
TYPE: Medical, dental, nursing
HOURS: Staffed Mon-Fri 9-5. Keys available at other times
READERS: Medical and dental staff, other users by appointment
STOCK POLICY: Books and journals discarded at varying intervals
LENDING: Books only. Photocopies provided
COMPUTER DATA RETRIEVAL: DATASTAR online - free

HOLDINGS: 2,300 books; 110 current journals
CLASSIFICATION: Barnard (modified)
PUBLICATIONS: Current awareness bulletins; Recent additions lists;
              General/specific information; Guide to the library
NETWORK: E Anglian NHS Region
BRANCH: Stamford Hospital, Stamford

528
ROYAL NATIONAL INSTITUTE FOR THE BLIND, LITERATURE TEAM
P O Box 173, Peterborough PE2 0WS
Tel: 0733 370777   Fax: 0733 371555
STAFF: Mrs L Riley ALA, JM Crampton BSc(Econ) DipLib ALA, Mrs K Dane
BA(Hons), M Jacques BA(Hons) DipLib, Miss A Lingwood BA(Hons),
Miss KS Medd BLib
TYPE: Material for the blind in braille and on tape
HOURS: Mon-Fri 9-5
READERS: Staff and other users
STOCK POLICY: Books discarded
LENDING: Braille, 2 & 4 track tapes to registered blind or
         visually handicapped
HOLDINGS: No letterprint books, 60,000 braille volumes; 17,500 tapes
CLASSIFICATION: DDC 20
PUBLICATION: Bookcase (in New Beacon)

Plymouth

529
PLYMOUTH HEALTH AUTHORITY DISTRICT LIBRARY SERVICE
Medical Library and Information Centre, Level 02,
Derriford Hospital, Derriford Rd, Plymouth PL6 8DH
Tel: 0752 792265
STAFF: Miss VM Trinder BEd CertEd ALA, Mrs A Jones BLib ALA
TYPE: Multidisciplinary
HOURS: Mon-Fri 9-5.
READERS: Staff, other users at Librarian's discretion
STOCK POLICY: Books discarded at varying intervals
LENDING: Books and AV material. Photocopies provided
COMPUTER DATA RETRIEVAL: DATASTAR online
HOLDINGS: c6,500 books; 350 journals, 300 current titles;
                3 tape/slides, 25 videotapes (VHS)
CLASSIFICATION: NLM
BRANCHES: Freedom Fields Hospital Staff Library; Mount Gould
   Hospital Staff Library; Moorhaven Hospital Medical Library;
   Several other small collections
NETWORK: SWEHSLinC; Plymouth Librarians Group; NHS Management
  Librarians Group; PLCS

530
PLYMOUTH HEALTH AUTHORITY DISTRICT LIBRARY SERVICE
South West College of Health Studies - Plymouth School of Nursing
North Friary House, Greenbank Terrace, Plymouth, PL4 8QQ
STAFF: Mrs D Lawer BA DipLib ALA
TYPE: Multidisciplinary
HOURS: Mon-Fri 8.30-4.30
READERS: Nursing and medical staff. Others users at Librarian's
                         discretion
STOCK POLICY: Books and journals selectively discarded
LENDING: Books and study packs. Photocopies provided
COMPUTER DATA RETRIEVAL: DATASTAR online - charged full cost
HOLDINGS: 10 ,000+ books ; 6 journals, 52 current titles;
CLASSIFICATION: NLM
SPECIAL COLLECTION: Plymouth School of Nursing Archives (65 vols)
BRANCH: Moorhaven Psychiatric Nurses Training Library,
  Ivybridge; School of Midwifery, Plymouth; Various small branch
    collections

Pontefract

531
POSTGRADUATE MEDICAL CENTRE LIBRARY
Pontefract General Infirmary, Southgate, Pontefract, West
  Yorkshire WF8 1PL
Tel: 0977 600600
STAFF: Miss J Smethurst BA ALA
FOUNDED: 1970
TYPE: Medical, paramedical
HOURS: Mon-Fri 9-5
READERS: Staff and other users
STOCK POLICY: Journals discarded after 15 years, previous editions
                         of books discarded
LENDING: Books, journals and AV material. Photocopies provided
HOLDINGS: 4,600 books; 140 journals, 120 current titles;
                         50 sets 35mm slides, 15 videotapes (VHS)
CLASSIFICATION: NLM
PUBLICATIONS: Library bulletin
NETWORK: Yorkshire Joint Medical Library Service
BRANCH: Castleford and Normanton District Hospital,
  Castleford

Pontypridd

532
EAST GLAMORGAN HOSPITAL, MEDICAL STAFFS LIBRARY
Church Village, near Pontypridd, Mid-Glamorgan CF38 1AB
Tel: 0443 204242 x6585
STAFF: Mrs PJ Evans ALA
TYPE: Medical
HOURS: Mon, Wed, Fri 8.30-5, Tues, Thurs 1-8

READERS: Medical staff
STOCK POLICY: Out of date books discarded
LENDING: Books, journals and AV material. Photocopies provided
COMPUTER DATA RETRIEVAL: DATASTAR online - free
HOLDINGS: 3,500 books; 160 journals, 142 current titles;
                 40 35mm slides, 35 videotapes (VHS)
CLASSIFICATION: DDC
PUBLICATIONS: New books lists; Introduction to library
NETWORK: AWHILES

Poole

533
EAST DORSET DISTRICT LIBRARY SERVICE
Poole General Hospital, Longfleet Road, Poole, Dorset BH15 2JB
Tel: 0202 675100 x2101
STAFF: JB Gill BScEcon ALA (District Librarian), 1 vacant post
TYPE: Multidisciplinary
HOURS: Mon-Fri 8.30-5.30
READERS: Staff, other users by prior application only
STOCK POLICY: Out of date books and journals discarded
LENDING: Books and journals. Photocopies provided
COMPUTER DATA RETRIEVAL: DATASTAR, BLAISE online - charged flat
                     rate contribution to cost. PRESTEL available
HOLDINGS: 10,000 books; 150 current journals; 60 tape/slides,
                 70 videotapes (VHS)
CLASSIFICATION: NLM (Wessex modification)
BRANCHES: Saint Ann's Hospital, Poole; Saint Leonard's
Hospital, Ringwood
NETWORKS: WRLIS; HATRICS

Portsmouth

PORTSMOUTH AND SE HANTS HEALTH AUTHORITY, DISTRICT LIBRARY SERVICES
District Librarian: D Bartholomew BA(Hons) ALA DMS MIInfSc
(based at St Mary's General Hospital: 0705 822331 x4855)

534
PORTSMOUTH SCHOOL OF NURSING
Queen Alexandra Hospital, Cosham, Portsmouth, Hants, PO6 3LY
Tel: 0705 379451 x2304
STAFF: Mrs E Dominguez BA(Hons)
FOUNDED: 1970
TYPE: Nursing
HOURS: Mon-Thu 8.30-5, Fri 8.30-4.30
READERS: Staff and other users
STOCK POLICY: Books and journals discarded
LENDING: Books only. Photocopies provided
COMPUTER DATA RETRIEVAL: Access to DATASTAR
HOLDINGS: c3,500 books; 46 journals, 42 current titles; 193 tape/
       slides
CLASSIFICATION: NLM (amended)
NETWORK: WRLIS

535
QUEEN ALEXANDRA HOSPITAL, STAFF LIBRARY
Postgraduate Centre, Cosham, Portsmouth, Hants PO6 3LY
Tel: 0705 379451 x2043
STAFF: Ms J Reeves BA(Hons), Mrs J Gavriel
FOUNDED: 1979
TYPE: Multidisciplinary
HOURS: Mon-Thurs 8.30-5 Fri 8.30-4
READERS: Staff only
STOCK POLICY: Books discarded after 15 years
LENDING: Books and journals. Photocopies provided
COMPUTER DATA RETRIEVAL: DATASTAR online - free
HOLDINGS: 4,000 books; 80 current journals
CLASSIFICATION: NLM (amended)
NETWORK: HATRICS; WRLIS

536
SAINT JAMES' HOSPITAL STAFF LIBRARY
Locksway Road, Portsmouth, Hants, PO4 8LD
Tel: 0705 822331 x4361
STAFF: Ms J Derbyshire BA(Hons) PGCE DipLib ALA (part time)
FOUNDED: Librarian appointed 1984 - previously staffed from General
         Hospital
TYPE: Multidisciplinary
HOURS: Access available at all times (Staffed mon-Fri 9-1)
READERS: Staff and other users
STOCK POLICY: Books and journals discarded as necessary
LENDING: Books, journals, videocassettes. Photocopies provided
COMPUTER DATA RETRIEVAL: Access to DATASTAR
HOLDINGS: c3,000 books; 30 journals, 22 current titles; 6 videotapes
         (VHS)
CLASSIFICATION: NLM (amended)
NETWORKS: WRLIS; PLCS

537
SAINT MARY'S GENERAL HOSPITAL STAFF LIBRARY
Education Centre, Milton Road, Portsmouth, Hants, PO3 6AD
Tel: 0705 822331 x4856
STAFF: Mrs B Pitman BA(Hons) DipLib ALA, Mrs P Morris
FOUNDED: 1963
TYPE: Multidisciplinary
HOURS: 24 hour access (Staffed Mon-Thu 8.30-5, Fri 8.30-4)
READERS: Staff, bona fide users for reference only
STOCK POLICY: Books discarded when appropriate
LENDING: Books and journals. Photocopies provided
COMPUTER DATA RETRIEVAL: DATASTAR online. Free
HOLDINGS: c4,000 books; c140 journals, c130 current titles
CLASSIFICATION: NLM (amended)
NETWORKS: WRLIS; HATRICS

Potters Bar

538
NATIONAL INSTITUTE FOR BIOLOGICAL STANDARDS AND CONTROL
Blanche Lane, South Mimms, Potters Bar, Herts, EN6 3QG
Tel: 0707 54753   Telex: 21911 NIBSAC G   Fax: 0707 46730
STAFF: Mrs L Anthony BSc MSc ALA, Ms D Macnamara BA
FOUNDED: 1976
TYPE: Medical
HOURS: 7-7 every day. Staffed Mon-Fri 9-5
READERS: Staff, other users by arrangement
LENDING: Books and journals. Photocopies provided
COMPUTER DATA RETRIEVAL: BLAISE, DATASTAR, DIALOG, ISTEL. CD-ROM
HOLDINGS: 3,000 books; 300 journals, 200 current titles;
                    10 videotapes (VHS)
CLASSIFICATION: NLM
PUBLICATIONS: Periodical holdings list; Newsletter
NETWORK: Medical Research Council

Prescot

539
RAINHILL HOSPITAL LIBRARY
Prescot, Merseyside L35 4PQ
Tel: 051 426 6511 x24
STAFF: J Bentley BA DipLib ALA DipEdTech, Ms C Benny BA
TYPE: Multidisciplinary
HOURS: Mon-Tue 9-7, Wed-Fri 9-5
READERS: Staff and other users
STOCK POLICY: Some out of date books discarded.
LENDING: Books and journals. Photocopies provided
COMPUTER DATA RETRIEVAL: DATASTAR online - charged full cost.
                          PRESTEL available.
HOLDINGS: 10,000 books; 100 journals, 65 current titles
CLASSIFICATION: DDC
NETWORKS: Mersey Region; PLCS; NW Libraries Group

540
SAINT HELENS AND KNOWSLEY POSTGRADUATE CENTRE
Whiston Hospital, Prescot, Merseyside L35 5DR
Tel: 051 426 0319
STAFF: Mrs T Jackson (part-time)
FOUNDED: 1974
TYPE: Multidisciplinary
HOURS: Mon-Fri 8.30-5
READERS: Staff only
STOCK POLICY: Books and journals discarded after 15 years
LENDING: Books only. Photocopies provided
COMPUTER DATA RETRIEVAL: Access to terminal. CD-ROM from 1990
HOLDINGS: 1,200 books; 50 current journals; 24 tape/slides,
                    videotapes (VHS)
CLASSIFICATION: Own
NETWORK: Merseyside NHS Region

541
LANCASHIRE POLYTECHNIC LIBRARY
Corporation Street, Preston PR1 2TQ
Tel: 0772 201201   Telex 677409 LANPOL   Fax: 0772 202073
STAFF: P Brophy JP BSc FLA MIInfSc, 18 other professional and 36
                  non-professional staff
TYPE: Multidisciplinary
HOURS: Mon-Thurs 8.45-9, Fri 8.45-8, Sat 9-1, Sun 10-2
              (Mon-Thurs 9-5.30, Fri 9-5 during vacation)
READERS: Staff and other users
LENDING: Books and videotapes only
COMPUTER DATA RETRIEVAL: Online terminal. CD-ROM from 1988.
                          PRESTEL available
HOLDINGS: 243,699 books; 1,715 current journals; 2,483 microfilms,
          48,157 35mm slides, tape/slides, 2195 videotapes
CLASSIFICATION: DDC
PUBLICATIONS: Various guides to services and bibliographical
                  subject guides

542
PRESTON SCHOOL OF NURSING
Watling Street Road, Fulwood, Preston, PR2 4DX
Tel: 0772 711446
STAFF: Ms D Phelps BA MA ALA
FOUNDED: c1984 as a professional service
TYPE: Nursing
HOURS: Mon-Fri 8.30-4.30 - not always staffed
READERS: Staff and other users
STOCK POLICY: Books over 10 years old discarded
LENDING: Books only. Photocopies provided
HOLDINGS: 6,000 books; 35 journals, 33 current titles
CLASSIFICATION: NLM
PUBLICATION: Library guide; Current contents page; New books list
BRANCH: Whittingham Psychiatric Hospital School of Nursing,
                  Preston
NETWORKS: NORWHSLA; North West Nursing Librarians Group

543
ROYAL PRESTON HOSPITAL DISTRICT LIBRARY
Sharoe Green Lane North, Fulwood, Preston PR2 4HT
Tel: 0772 710763
STAFF: Ms A Strange BA ALA (District Librarian)
FOUNDED: 1986
TYPE: Multidisciplinary
HOURS: Staffed Mon 9-5, Tue 1-7, Wed 4-6, Thu 2.30-5, Fri 11-5.
              Key available at other times
READERS: Staff, other users by arrangement
STOCK POLICY: Books and journals discarded at varying intervals

LENDING: Books and non-current journals. Photocopies provided
COMPUTER DATA RETRIEVAL: Access to terminal. Free. PRESTEL
                         available at other library
HOLDINGS: 1,100 books; 45 journals, 28 current titles
CLASSIFICATION: NLM
PUBLICATIONS: Library guides; Newsletter
NETWORK: NORWHSLA
BRANCH: Royal Preston Hospital, Sharoe Green Lane North,
 Fulwood, Preston

544
POSTGRADUATE MEDICAL CENTRE LIBRARY
Sharoe Green Hospital, Watling Street Rd, Fulwood, Preston PR2 4DY
Tel: 0772 711763
STAFF: Ms A Strange BA ALA, Mrs D Bradley BA (part time)
TYPE: Medical
HOURS: Mon-Fri 9-11, Sat 9-1. Staffed: Mon 9-2.30, Wed 9-4,
    Thu 9-12.30, Fri 9-11. Access at other times for Centre Members
READERS: Staff and other users
STOCK POLICY: Books and journals discarded at varying periods
LENDING: Books, videos, non-current journals. Photocopies provided
COMPUTER DATA RETRIEVAL: Access to terminal. PRESTEL available
HOLDINGS: 500 books; 40 journals, 37 current titles;
                       18 videotapes (VHS)
CLASSIFICATION: NLM
PUBLICATIONS: Guide to the District Library Service; Newsletters
NETWORK: NORWHSLA

545
WHITTINGHAM HOSPITAL MEDICAL LIBRARY
Whittingham, Preston PR3 2JH
Tel: 0772 865531
STAFF: Mrs N Blackburn ALA (part time)
TYPE: Medical, Psychiatric
HOURS: Staffed Mon-Fri 9.30 until lunch
READERS: Staff, other users occasionally for reference
STOCK POLICY: Books and journals discarded at varying periods
LENDING: Books, videos only.Photocopies provided
COMPUTER DATA RETRIEVAL: Access to terminal. .
HOLDINGS:1,300 books; 40 current journals; videotapes (U-matic, VHS)
CLASSIFICATION: NLM
PUBLICATIONS: Quarterly recent additions list; Library guide
NETWORKS: NORWHSLA; PLCS

Radlett

546
HARPERBURY HOSPITAL MEDICAL LIBRARY
Harper Lane, Shenley, Radlett, Herts, WD7 4HQ
Tel: 0923 854861
STAFF: Mrs JE Jolley BA(Hons) ALA (part time)
FOUNDED: 1963
TYPE: Multidisciplinary
HOURS: Mon, Tue, thu 9-5, Wed, Fri 9-1. Key available at other times
READERS: Staff and other users
STOCK POLICY: Books and journals discarded at varying periods
LENDING: Books, AV material. Photocopies provided
COMPUTER DATA RETRIEVAL: Access to terminal. CD-ROM from 1983
HOLDINGS: 42 journals; 28 tape/slides, 20 videotapes (VIS)
CLASSIFICATION: NLM
SPECIAL COLLECTION: Mental handicap (c500 vols)
PUBLICATIONS: Library guide; Bulletin
NETWORKS: NWThames; PLCS

547
SHENLEY HOSPITAL NURSE EDUCATION CENTRE
Shenley, Radlett, Herts WD7 9HB
Tel: 0923 855631
No furthur information available

Reading

548
AFRC INSTITUTE OF FOOD RESEARCH
Church Lane, Shinfield, Reading RG2 9AT
Tel: 0734 883103   Telex 9312102022 LBG   Fax: 0734 884763
STAFF: Ms A Cox
 staff
TYPE: Science and technology
HOURS: Mon-Thurs 8.30-5.30, Fri 8.30-5
READERS: Staff and other users
STOCK POLICY: Journals discarded after 40 years
LENDING: Books and journals. Photocopies provided
COMPUTER DATA RETRIEVAL: DIMDI, DIALOG online - other libraries
                charged full cost
HOLDINGS: c5,500 books; 600 journals, 300 current titles
CLASSIFICATION: UDC

549
BRYN THOMAS MEMORIAL LIBRARY
Postgraduate Medical Education Centre, Royal Berkshire
 Hospital, Reading, Berks RG1 5AN
Tel: 0734 8778 48 or 0734 877849

STAFF: Dr AM Barr FFARCS (Honorary Librarian), Ms E Forsyth BSc
    DipLib ALA MIInfSc (District Librarian), Mrs P Smalley
    (Psychiatric Librarian), Mrs M Coleman (Asst Librarian)
TYPE: Multidisciplinary
HOURS: Access available at all times. Staffed Mon-Fri 9-5
READERS: Staff and other users
STOCK POLICY: All pre-1960 material relegated to RPS
 Library
LENDING: Books only. Photocopies provided
COMPUTER DATA RETRIEVAL: DATASTAR, BLAISE, DIALOG online.
        CD-ROM from 1983
HOLDINGS: 2,500 books; c250 current journals. 35mm slides
SPECIAL COLLECTIONS: Hamilton Fairley (Tropical medicine)
 (200 vols); Keith Lyle (Ophthalmology) (100 vols); Bryn
 Thomas (History of medicine and anaesthesia) (400 vols);
 autographs and lectures of medical men; historical
 material; hospital archives
CLASSIFICATION: NLM and own
PUBLICATIONS: Acquisitions list; library guide ; Current awareness
NETWORK: Oxford Region Library and Information Service
BRANCHES: Reading Pathological Society Library (opened
 1882; 10,000 vols, all pre-1960); Mary Ambrose Library
 (Ophthalmology), Royal Berks Hospital, Reading; Battle
 Hospital, Reading; Fairmile Hospital, Cholsey nr
 Wallingford; Borocourt Hospital, Wyfold nr Reading

550
WEST BERKSHIRE SCHOOL OF NURSING
Nurse Education Centre, Royal Berkshire Hospital, London Road,
 Reading, Berks, RG1 5AN
Tel: 0734 877657
STAFF: Miss S Lerch BA
TYPE: Nursing
HOURS: Mon-Thu 8.30-5, Fri 8.30-4.30
READERS: Staff and other users
STOCK POLICY: Jounals discarded from 1-10 years (depending on
        journal). Books discarded after 10 years in consultation
        with teaching staff
LENDING: Books and videos only to HA staff. photocopies provided
COMPUTER DATA RETRIEVAL: Access to DATASTAR, BLAISE, DIALOG -
        charged. Access to CD-ROM from 1983
HOLDINGS: 7,000 books; 85 journals, 67 current titles;
 58 tape/slides, 83 videotapes (VHS)
CLASSIFICATION: NLM
SPECIAL COLLECTIONS: Geriatrics, Research methods; Mental handicap
PUBLICATIONS: Book lists; annual report
NETWORK: Oxford Region Library and Information Service

Redditch

551
MID-WORCESTERSHIRE SCHOOL OF NURSING LIBRARY
Alexandra Hospital, Woodrow Drive, Redditch, Worcs, B98 7UB
Tel: 0527 503030 x4618
STAFF: Mrs M Morris
TYPE: Nursing, psychiatry
HOURS: Mon-Fri 8.30-4.30
READERS: Nurses in district and in training
COMPUTER DATA RETRIEVAL: Access to terminal
HOLDINGS: 5,000 books; 10 current journal; AV material
CLASSIFICATION: RCN
NETWORK: West Midlands

552
WYNNE DAVIES POSTGRADUATE MEDICAL CENTRE
Alexandra Hospital, Woodrow Drive, Redditch, Worcs, B98 7UB
Tel: 0527 503030
STAFF: Mrs A Preston (part time), Mrs P Smith (part time)
FOUNDED: 1972
TYPE: Medical
HOURS: 24 hour access (Staffed Mon-Fri 9-5)
READERS: Staff and other users
STOCK POLICY: Journals discarded after 10 years
LENDING: Reference only. Photocopies provided
COMPUTER DATA RETRIEVAL: Access to terminal. Charged full cost
HOLDINGS: 600 books; 50 current journals
CLASSIFICATION: DDC
NETWORK: West Midlands

Redhill

553
ESHA DISTRICT HEALTH SERVICES LIBRARY AND INFORMATION SERVICE
East Surrey Hospital, Three Arch Rd, Redhill, Surrey RH1 5RH
Tel: 0737 765030 x2188
STAFF: Mrs BP Saich BA ALA, Mrs F Knight ALA, Mrs E Luker
FOUNDED: 1979
TYPE: Multidisciplinary
HOURS: Staffed Mon-Fri 9-4. Key access at other times
READERS: Hospital staff and other users
STOCK POLICY: Out of date books discarded
LENDING: Books only. Photocopies provided
COMPUTER DATA RETRIEVAL: DATASTAR online - free
HOLDINGS: 3,000 books; 140 journals, 120 current titles;
                         Tape/slides
CLASSIFICATION: NLM
PUBLICATIONS: Readers Guide; New books list
BRANCHES: Redhill Hospital; Dorking Hospital
NETWORK: SW Thames Regional Library and Information Service

Reigate
554
SMITHKLINE BEECHAM PHARMACEUTICALS
Headquarters Medical Department, 47-49 London Road, Reigate, Surrey,
RH2 9PQ
Tel: 0737 364870   Telex: 927338   Fax: 0737 364990
STAFF: K De-Voy BSc MSc (Senior Medical Information Officer)
TYPE: Medical, pharmaceutical
HOURS: Mon-Fri 9-5.15
READERS: Staff only
LENDING: Staff only. Photocopies provided
COMPUTER DATA RETRIEVAL: DATASTAR, DIALOG online.
HOLDINGS: 100 books; 45 current journals; 34,000 microfiche
CLASSIFICATION: UDC

Rhyl
555
YSBYTY GLAN CLWYD
Bodelwyddan, Rhyl, Clwyd LL18 5UJ
Tel: 0745 583910   Fax: 0745 583143
STAFF: KJ Bladon BA FLA, Mrs EM Smith (Librarian-Nurse Education),
          Mrs H Vickers
FOUNDED: 1980
TYPE: Multidisciplinary
HOURS: Mon-Fri 9-5
READERS: Staff only
STOCK POLICY: Ephemeral material discarded
LENDING: Reference only. Photocopies provided
COMPUTER DATA RETRIEVAL: DATASTAR, BLAISE online - other libraries
             charged full cost
HOLDINGS: 4,000 books; 140 current journals;
                     Tape/slides, videotapes (VHS)
CLASSIFICATION: NLM
PUBLICATION: Library guide
BRANCHES: Abergele Hospital; HM Stanley Hospital, Saint Asaph
NETWORK: AWHILES

Rochdale
556
THE BATEMAN CENTRE FOR POSTGRADUATE MEDICAL STUDIES
Birch Hill Hospital, Rochdale OL12 9QB
Tel: 0706 70403
STAFF: Mrs SM Chetwynd (part-time), Miss B Hardy (part time)
FOUNDED: 1968
TYPE: Medical
HOURS: Mon-Fri 8-11. Staffed Mon-Fri 9-5
READERS: Medical and dental staff
STOCK POLICY: Books discarded after 10 years
LENDING: Books, AV material. Photocopies provided
COMPUTER DATA RETRIEVAL: Access to terminal.
HOLDINGS: 1,500 books; 190 current journals;
                     40 tape/slides, 53 videotapes (VHS)
CLASSIFICATION: DDC (modified)
NETWORK: NORWHSLA

Romford

557
ROMFORD MEDICAL ACADEMIC CENTRE
Oldchurch Hospital, Romford, Essex RM7 0BE
Tel: 0708 46090 x3101
STAFF: Mrs TM Williams (part-time)
FOUNDED: 1967
TYPE: Medical, dental
HOURS: Always open. Staffed Mon-Fri 10.30-3
READERS: Staff and other users (except nursing staff)
LENDING: Books only. Photocopies provided
HOLDINGS: 2,000 books; 120 current journals
CLASSIFICATION: NLM
NETWORK: NE Thames Regional Library and Information Service

Roslin

558
AFRC INSTITUTE OF ANIMAL PHYSIOLOGY AND GENETICS RESEARCH
Edinburgh Research Station, Roslin, Midlothian EH25 9PS
Tel: 031 440 2726   Fax: 031 440 0434
STAFF: M McKeen DMS ALA
FOUNDED: 1947 (as Poultry Research Centre)
TYPE: Animal genetics/breeding
HOURS: Mon-Fri 9-5
READERS: Staff, other users subject to approval
LENDING: Books and journals. Photocopies provided
COMPUTER DATA RETRIEVAL: DIALOG online
HOLDINGS: c10,000 books; 350 journals, 250 current titles
CLASSIFICATION: Own
NETWORK: Agriculture & Food research Service; Scottish Agricultural
                    Libraries Group

Rotherham

559
ROTHERHAM HEALTH AUTHORITY STAFF LIBRARY AND INFORMATION
  SERVICE
Rotherham District General Hospital, Moorgate Road,
  Rotherham, South Yorkshire S60 2UD
Tel: 0709 824525 or 0709 820000 x4525
  Fax: 0709 820007 (specify library)
STAFF: GL Matthews ALA (Principal Librarian), GR Wade BA MLS ALA
    (Senior Librarian), 2 other (full-time), 1 (part-time) staff
TYPE: Multidisciplinary
HOURS: Mon 11-8, Tue-Thu 9-8, Fri 9-4.30, Sat 9.30-1
READERS: Staff and other users
STOCK POLICY: Journals discarded after 5-10 years, books discarded
                    after varying intervals
LENDING: Books, pre-current journals, AV material. Photocopies
                    provided
COMPUTER DATA RETRIEVAL: DATASTAR online - free. PRESTEL available

HOLDINGS: 15,000 books; 200 current journals; 190 tape/slides,
                    3,000 35mm slides, 14 videotapes (VHS)
CLASSIFICATION: NLM modified
SPECIAL COLLECTION: Health information (2,100 vols)
PUBLICATIONS: Current awareness bulletins; Health & social
 service briefing; HMSO briefing; Parliamentary briefing
BRANCH: Badsley Moor Lane Hospital
NETWORK: Yorkshire Joint Medical Libraries Service; SINTO
The Staff Library and Information Service is a jointly
 funded co-operative venture between Rotherham Health
 Authority and Rotherham Metropolitan Borough Council,
 Department of Libraries, Museum and Arts. The Service is
 operated by the Libraries Department as agents for the
 Health Authority, and is open to all bona fide
 practitioners and students of health care in the Rotherham
 locality.

Rugby

560
EDYVEAN-WALKER MEDICAL LIBRARY
Hospital of Saint Cross, Barby Road, Rugby, Warwickshire, CV22 5PX
Tel: 0788 72831
Mrs EM Hunter ALA (part-time)
FOUNDED: 1976
TYPE: Medical
HOURS: Mon, Tues, Wed 8.40-10.40, Fri 1.20-3.20
READERS: Medical staff only
STOCK POLICY: Journals discarded after 2 years, books discarded
                    after c30 years
HOLDINGS: 2,000 books; 30 current journals
CLASSIFICATION: DDC

St Albans

561
BARNET COMMUNITY HEALTH SERVICES LIBRARY AND INFORMATION SERVICE
Napsbury Hospital, Shenley Lane, St Albans, Herts, AL2 1AA
Tel: 0727 23333   Fax: 0727 26245
STAFF: Ms P Shapland-Howes BA ALA and Ms A John BA ALA (job share)
TYPE: Multidisciplinary
HOURS: Mon-Fri 9-5
READERS: Staff and other users
STOCK POLICY: Books and journals discarded after varying periods
LENDING: Books, journals, videos. Photocopies provided
COMPUTER DATA RETRIEVAL: DATASTAR online - free. CD-ROM
HOLDINGS: c5,000 books; c70 journals, c65 current titles;
                    50 tape/slides, 12 videotapes (VHS)
CLASSIFICATION: NLM
PUBLICATIONS: Monthly current awareness bulletin
NETWORKS: NW Thames; Herts County Library Service; PLCS

562
HILL END HOSPITAL
Hill End Lane, Saint Albans, Herts AL4 0RB
Tel: 0727 855555 x3313
STAFF: Ms D Levey BEd DipLib ALA (part time)
TYPE: Multidisciplinary
READERS: Staff, other users by special arrangement
LENDING: Books, journals and non-book material for use with
               patients. Photocopies provided
COMPUTER DATA RETRIEVAL: DATASTAR online - free. CD-ROM
HOLDINGS: 3,500 books; 55 journals,48 current titles.
CLASSIFICATION: NLM
PUBLICATIONS: Library bulletin; Guide to the library
NETWORK: NW Thames; PLCS; Hertfordshire County Library Service

563
SAINT ALBANS CITY HOSPITAL
Normandy Road, Saint Albans, Herts AL3 5PN
Tel: 0727 66122
STAFF: Mrs L Trounce BA ALA
TYPE: Multidisciplinary
HOURS: Mon-Fri 9-5. Key access at other times
READERS: Staff, other users for reference only
STOCK POLICY: Books discarded after varying periods
LENDING: Books only. Photocopies provided
COMPUTER DATA RETRIEVAL: DATASTAR online - free. CD-ROM from 1983
HOLDINGS: 1,176 books; 142 journals, 120 current titles
CLASSIFICATION: NLM
PUBLICATION: Library guide; Bi-monthly bulletin
NETWORKS: NW Thames; Herts County Library Service

St Andrews

564
SAINT ANDREWS UNIVERSITY LIBRARY
North St, St Andrews, Fife, KY16 9TR
Tel: 0334 76161   Telex: 9312110846 SA G   Fax: 0334 75851
Electronic mail: Telecom Gold 79:LLA1002
STAFF: Librarian post vacanct, NF Dumbleton BA MA
FOUNDED: 1612
TYPE: Multidisciplinary
READERS: Staff and other users
STOCK POLICY: No stock discarded
LENDING: Books and journals. Photocopies supplied
COMPUTER DATA RETRIEVAL: BLAISE, DIALOG etc, online - charged
               CD-ROM from 1986
HOLDINGS: c30,000 books; 480 journals, 180 current titles
CLASSIFICATION: LC
PUBLICATION: Current serials list

St Helier

565
Jersey General Hospital
St Helier, Jersey, Channel Islands
Tel: 0534 59000 x2664 (Direct line: 0534 34362)   Telex: 4192538
Fax: 0534 59805
STAFF: Mrs S Tillman ALA
FOUNDED: 1985
TYPE: Multidisciplinary
HOURS: Mon-Thu 9-5.30, Fri 9-5
READERS: Staff and other users
STOCK POLICY: Books discarded after 10 years
LENDING: Books, journals, videos. Photocopies supplied
COMPUTER DATA RETRIEVAL: DATASTAR online - free
HOLDINGS: 2,500 books; 170 journals, 160 current titles;
        30 videotapes (VHS)
CLASSIFICATION: NLM
NETWORK: WRLIS

St Martin's

566
EMMA FERBRACHE SCHOOL OF NURSING LIBRARY
Rondel House, Oberlands, St Martin's, Guernsey, Channel Islands
Tel: 0481 25241 x4304   Fax: 0481 35988
STAFF: Mrs S Graham SRN C&G
FOUNDED: 1985 (Librarian appointed 1987)
TYPE: Midwifery, nursing, psychiatric
HOURS: Mon-Fri 9-12, 1-4
READERS: Staff, other users for reference only
LENDING: Books only. Photocopies provided
COMPUTER DATA RETRIEVAL: In-house terminal
HOLDINGS: 17 current journals
CLASSIFICATION: NLM (WRLIS modification)
NETWORK: WRLIS

567
PRINCESS ELIZABETH HOSPITAL, MEDICAL STAFF LIBRARY
Le Vauquiedor, St Martin, Guernsey, Channel Islands
Tel: 0481 25241
STAFF: Dr FH Degnen MRCP
FOUNDED: 1980
TYPE: Medical
HOURS: 9-5
READERS: Staff and other users
STOCK POLICY: Books discarded after 5 years, journals discarded
        after 10 years
LENDING: Books and journals
HOLDINGS: 14 current journals; 500 slides, 120 videotapes (VHS)
CLASSIFICATION: Own

Salford

568
FRANK RIFKIN POSTGRADUATE MEDICAL CENTRE
Hope Hospital, Eccles Old Road, Salford, Manchester M6 8HD
Tel: 061 789 7373 x5405
STAFF: Ms SE Stephens BSc ALA, M McCormack BA (part time)
TYPE: Multidisciplinary
HOURS: Mon-Fri 9.15-8
READERS: Staff, other users for reference only
LENDING: Books, journals and AV material. Photocopies provided
COMPUTER DATA RETRIEVAL: DATASTAR online - charged full cost
HOLDINGS: 4,500 books; 400 journals, 300 current titles; 30 sets
          tape/slides, 100 audiocassettes, 6 sets 35mm slides,
          10 videotapes (VHS)
CLASSIFICATION: NLM
SPECIAL COLLECTIONS: Orthopaedics, Gastroenterology, Surgery
PUBLICATIONS: Library news; recent additions;library guide;
         periodicals list
BRANCHES: Salford Royal Hospital
NETWORK: NORWHSLA

569
BOLTON & SALFORD AREA COLLEGE OF MIDWIFERY & NURSING
10th Floor, Peel House, Albert Street, Eccles, Manchester, M30 ONJ
Tel: 061 789 7373
STAFF: Mrs BC Pye BA ALA, Mrs J Garnett, Mrs M Todd
FOUNDED: 1974
TYPE: Multidisciplinary
HOURS: Mon-Fri 8.30-4.30
READERS: Staff only
STOCK POLICY:Books discarded after 15 years, journals after 10 years
LENDING: Books only. Photocopies provided
COMPUTER DATA RETRIEVAL: Access to terminal
HOLDINGS: 6,000 books; 42 current journals; microfilms, tape/slides,
          35mm slides
CLASSIFICATION: Own
PUBLICATIONS: Library Guide; How to do a literature search

570
SALFORD COLLEGE OF TECHNOLOGY
Frederick Road, Salford, M6 6PU
Tel: 061 736 6541
STAFF: S Smith BA, S Chester BSc DipLib, D Hall BA, G McGoukin BA,
    M Groen BA DipLib, S Slade BA DipLib, L Sharma BA, L O'Neill BA
    MPhil
FOUNDED: 1967
TYPE: Multidisciplinary
HOURS: Mon-Thu 8.45-8, Fri 8.45-5
READERS: Staff and other users
STOCK POLICY: Books and journals discarded when appropriate
LENDING: Books and journals. Photocopies supplied

COMPUTER DATA RETRIEVAL: DIALOG online
HOLDINGS: 480 journals, 460 current titles; 20 tape/slides, 260
          videotapes (VHS), 8 interactive videos
CLASSIFICATION: UDC
BRANCH: Adelphi

571
SALFORD ROYAL HOSPITAL MEDICAL LIBRARY
Chapel Street, Salford M60 9EP
Tel: 061 789 7373 x3400/3401
STAFF: Mrs HE Hopkins BA BEd SRN (part-time)
FOUNDED: c1970
TYPE: Multidisciplinary
HOURS: Staffed Mon-Fri 9.15-3.15. Key access at other times
READERS: Staff and other users
STOCK POLICY: Books discarded after 15 years
LENDING: Books and journals. Photocopies provided
COMPUTER DATA RETRIEVAL: DATASTAR online - charged computer time
                         only
HOLDINGS: 2,500 books; 130 journals, 46 current titles
CLASSIFICATION: NLM
PUBLICATION: Bi-monthly bulletin
NETWORK: Salford District Health Authority Libraries; NORWHSLA

Salisbury

572
SALISBURY HEALTH AUTHORITY LIBRARY AND INFORMATION SERVICE
Postgraduate Medical Centre, Salisbury General Infirmary,
 Fisherton Street, Salisbury, Wilts SP2 7SX
Tel: 0722 336212 x601
STAFF: Miss S Henshaw MA DipLib (District Librarian),
 W Alexander MA DipLib, Miss S Brain BA(Hons) DipLib
TYPE: Multidisciplinary
HOURS: Mon-Fri 8-10.30. Staffed Mon-Thurs 9-5.30, Fri 9-5
READERS: Staff and other users
STOCK POLICY: Books and journals discarded
LENDING: Books, journals and AV material. Photocopies provided
COMPUTER DATA RETRIEVAL: DATASTAR online - free. CD-ROM from
                         1982. PRESTEL available
HOLDINGS: 14,000 books; 280 current journals; 25 Tape/slides,
                         47 videotapes (VHS)
CLASSIFICATION: NLM (Wessex adaptation)
BRANCHES: Odstock Hospital, Salisbury; Old Manor Hospital,
 Salisbury; Salisbury School of Nursing
NETWORKS: WRLIS; WILCO; HATRICS; PLCS

Scarborough

573
SCARBOROUGH HEALTH AUTHORITY DISTRICT LIBRARY
Scarborough Hospital, Scalby Road, Scarborough, North Yorkshire
    YO12 6QL
Tel: 0723 368111 x2075   Fax: 0723 377233
STAFF: Ms A Ray BA MA DipLib ALA MIInfSc
FOUNDED: 1985
TYPE: Multidisciplinary
HOURS: Staffed Mon-Fri 9-5. Members have 24 hour access via keypad
READERS: Staff, other users at discretion of Librarian
STOCK POLICY: Books discarded after 10 years
LENDING: Books, videos, tape/slide sets. Photocopies provided
COMPUTER DATA RETRIEVAL: BLAISE online - free
HOLDINGS: 3,000 books; 166 journals, 80 current titles;
        12 tape/slides, 10 35mm slides, videotapes (2 U-matic,
        2 Betamax, 96 VHS)
CLASSIFICATION: NLM
SPECIAL COLLECTION: History of SHA hospitals
BRANCHES: Bench book collections at Whitby Hospital and Malton
                        Hospital;
NETWORKS: YRAHCLIS; NIS

Selkirk

574
BORDERS HEALTH BOARD
Thornfield, Selkirk TD7 4DT
Tel: 0750 20212
No furthur information available

Sheffield

575
HEALTH AND SAFETY EXECUTIVE LIBRARY AND INFORMATION SERVICES
Broad Lane, Sheffield S3 7HQ
Tel: 0742 768141 x3113   Telex 54556 (HSE RLS G)
Fax: 0742 755792
STAFF: Mrs S Pantry BA FLA Head of Library & Information Services
FOUNDED: In present form 1975, but earlier (1920s) as Safety in
                        Mines Establishment
TYPE: Health administration, health & safety at work
HOURS: Open Mon-Fri 10-3 for the public
READERS: Staff and other users
STOCK POLICY: Some stock discarded if out of date
LENDING: Books and journals through organised libraries.
                Photocopies provided to organisations

COMPUTER DATA RETRIEVAL: Online: ESA/IRS, DATASTAR, MERIDION,
        DIALOG, etc.; CD-ROM (also an information provider - OSHROM)
HOLDINGS: c2,000 journals, c1,700 current titles
SPECIAL COLLECTION: All aspects of occupational health, mining,
                nuclear, etc
CLASSIFICATION: UDC
PUBLICATIONS: Current periodicals holdings list (annual);
 subject index to the HSE periodical holdings list (annual);
 publications in series (bi-annual); HSL bibliography
 (annual); bibliographies on specific subjects (on demand);
 translations bulletin (quarterly; Prestel directory
BRANCHES : 5 main branches and 24 minor branches
NETWORKS: BLDSC backup library; SINTO; CICRIS; LADSIRLAC

576
TRENT REGIONAL HEALTH AUTHORITY HEADQUARTERS LIBRARY
Fulwood House, Old Fulwood Road, Sheffield S10 3TH
Tel: 0742 630300   Telex 547246 (TRHA G)   Fax: 0742 306956
STAFF: Mrs G Roddis, Mrs A Cobb (part time)
FOUNDED: 1965
TYPE: Health administration
HOURS: Mon-Fri 9-5
READERS: Staff, other users by appointment
STOCK POLICY: Journals discarded after 5 years
LENDING: Books only. Photocopies provided
HOLDINGS: 10,000 books; 180 current journals
CLASSIFICATION: DDC

577
UNIVERSITY OF SHEFFIELD MEDICAL AND DENTAL LIBRARY
Northern General Hospital, Herries Road, Sheffield S5 7AU
Tel: 0742 434343 x4902
STAFF: Dr SE Nicholls BSc PhD MIInfSc (Assistant Librarian)
FOUNDED: 1980
TYPE: Multidisciplinary
HOURS: Mon-Thu 9-7, Fri 9-5
READERS: Staff, other users on application to Librarian
STOCK POLICY: Multiple copies of superseded editions discarded.
LENDING: Books, journals overnight only. Photocopies provided
COMPUTER DATA RETRIEVAL: DIALOG online - free. CD-ROM: CINAHL,
                OSH-ROM
HOLDINGS: 5,000 books; 220 current journals; tape/slides,
                videotapes (U-matic, VHS)
CLASSIFICATION: NLM
PUBLICATION: Recent accessions; Subject accessions; Newsletter
NETWORK: SINTO, BLCMP

578
UNIVERSITY OF SHEFFIELD MEDICAL AND DENTAL LIBRARY
Royal Hallamshire Hospital, Glossop Road, Sheffield, S10 2JF
Tel: 0742 766222 x2030   Fax: 0742 739826
Electronic mail: Janet MD1ML @ UK.AC.SHEFFIELD.PRIMEA
STAFF: MJ Lewis MA ALA, Ms FD Macgillivray BA DipLib, Dr SE
 Nicholls BSc PhD MIInfSc, JM Clarke BA DipLib, Ms K Burkinshaw
 BA DipLib
TYPE: Multidisciplinary
HOURS: Mon-Thu 9-9.30, Fri 9-7, Sat 9-1 (Mon-Fri 9-7, Sat 9-12.30
            during Summer vacation)
READERS: Staff, other users on application to Librarian
STOCK POLICY: Multiple copies of superseded editions discarded
LENDING: Books, journals overnight only. Photocopies provided
COMPUTER DATA RETRIEVAL: DIALOG, ESA/IRS online - free to University
 and NHS staff. CD-ROM: MEDLINE (latest 4 years)
HOLDINGS: 20,000 books; 450 current journals; tape/slides,
                    videotapes (200 U-matic, 20 VHS)
CLASSIFICATION: NLM
SPECIAL COLLECTION: Sheffield Infirmary collection (500 early
                    medical works housed in main University library)
PUBLICATIONS: Recent accessions; Subject accessions; Newsletter
BRANCH: Northern General Hospital
NETWORKS: SINTO; BLCMP

579
WESTON PARK HOSPITAL
Whitham Road, Sheffield S10 2SJ
Tel: 0742 670222
STAFF: Prof BW Hancock MD FRCP (Honorary Librarian), Ms J Warnock
            (part time)
FOUNDED: c1960
TYPE: Oncology
HOURS: Mon-Fri 9-5. Available for emergency referral out of hours
READERS: Staff and other users
STOCK POLICY: No stock discarded
LENDING: Books only
HOLDINGS: c1355 bound journals, c1250 current titles
CLASSIFICATION: Own

Shotts

580
HARTWOOD HOSPITAL DIVISION OF PSYCHIATRY
Hartwood, Shotts, Lanarkshire ML7 4LA
Tel: 0501 23366
STAFF: J Hodgson BMus ALA
TYPE: Psychiatric
HOURS: Always open to staff, staffed Fridays
READERS: Medical staff only
LENDING: Books only. Photocopies supplied

HOLDINGS: 1,100 books; 22 current journals; 4 tape/slides,
           videotapes (6 Betamax, 18 VHS)
CLASSIFICATION: Royal College of Psychiatrists
NETWORKS: PLCS; ASHSL

Shrewsbury

581
HEALTH EDUCATION DEPARTMENT, SHROPSHIRE HEALTH AUTHORITY
Health Authority District HQ, Cross Houses, Shrewsbury SY5 6JN
Tel: 0743 75242   Fax: 0743 75601
STAFF: None, the library is the responsibility of the Resources
           Manager
TYPE: Multidisciplinary
HOURS: Mon-Fri 8.45-3.45
READERS: Staff and other users
STOCK POLICY: Journals discarded after 5 years, books discarded
           when appropriate
LENDING: Books, teaching packs on health education. Photocopies
           provided
HOLDINGS: 600 books; 10 current journals; 160 videotapes (VHS)
CLASSIFICATION: Own

582
ROYAL SHREWSBURY HOSPITAL - SHELTON
Shelton Hospital, Bicton Heath, Shrewsbury, Shropshire SY3 8DN
Tel: 0743 231122
STAFF: Mrs MJ Nicholls (part-time)
TYPE: Psychiatric
HOURS: Mon-Fri 9-5. Staffed Mon-Fri 9-2
READERS: Medical staff.
LENDING: Books only. Photocopies supplied
HOLDINGS: 300 books; 20 current journals.
CLASSIFICATION: NLMC
NETWORK: West Midlands Regional Health Libraries

583
SHREWSBURY MEDICAL INSTITUTE LIBRARY
Royal Shrewsbury Hospital (South), Mytton Oak Road,
 Shrewsbury, Shropshire SY3 8XF
Tel: 0743 231122
STAFF: Mrs C Carr BA DipLib
TYPE: Medical
HOURS: Mon-Fri 9-5
READERS: Staff only (some restrictions)
STOCK POLICY: Journals discarded after 10 years
LENDING: Books to staff only
COMPUTER DATA RETRIEVAL: Access to terminal -all charged full cost
HOLDINGS: 2,300 books; 100 journals, 80 current titles
CLASSIFICATION: NLM
NETWORK: West Midlands Regional Health Libraries

584
ROYAL SHREWSBURY HOSPITAL SCHOOL OF NURSING
Royal Shrewsbury Hospital (North), Education Centre,
 Mytton Oak Road, Shrewsbury, Shropshire SY3 8XQ
Tel: 0743 231122 x3859
STAFF: Ms E Tilley MA(Hons) DipLib ALA
FOUNDED: 1983
TYPE: Nursing
HOURS: Mon-Thu 8.30-5, Fir 9.30-4.30
READERS: Staff and other users
STOCK POLICY: Books and journals discarded after varying intervals
LENDING: Books only. Photocopies provided
HOLDINGS: 6,000 books; 65 journals, 60 current titles.
CLASSIFICATION: NLM
PUBLICATIONS: Library guides; Accessions bulletin; current
                awareness bulletin
NETWORK: West Midlands Regional Health Libraries

Sidcup

585
QUEEN MARY'S HOSPITAL, CHARNLEY LIBRARY
Frognal Centre for Medical Studies, Sidcup, Kent DA14 6LT
Tel: 081 302 2678 x4439   Fax: 081 308 0457
STAFF: Mrs VJ Jennings ALA
FOUNDED: 1986 (absorbed old medical library founded 1974)
TYPE: Medical, paramedical
HOURS: Access by key at all times. Staffed Mon-Fri 9.30-5.30
READERS: Staff and other users
STOCK POLICY: Journals discarded after 10 years, books discarded
                after 10-15 years
LENDING: Books, videos to medical staff only. Photocopies provided
COMPUTER DATA RETRIEVAL: DATASTAR online - outsiders charged cost
                of computer time
HOLDINGS: 1,600 books; 109 journals, 105 current titles;
                2,000 35mm slides, 20 tape/slides, 45 videotapes (VHS)
CLASSIFICATION: NLM
PUBLICATIONS: Journal holdings; Users guide
NETWORK: SE Thames Regional Library and Information Service

Sleaford

586
RAUCEBY HOSPITAL STAFF LIBRARY
Sleaford, Lincs NG34 8PP
Tel: 05298 241 x302
STAFF: Mrs SL Taylor ALA (part time)
FOUNDED: 1981
TYPE: Multidisciplinary
HOURS: Mon-Thu 9-4.30, Fri 9-3.30

READERS: Health Service staff. Other bona fide users for reference
STOCK POLICY: Books and journals selectively discarded
LENDING: Books only. photocopies provided
HOLDINGS: 3,000 books; 60 journals, 57 current titles
CLASSIFICATION: DDC
PUBLICATION: Additions to stock
NETWORK: South Lincolnshire Health District Library Service;
Lincolnshire County Library

Slough

587
EAST BERKSHIRE NURSING AND MIDWIFERY EDUCATION CENTRE
Wexham Park Hospital, Slough, Berks SL2 4HL
Tel: 0753 34567
STAFF: Ms AG Allison MA(Hons) DipILS ALA, 1 other (part time) staff
TYPE: Nursing
HOURS: Mon-Fri 8-4
READERS: Nursing staff
STOCK POLICY: No stock discarded
LENDING: Books only. Photocopies supplied
COMPUTER DATA RETRIEVAL: DATASTAR online - free
HOLDINGS: c6,000 books; 63 journals, 59 current titles;
                10 microfilms, 90 tape/slides, 15 35mm slides,
                120 videotapes (VHS), medical models
CLASSIFICATION: Own (changing to NLM)
BRANCHES: Church Hill House Hospital, Bracknell; Heatherwood
                Hospital, Ascot
NETWORK: Oxford Region

588
WEXHAM PARK HOSPITAL MEDICAL LIBRARY
Slough, Berks SL2 4HL
Tel: 0753 34567 x4020 or x4021
STAFF: Mrs H Mills BA DipLib (part time)
TYPE: Medical
HOURS: Always open. Staffed Mon-Fri 10-2
READERS: Staff and other users
STOCK POLICY: Books and journals discarded at variable intervals
LENDING: Books and journals. Photocopies provided
COMPUTER DATA RETRIEVAL: DATASTAR online - free
HOLDINGS: 500 books; 60 current journals
CLASSIFICATION: NLM
NETWORK: Oxford Region Library and Information Service

Solihull

589
EDUCATION CENTRE, SOLIHULL HEALTH AUTHORITY
Brook House, 21 Lode Lane, Solihull, West Midlands B91 2AB
Tel: 021 704 5191   Fax: 021 705 9541
STAFF: Ms J Whitaker BA(Hons)
TYPE: Multidisciplinary
HOURS: Mon-Fri 9-1, 2-5
READERS: Staff only
STOCK POLICY: Some journals discarded
LENDING: Books only. Photocopies provided
COMPUTER DATA RETRIEVAL: In-house terminal
HOLDINGS: 988 books; 32 current journals; tape/slides,35mm slides,
                   videotapes (36 U-matic, 22 VHS)
CLASSIFICATION: LC

South Shields

590
SOUTH SHIELDS POSTGRADUATE MEDICAL CENTRE
General Hospital, South Shields, Tyne and Wear NE34 0PL
Tel: 091 4548888 x2572
STAFF: Mrs M Duffy ALA (part-time)
FOUNDED: 1972
TYPE: Medical
HOURS: Mon-Fri 9-5. Staffed 10-2.30. Key available at other times
READERS: Medical and dental staff only
STOCK POLICY: Books discarded after 10 years
LENDING: Books, AV material,(journals in special circumstances).
                   Photocopies provided
COMPUTER DATA RETRIEVAL: DATASTAR online - free
HOLDINGS: 2,200 books; 153 journals, 107 current titles;
 5 sets 35mm slides, 21 videotapes (VHS), 10 sets audiotapes
CLASSIFICATION: DDC
BRANCH: Ingham Infirmary Library, South Shields
NETWORK: Northern Regional Association of Health Service
 Librarians

Southall

591
EALING DISTRICT SCHOOL OF NURSING
Ealing Hospital, Uxbridge Road, Southall, Middlesex UB1 3HW
Tel: 081 574 2444 x628
No furthur information available

592
EALING HOSPITAL (SAINT BERNARD'S WING), COOMBS MEDICAL LIBRARY
Uxbridge Road, Southall, Middlesex UB1 3EU
Tel: 081 574 2444 x2135
STAFF: P Valentine BA ALA
TYPE: Multidisciplinary

HOURS: Mon-Fri 9-5
READERS: Staff and other users
STOCK POLICY: Books discarded after 10 years
LENDING: Books only. Photocopies provided
COMPUTER DATA RETRIEVAL: DATASTAR online - charged computer time
                  only. CD-ROM: MEDLINE (Silver Platter) from 1983
HOLDINGS: 2,900 books; 67 journals, 56 current titles;
                  23 Videotapes (VHS)
SPECIAL COLLECTION: Psychiatry (1,200 vols)
CLASSIFICATION: NLM
PUBLICATIONS: Library guide; new accessions/current
 literature list
NETWORK: NW Thames Regional Library and Information Service;
                  London Borough of Ealing

Southampton

593
HELP FOR HEALTH INFORMATION SERVICE (WRLIS)
Grant Building, Southampton General Hospital, Southampton SO9 4XY
Tel: 0703 779091
RE Gann BA DipLib ALA, 1 other staff
FOUNDED: 1980
TYPE: Multidisciplinary
HOURS: Mon-Fri 9-4.30
READERS: Staff and other users
STOCK POLICY: Journals discarded after 1 year, books discarded
                  after 5 years
COMPUTER DATA RETRIEVAL: In-house terminal for Help for
 Health data (no on-line access). CD-ROM from 1989
HOLDINGS: 3,000 books; 150 current journals; 30 videotapes (VHS)
SPECIAL COLLECTIONS: Patient information; voluntary
 organisations and self help groups
CLASSIFICATION: NLM (modified)
PUBLICATIONS: Newsletter; Publicity leaflets; reports
NETWORK: WRLIS

594
ROYAL SOUTH HANTS HOSPITAL STAFF LIBRARY
Newtown, Southampton SO9 4PE
Tel: 0703 634288 x2491/2714
STAFF: Ms R Noyes BA DipLib, Mrs D Stratford
FOUNDED: 1974
TYPE: Multidisciplinary
HOURS: Mon-Fri 9-5.30
READERS: Staff and other users
STOCK POLICY: Out of date books and journals discarded
LENDING: Books, journals and AV material. Photocopies provided
COMPUTER DATA RETRIEVAL: DATASTAR, BLAISE online - free
HOLDINGS: 12,000 books; 350 journals, 274 current titles
CLASSIFICATION: NLM (WRLIS modification)
BRANCHES: 4
NETWORK: HATRICS; WRLIS

595
UNIVERSITY OF SOUTHAMPTON, DEPARTMENT OF TEACHING MEDIA
Audiovisual Resources Unit, South Academic Block, Southampton
General Hospital, Southampton, SO9 4XY
Tel: 0703 777222 x3764
STAFF: Miss M McKenna BA(Hons) DipLib
FOUNDED: 1969
TYPE: Multidisciplinary
HOURS: Mon-Fri 9-5
READERS: NHS Staff in Wessex Region only
LENDING: AV material
COMPUTER DATA RETRIEVAL: Access to terminal.
HOLDINGS: 5,000 35mm slides, 284 tape/slides, 380 videotapes (VHS)
               182 slide sets, 81 Overhead transparencies
CLASSIFICATION: NLM
NETWORK: WRLIS

596
UNIVERSITY OF SOUTHAMPTON, WESSEX MEDICAL LIBRARY (GENERAL
  HOSPITAL BRANCH)
Southampton General Hospital, Tremona Road, Southampton, SO0 4XY
Tel: 0703 777222 x3758   Fax: 0703 593939
Electronic mail: LBI007 @ UK.AC.SOTON.IBM
STAFF: TA King BA ALA, Miss J Welch BA MIInfSci (part time),
           P Boagey ALA, Miss S Dawson
FOUNDED: 1970
TYPE: Multidisciplinary
HOURS: Mon-Thu 9-10, Fri 9-6, Sat 9-5, Sun 2-5. Staffed Mon-Fri
              9-6, Sat 9-12.30
READERS: Staff, members of Southampton University and NHS personnel
  within the Wessex Region. Other users on application to Librarian
STOCK POLICY: No stock discarded
LENDING: Books and A/V material only. Photocopies provided
COMPUTER DATA RETRIEVAL: DATASTAR online - free to NHS staff,
               others charged full cost. CD-ROM from 1989
HOLDINGS: 13,000 books; 700 journals, 570 current titles
CLASSIFICATION: NLM and LC
PUBLICATIONS: Guides for newly qualified staff; guide for
  nurses
NETWORK: HATRICS; S3RBK; WRLIS

597
UNIVERSITY OF SOUTHAMPTON, WESSEX MEDICAL LIBRARY   (UNIVERSITY
  BRANCH)
Medical & Biological Sciences Building, Bassett Crescent East,
  Southampton SO9 3TU
Tel: 0703 594217   Telex 477057   Fax: 0703 593939
Electronic mail: LBI007 @ UK.AC.SOTON.IBM
STAFF: TA King BA ALA, Miss A Norman BA DipLib ALA, Mrs K Nelson
  MA ALA, Mrs JM Springer BA DipLib ALA (part time)

FOUNDED: 1970
TYPE: Multidisciplinary
HOURS: Mon-Thu 9-10, Fri 9-6, Sat 9-5, Sun 2-5. Staffed Mon-Fri
9-6, Sat 9-12.30
READERS: Members of staff of Southampton University and NHS
personnel within the Wessex Region. Other users on approval
of application to Librarian
STOCK POLICY: No stock discarded
LENDING: Books only. Photocopies provided
COMPUTER DATA RETRIEVAL: DATASTAR, DIALOG online - charged full
cost
HOLDINGS: 20,000 books; 800 journals, 650 current titles
CLASSIFICATION: NLM and LC
PUBLICATION: Guide for new users
NETWORK: HATRICS; S3RBK; WRLIS
Wessex Medical Library is a section of Southampton
University Library (Librarian: B Naylor, MA DipLib). The
two branches are complementary, the General Hospital Branch
holding mainly clinical and nursing material, the
University Branch mainly pre-clinical and biological.

598
WESSEX REGIONAL LIBRARY AND INFORMATION SERVICE
Regional Office, South Academic Block, Southampton General
Hospital, Southampton SO9 4XY
Tel: 0703 777222 x3750   Fax: 0703 785648
STAFF: RB Tabor MIInfSc,Mrs J Stephenson BLib ALA (part time)
FOUNDED: 1967
HOURS: Mon-Fri 9-5
CLASSIFICATION: NLM
PUBLICATIONS: Directory of WRLIS libraries
NETWORK: WRLIS; HATRICS

Stafford

599
MID-STAFFORDSHIRE HEALTH AUTHORITY LIBRARY AND INFORMATION UNIT
Mellor House, Corporation Street, Stafford ST16 3SR
Tel: 0785 52233   Fax: 0785 54640
STAFF: Mrs CA Phillips (part time)
FOUNDED: 1974
TYPE: Health administration
HOURS: Mon-Fri 9.30-12.30, 1.30-4
READERS: Staff and other users
STOCK POLICY: Books discarded
LENDING: Books only. Photocopies provided
COMPUTER DATA RETRIEVAL: Access to terminal.
HOLDINGS: c2,000 books; 20 current journals. ,
CLASSIFICATION: Own
PUBLICATION: Publications received list (monthly)
NETWORKS: West Midlands Regional Health Libraries; FIRST

600
MID-STAFFORDSHIRE HEALTH AUTHORITY, TRAINING & DEVELOPMENT LIBRARY
David Hollin Building, Staffordshire General Infirmary,
Stafford, ST16 1BB
Tel: 0785 58251 x3557
STAFF: Mrs W Bastable BA(Hons) ALA, Ms C Boulton BA
FOUNDED: Centralised in 1986
TYPE: Health administration, nursing, paramedical
HOURS: Mon, Wed, Thu 8.30-5, Tue 8.30-6, Fri 8.30-4
READERS: Staff, other users for reference only
STOCK POLICY: Books discarded after 10 years
LENDING: Books and AV material. Photocopies provided
COMPUTER DATA RETRIEVAL: Access to terminal
HOLDINGS: c7,000 books; 60 current journals; 6 tape/slides,
          150 study packs, videotapes (25 Betamax, 30 VHS)
CLASSIFICATION: LC
NETWORK: West Midlands Regional Health Libraries

601
SAINT GEORGE'S HOSPITAL MEDICAL LIBRARY
Corporation St, Stafford, ST16 3AG
Tel: 0785 57888 x5509
STAFF: Miss V Horne (part time)
TYPE: Psychiatric
HOURS: Always open
READERS: Staff, other users by arrangement
LENDING: Books and journals
COMPUTER DATA RETRIEVAL: Access to terminal
HOLDINGS: 26 current journals
CLASSIFICATION: DDC
NETWORK: West Midlands Region Health Libraries

602
SHROPSHIRE AND STAFFORDSHIRE COLLEGE OF NURSING and MIDWIFERY
David Hollin Building, Staffordshire General Infirmary,
 Foregate Street, Stafford ST16 2PA
Tel: 0785 58251 x3557
STAFF: Mrs W Bastable BA(Hons) ALA, Ms C Boulton BA
FOUNDED: 1986
TYPE: Nursing, paramedical, psychiatric
HOURS: Mon, Wed, Thu 8.30-5, Tue 8.30-6, Fri 8.30-4.30
READERS: Staff and other users
STOCK POLICY: Some books discarded after 10 years
LENDING: Books and AV material only. Photocopies provided
COMPUTER DATA RETRIEVAL: Access to terminal
HOLDINGS: 7,000 books; 70 journals, 60 current titles;
          tape/slides, 35mm slides, videotapes (20 Betamax, 50 VHS)
CLASSIFICATION: LC
PUBLICATION: Guide to the library
NETWORK: West Midlands Regional Health Libraries

603
STAFFORD DISTRICT GENERAL HOSPITAL, LUCY WILMORE MEMORIAL LIBRARY
Postgraduate Medical Centre, Weston Road, Stafford, ST16 3SA
Tel: 0785 57731 x4633
STAFF: Miss EA Hanley C&G LibAsstCert
TYPE: Multidisciplinary
HOURS: Open 24 hours (Staffed Mon-Fri 9-5)
READERS: Staff and other users
STOCK POLICY: No stock discarded
LENDING: Books and journals. Photocopies provided
HOLDINGS: c1,800 books; 62 journals, c55 current titles;
             35mm slides, 80 videotapes (VHS)
CLASSIFICATION: NLM
SPECIAL COLLECTION: Speech therapy (120 vols)
BRANCH: Staffordshire General Infirmary
NETWORK: West Midlands regional Health Libraries

604
STAFFORDSHIRE GENERAL INFIRMARY, MEDICAL LIBRARY
Staffordshire General Infirmary, Foregate Street, Stafford, ST16 2PA
Tel: 0785 58251 x3410
STAFF: Dr FJ Pick (Honorary Librarian), Mrs CM Prescott (part time)
TYPE: Medical
HOURS: Always open. Staffed Tue 9-12, Wed 2-5
READERS: Staff only
STOCK POLICY: Journals over 10 years old discarded
LENDING: Books and journals
COMPUTER DATA RETRIEVAL: Access to terminal
HOLDINGS: 750 books; 80 current journals
CLASSIFICATION: NLM
NETWORK: West Midlands Region Health Libraries

Stanmore

605
ROYAL NATIONAL ORTHOPAEDIC HOSPITAL, NURSE EDUCATION LIBRARY
Brockley Hill, Stanmore, Middlesex, HA7 4LP
Tel: 081 954 2300 x216
STAFF: Mrs HC Isham BSc ALA (part time)
FOUNDED: 1960
TYPE: Nursing, paramedical
HOURS: Mon-Fri 8-5 (Staffed Mon-Wed 10-5)
READERS: Staff, other users by written request
STOCK POLICY: Books discarded after 10 years
LENDING: Books and bones. Photocopies provided
COMPUTER DATA RETRIEVAL: Access to terminal
HOLDINGS: 3,000 books; 40 journals, 35 current titles
CLASSIFICATION: NLM
NETWORK: NE Thames

606
NORTH HERTS HEALTH AUTHORITY, DISTRICT LIBRARY
Lister Hospital, Corey's Mill Lane, Stevenage SG1 4AD
Tel: 0438 314333 x520/431
STAFF: Mrs S Knight JP ALA, Ms L Collings BLib ALA, Ms J Mackenzie
       SEN, Ms C Parr ALA
FOUNDED: 1972
TYPE: Multidisciplinary
HOURS: Mon-Fri 9.30-12.30, 1.15-5.30. Key available to staff
READERS: Staff and other users
STOCK POLICY: Superseded editions of books and journals over
               10 years old discarded
LENDING: Books and noncurrent journals. Photocopies provided
COMPUTER DATA RETRIEVAL: DATASTAR online - free. CD-ROM from 1988
HOLDINGS: 2,000 books; 110 current journals
CLASSIFICATION: NLM
PUBLICATIONS: Library bulletin; new books list
NETWORK: NW Thames; Herts County Library service

Stockport

607
STEPPING HILL HOSPITAL POSTGRADUATE MEDICAL LIBRARY
Poplar Grove, Stockport, Cheshire SK2 7JE
Tel: 061 419 5672
STAFF: Mrs J Fantom (part time), Mrs J Thorpe (part time)
TYPE: Medical
HOURS: Mon-Thurs 8.30-5.30, Fri 8.30-5
READERS: Medical staff and nursing staff only.
STOCK POLICY: No stock discarded
LENDING: Books, journals and AV material. Photocopies provided
COMPUTER DATA RETRIEVAL: In-house terminal
HOLDINGS: 1,500 books; 70 current journals
CLASSIFICATION: Own
NETWORK: NORWHSLA

Stockton-on-Tees

608
NORTH TEES GENERAL HOSPITAL MEDICAL LIBRARY
Hardwick, Stockton-on-Tees, Cleveland TS19 8PE
Tel: 0642 672122 x603
STAFF: Mrs E Clemo BA ALA

FOUNDED: 1974
TYPE: Multidisciplinary
HOURS: Mon-Wed 9-6, Thurs, Fri 9-5
READERS: Staff and other users
STOCK POLICY: Out of date editions of books discarded, journals
              discarded after 5 years
LENDING: Books and journals. Photocopies supplied
HOLDINGS: 11,000 books; 260 journals, 200 current titles
CLASSIFICATION: DDC 18
PUBLICATIONS: Accessions list; library guide
NETWORK: NORWHSLA

609
WINTERTON HOSPITAL TEACHING CENTRE LIBRARY
Sedgefield, Stockton-on-Tees, Cleveland TS21 3EJ
Tel: 0740 20521 x2931
STAFF: Mrs S Bass ALA
FOUNDED: 1974
TYPE: Multidisciplinary
HOURS: Mon-Fri 8.30-5
READERS: Medical, nursing and paramedical staff
LENDING: Books only. Photocopies provided
COMPUTER DATA RETRIEVAL: DATASTAR online - free
HOLDINGS: 5,250 books; 45 current journals; 100 tape/slides,
           30 CAL discs
CLASSIFICATION: DDC
NETWORK: PLCS

Stoke-on-Trent

610
NORTH STAFFORDSHIRE COLLEGE OF NURSING AND MIDWIFERY
City General Hospital, Newcastle Road, Stoke-on-Trent, ST4 6QG
Tel: 0782 621133 x2949
STAFF: DT Bird MA
TYPE: Nursing, midwifery
HOURS: Mon, Tue, Thu 8.30-5, Wed 8.30-6, Fri 8.30-4.30
READERS: Staff and other users
STOCK POLICY: Out of date books discarded
LENDING: Books only. Photocopies provided
COMPUTER DATA RETRIEVAL: Access to terminal
HOLDINGS: 15,000 books; 206 journals, 144 current titles
CLASSIFICATION: LC
BRANCHES: Two (Mental handicap, mental illness)
NETWORKS: West Midlands Regional Health Libraries; FIRST

611
THE NORTH STAFFORDSHIRE MEDICAL INSTITUTE
Hartshill, Stoke-on-Trent ST4 7NY
Tel: 0782 49144 x4198
STAFF: Mrs I Fenton ALA
FOUNDED: 1965
TYPE: Multidisciplinary
HOURS: Mon-Fri 8.30-8.30, (weekend access by arrangement).
            Staffed Mon-Fri 9-5
READERS: Staff, other users for reference only
STOCK POLICY: Out of date books discarded.
LENDING: Books, videotapes only. Photocopies provided
COMPUTER DATA RETRIEVAL: DATASTAR online - standard charge
HOLDINGS: 2,241 books; 350 journals, 305 current titles;
                        40+ videotapes (VHS)
SPECIAL COLLECTION: Historical medical/Andrew Meiklejohn collection
                of industrial medicine (963 vols)
CLASSIFICATION: LC
BRANCHES: St Edward's Hospital, Cheddleton; Stallington Hospital,
                        Blythe Bridge
NETWORK: West Midlands Regional Health Libraries; PLCS

Stourbridge

612
CORBETT HOSPITAL, MEDICAL SERVICES CENTRE LIBRARY
Stourbridge, West Midlands, DY8 4JB
Tel: 0384 371233
STAFF: Dr AM Zalin (honorary Librarian), Mrs Y Price (General
                Administrator)
HOURS: Mon-Fri 8-5.30. Key available at other times
READERS; all NHS staff from hospital and district
COMPUTER DATA RETRIEVAL; Access to terminal
HOLDINGS: 1,700 books; 40 current journals
CLASSIFICATION: NLM
NETWORK: West Midlands

613
WORDSLEY HOSPITAL MEDICAL LIBRARY
Stream Road, Stourbridge, West Midlands DY8 5QX
Tel: 0384 288778
See entry no 668

Sutton Coldfield

614
BIRMINGHAM COLLEGE OF NURSE EDUCATION
Good Hope General Hospital, Rectory Road, Sutton Coldfield,
  West Midlands B75 7RR

Tel: 021 378 2211 x2093
STAFF: Librarian post vacant
FOUNDED: 1961
TYPE: Nursing, psychiatric
HOURS: Mon-Fri 9-5
READERS: Nursing staff and students. Other users by arrangement
STOCK POLICY: No stock discarded
LENDING: Books only. Photocopies provided
COMPUTER DATA RETRIEVAL: Access to terminal.
HOLDINGS: 9,000 books; 24 current journals; videotapes (50 U-matic,
                    120 VHS)
CLASSIFICATION: LC
NETWORK: West Midlands Regional Health Libraries

615
GOOD HOPE DISTRICT GENERAL HOSPITAL POSTGRADUATE MEDICAL CENTRE
Rectory Road, Sutton Coldfield, West Midlands B75 7RR
Tel: 021 378 2211 x2625
STAFF: Mrs SA Hannington (part time), Mrs PM Winder (part time)
FOUNDED: 1967
TYPE: Multidisciplinary
HOURS: Mon-Fri 9-5. Key available at other times
READERS: Hospital medical staff, GPs and health workers
STOCK POLICY: Books discarded occasionally
LENDING: Books and journals. Photocopies provided
COMPUTER DATA RETRIEVAL: Access to terminal.
HOLDINGS: 1,400 books; 80 current journals; 12 tape/slides,
                    24 videotapes (VHS)
CLASSIFICATION: LC
NETWORK: West Midlands Regional Health Libraries

616
WEST MIDLANDS DRUG INFORMATION SERVICE
Good Hope General Hospital, Rectory Road, Sutton Coldfield,
 West Midlands B75 7RR
Tel: 021 378 2211 x3565
STAFF: Miss E Grant BPharm MSc MPS MCPP (Principal Pharmacist),
    Mrs DE Frost BSc(Pharm) MPS ALA (Staff Pharmacist)
TYPE: Multidisciplinary
HOURS: Mon-Fri 8.30-5
READERS: Staff only
COMPUTER DATA RETRIEVAL: In-house terminal. Free to Health
 Service personnel
HOLDINGS: 180 books; 30 current journals
PUBLICATIONS: Drug inform; Drug information letter (within
 West Midlands RHA)
NETWORK: West Midlands Regional Health Libraries

617
MORRISTON HOSPITAL POSTGRADUATE CENTRE MEDICAL LIBRARY
Swansea, West Glamorgan, SA6 6NL
Tel: 0792 703131
STAFF: Ms JR Rees ALA
FOUNDED: 1989
TYPE: Medical, dental
HOURS: Mon-Thu 9-5, Fri 9-4.30
READERS: Staff and other users
LENDING: Books and journals. Photocopies provided
COMPUTER DATA RETRIEVAL: DATASTAR online - free
HOLDINGS: c1,500 books; 90 current journals
CLASSIFICATION: NLM
NETWORKS: AWHILES ; West Glamorgan District

618
WEST GLAMORGAN COLLEGE OF NURSING AND MIDWIFERY
Parc Beck, Sketty Road, Swansea, SA2 9DX
Tel: 0792 201939 x26
STAFF: S Storey BSc (Hons) DipLib
FOUNDED: approximately 1947
TYPE: NURSING
HOURS: Mon-Thu 8.30-4.30, Fri 8.30-4
READERS: Staff and other users
LENDING: Books only. Photocopies provided
COMPUTER DATA RETRIEVAL: DATASTAR online - free
HOLDINGS: 10,000 books on 5 sites; 95 journals, 85 current titles
CLASSIFICATION: NLM (Wessex modification)
NETWORK: AWHILES

619
WEST GLAMORGAN HEALTH AUTHORITY DISTRICT LIBRARY SERVICE
Singleton Hospital, Sketty, Swansea, West Glamorgan SA4 2GL
Tel: 0792 205666 x5281   Fax: 0792 208647
STAFF: CD Engel BA DipLib ALA, Mrs M Greer MLS MIInfSc (part time),
          Mrs A Powell BA DipLib ALA (part time), Mrs R Rees ALA
FOUNDED: 1973
TYPE: Multidisciplinary
HOURS: Mon-Fri 8.30-5
READERS: Staff only
STOCK POLICY: Books and journals discarded at Librarian's discretion
LENDING: Books and journals. Photocopies provided
COMPUTER DATA RETRIEVAL: DATASTAR online - outside users charged
                full cost. CD-ROM from 1976
HOLDINGS: 1,000 books; 300 journals, 280 current titles;
                    12 videotapes (VHS)
CLASSIFICATION: NLM

BRANCHES: Cefn Coed Psychiatric Hospital, Swansea; Morriston
            Hospital, Swansea; Neath General Hospital
NETWORK: AWHILES

Swindon

620
PRINCESS MARGARET HOSPITAL
Okus Road, Swindon, Wiltshire SN1 4JU
Tel: 0793 536231 x3200
STAFF: Miss HL Spurrier ALA
FOUNDED: 1964
TYPE: Multidisciplinary
HOURS: Always open. Staffed Mon-Fri 9-5.15
READERS: Staff, other users at discretion of librarian
STOCK POLICY: Books and journals discarded at varying intervals
LENDING: Books and journals. photocopies provided
COMPUTER DATA RETRIEVAL: Access to DATASTAR online
HOLDINGS: 4,000 books; 210 journals, 160 current titles;
            33 tape/slides, 5 videotapes (VHS)
CLASSIFICATION: NLM
NETWORK: WILCO; WRLIS

Taunton

621
NUFFIELD LIBRARY, SOMERSET POSTGRADUATE CENTRE
Musgrove Park Hospital, Taunton, Somerset TA1 5DA
0823 73444 x4230
Mrs S McEnroe ALA (Locum Librarian)
TYPE: Multidisciplinary
HOURS: Always open. Staffed Mon-Fri 9-5.30
READERS: Medical, dental practitioners and ophthalmists in
 hospital and local area
STOCK POLICY: Out of date books and ephemeral material
 discarded
LENDING: Books and journals
HOLDINGS: 1,200 books, 1,860 bound journals; 150 current
 journals. Tape/slides, 35mm slides, cassettes
CLASSIFICATION: Own
NETWORK: SWEHSLinC

622
SOMERSET SCHOOL OF NURSING
Musgrove Park Hospital, Taunton, Somerset TA1 5DA
Tel: 0823 333444 x2465
STAFF: Miss L Crecy BA(Hons) DipLib, Mrs L Sadler (part time)
TYPE: Nursing
HOURS: Mon-Fri 8.15-5
READERS: Nursing staff and other users
STOCK POLICY: Books discarded after 10-12 years
LENDING: Books only
COMPUTER DATA RETRIEVAL: In-house terminal
HOLDINGS: 1,991 books; 20 current journals;
125 videotapes (VHS)
CLASSIFICATION: RCN
BRANCHES: Mendip Nursing School, Wells; Sandhill Park Nursing
School, Taunton; Tone Vale Nursing School, Taunton;
Yeovil Nursing School, Yeovil
NETWORK: SWEHSLinC

Telford

623
TELFORD HOSPITAL LIBRARY EDUCATION CENTRE
Apley Castle, Telford, Shropshire, TF6 6TF
Tel: 0952 641222 x4440
STAFF: Miss AR Edwards MA ALA
FOUNDED: 1989
TYPE: Multidisciplinary
HOURS: Mon-Thu 8.30-5, Fri 8.30-4
READERS: All Shropshire Health Authority staff
LENDING: Books and journals. Photocopies provided
COMPUTER DATA RETRIEVAL: Access to terminal
HOLDINGS: c1,600 books; 100 current journals
CLASSIFICATION: NLM
NETWORK: West Midlands

Torquay

624
TORBAY HOSPITAL DISTRICT LIBRARY
Medical Centre, Torbay Hospital, Torquay, Devon TQ2 7AA
Tel: 0803 614567 x4704
STAFF: Mrs PK Prior BSc CertEd ALA, Mrs D Smurthwaite BLib,
Mrs A Bradley (part time), Mrs J Jackson BA (part time)

TYPE: Multidisciplinary
HOURS: Mon-Fri 8-5.15
READERS: Staff and other users
STOCK POLICY: Journals discarded after 15 years, old editions of
             books discarded
LENDING: Books and videotapes. Photocopies provided
COMPUTER DATA RETRIEVAL: DATASTAR online - charged full cost
HOLDINGS: 1,000 books; 150 journals, 125 current titles;
          10 tape/slides, 10 videotapes (VHS)
CLASSIFICATION: NLM
NETWORK: SWEHSLinC

Truro

625
CORNWALL POSTGRADUATE CENTRE, DISTRICT LIBRARY SERVICE
Royal Cornwall Hospital (Treliske), Truro, Cornwall TR1 3LJ
Tel: 0872 73369 x2610   Fax: 0872 222838
STAFF: Mrs PW Kitch ALA, Mrs S Richards BA
FOUNDED: Opened 1983
TYPE: Health administration, Medical, Paramedical
HOURS: Mon-Fri 9-5 (Wed 10-8)
READERS: Staff and other users
STOCK POLICY: Stock selectively discarded
LENDING: Books, journals and AV material. Photocopies provided
COMPUTER DATA RETRIEVAL: DATASTAR online - free. CD-ROM from 1990
HOLDINGS: 2,000 books; 170 journals, 140 current titles;
          tape/slides, videotapes (VHS)
CLASSIFICATION: NLM
NETWORK: SWEHSLinC

Tunbridge Wells

626
PEMBURY HOSPITAL MEDICAL LIBRARY
Pembury, Tunbridge Wells, Kent TN2 4QJ
Tel: 0892 82 3535
STAFF: Mrs JM Hurst ALA, Mrs J Barker (part time)
TYPE: Multidisciplinary
HOURS: Mon-Fri 8.30-4.30
READERS: Staff and other users
STOCK POLICY: Books and journals selectively discarded
LENDING: Books and journals. Photocopies provided
COMPUTER DATA RETRIEVAL: DATASTAR, BLAISE online - free
HOLDINGS: 300 books; 51 current journals
 journals
CLASSIFICATION: NLM
NETWORK: SE Thames Regional Library and Information Service

627
PEMBURY HOSPITAL NURSE EDUCATION LIBRARY
Pembury, Tunbridge Wells, Kent TN2 4QJ
Tel: 0892 82 3535 x3119
Mrs PM Maxwell
FOUNDED: 1972
TYPE: Nursing
HOURS: Mon-Thu 8.30-4.30, Fri 8.30-4. Key available outside hours
READERS: Staff and other users
STOCK POLICY: Out of date books selectively discarded
LENDING: Books and journals. Photocopies supplied
COMPUTER DATA RETRIEVAL: Access to terminal.
HOLDINGS: 3,500 books; 23 current journals; 70 videotapes (VHS)
CLASSIFICATION: NLM
NETWORK: SE Thames Regional Library and Information Service;
                    Tunbridge Wells Health Libraries

628
TUNBRIDGE WELLS POSTGRADUATE MEDICAL CENTRE LIBRARY
Kent and Sussex Hospital, Tunbridge Wells, Kent TN4 8AT
Tel: 0892 26111 x2384
STAFF: Miss M Montague BEd(Hons) DipLib
Founded: 1973
TYPE: Multidisciplinary
HOURS: Mon-Fri 9-5
READERS: Staff and other users
STOCK POLICY: Books and journals discarded at varying intervals
LENDING: Books and journals. Photocopies provided
COMPUTER DATA RETRIEVAL: DATASTAR, BLAISE, DIALOG online - free
HOLDINGS: 2,700 books; 150 journals, 120 current titles;
                    15 tape/slides, 10 videotapes (VHS)
CLASSIFICATION: NLM
PUBLICATIONS: Recent additions
NETWORK: SE Thames Regional Library and Information Service

Upton

629
WIRRAL SCHOOL OF NURSING
Arrowe Park Hospital, Upton, Wirral L49 5PE
Tel: 051 678 5111 x2115
STAFF: Ms S Hornby BA DipLib
FOUNDED: 1981
TYPE: Nursing
HOURS: Mon-Fri 8.30-4.30
READERS: Staff and students only

STOCK POLICY: Out of date books discarded
LENDING: Books only. Photocopies provided
COMPUTER DATA RETRIEVAL: In-house terminal. CD-ROM from 1989
HOLDINGS: 17,288 books; 40 journals, 34 current titles
CLASSIFICATION: NLM
NETWORK: Mersey Region

Uxbridge

630
HAREFIELD, HILLINGDON & MOUNT VERNON EDUCATION DIVISION
The Furze, Hillingdon Hospital, Uxbridge, Middx, UB8 3NN
Tel: 0895 57944 x215
STAFF: Librarian post vacant
TYPE: Nursing, midwifery
HOURS: Mon-Fri 8.30-4.30
READERS: Staff and students
STOCK POLICY: Books discarded
LENDING: Books only. Photocopies provided
COMPUTER DATA RETRIEVAL: Access to terminal
HOLDINGS: 93 journals, 69 current titles
CLASSIFICATION: DDC modified
BRANCH: Mount Vernon
NETWORK: NW Thames

631
HILLINGDON HOSPITAL MEDICAL LIBRARY
Post Graduate Centre, Hillingdon Hospital, Uxbridge, Middx, UB8 3NN
Tel: 0895 38282 x3250
STAFF: P Lovegrove BA DipLib ALA
FOUNDED: 1989
TYPE: Medica
HOURS: Mon-Fri 9-5
READERS: Staff and other users
STOCK POLICY: Books discarded after 10 years
LENDING: Books only. Photocopies provided
COMPUTER DATA RETRIEVAL; In-house terminal. CD-ROM
HOLDINGS: 50+ current titles
CLASSIFICATION: NLM
NETWORK: NW Thames

Wakefield

632
WAKEFIELD INFORMATION AND EDUCATION SERVICES
Pinderfields General Hospital, Aberford Road, Wakefield,
West Yorkshire WF1 4DG
Tel: 0924 375217 x2391   Fax: 0924 372079
STAFF: Mrs MM Ward BSc ALA, M Saunders BSc DipLib ALA, P Wiehl BA,
       1 vacant post
FOUNDED: 1971
TYPE: Multidisciplinary
HOURS: Mon-Fri 8.30-5
READERS: Staff and other users. National Demonstration
Centre only open to general public and NHS
STOCK POLICY: Out of date editions of books discarded, journals
                 discarded after 10 years
LENDING: Books, journals and videotapes. Photocopies provided
COMPUTER DATA RETRIEVAL: DATASTAR online - other libraries charged
                 computer time only
HOLDINGS: 7,000 books; 250 current journals; tape/slides, 35mm
                 slides, videotapes (U-matic, VHS)
SPECIAL COLLECTION: Rehabilitation (1,000 vols)
CLASSIFICATION: NLM adapted
PUBLICATION: Rehabilitation bulletin
NETWORK: Yorkshire Joint Medical Library Service
SPLIT SITE: Wakefield Postgraduate Medical Centre (Medicine
and Administration); National Demonstration Centre
(Rehabilitation and Nursing), Wakefield

Walsall

633
MANOR HOSPITAL POSTGRADUATE MEDICAL CENTRE
Moar Road, Walsall, West Midlands WS2 9PS
Tel: 0922 721172
STAFF: Mrs DM Hollingsworth MCSP (Honorary Librarian)
       Mrs C Thomas BSc(Hons) (part time)
FOUNDED: 1970
TYPE: Medical
HOURS: Always open. Staffed Mon-Fri 9-5
READERS: Qualified medical staff
STOCK POLICY: Out of date books discarded
LENDING: Reference only. Photocopies provided
COMPUTER DATA RETRIEVAL: Access to DATASTAR
HOLDINGS: 1,200 books; 210 journals, 92 current titles;
                 200 35mm slides, 34 videotapes (VHS)
CLASSIFICATION: Own
PUBLICATION: Recent acquisitions
NETWORK: West Midlands Region Health Libraries; BCLIP

634
SAINT MATTHEW'S HOSPITAL MEDICAL LIBRARY
Burntwood, Walsall, West Midlands WS7 9ES
Tel: 054 36 5511 x58   Fax: 054 36 73860

STAFF: Mrs R Pitt (part-time)
FOUNDED: 1979
TYPE: Psychiatric
HOURS: Open 24 hours. Staffed Mon-Fri 10-4
READERS: Staff and other users
STOCK POLICY: No stock discarded
LENDING: Books and auudiocassettes only. Photocopies provided
COMPUTER DATA RETRIEVAL: Access to terminal.
HOLDINGS: 1,400 books; 40 current journals; 20 audiotapes,
                19 videotapes (VHS)
CLASSIFICATION: Own
PUBLICATIONS: Information bulletins, library guide
NETWORK: PLCS; West Midlands Regional Health Libraries

635
ST MATTHEWS HOSPITAL NURSE EDUCATION CENTRE
St Matthews Hospital, Burntwood, Walsall, Staffs, WS7 9ES
Tel: 05436 5511 x47
STAFF: Mrs H Kendall
FOUNDED: 1984
TYPE: Health administration, nursing, psychiatry
HOURS: Mon-Fri 8.30-5
READERS: Staff and students
STOCK POLICY: Journals discarded after 6 years
LENDING: Books, resource files. Photocopies provided
HOLDINGS: 18 journals, 16 current titles; 20 sets 35mm slides,
           5 tape/slides, 4 audio tapes, 5 videotapes (VHS)
CLASSIFICATION: LC
BRANCH: Part of 100
NETWORK: West Midlands

636
SISTER DORA SCHOOL OF NURSING
Manor Hospital, Moat Road, Walsall, West Midlands WS2 9PS
Tel: 0922 721172
STAFF: Mrs P Jones (library clerk) (part-time)
FOUNDED: 1979
TYPE: Nursing
HOURS: Mon-Fri 8-4.15. Staffed Mon-Thurs 10.45-4.15, Fri
  10.30-4
READERS: Nursing staff
STOCK POLICY: Journals discarded after 10 years, books
                    discarded occasionally
LENDING: Books and journals. Photocopies provided
HOLDINGS: 3,025 books; 47 journals, 40 current titles;
                 c100 tape/slides, 136 videotapes (VHS)
CLASSIFICATION: DDC (modified)

Warley

637
MIDLAND CENTRE FOR NEUROSURGERY AND NEUROLOGY
Holly Lane, Smethwick, Warley, West Midlands B67 7JX
Tel: 021 558 3232 x350
STAFF: Mrs J Moore BA ALA
FOUNDED: c1950
TYPE: Medical
HOURS: Always open. Staffed Mon-Fri 8.30-5
READERS: Staff and other users
STOCK POLICY: Books selectively discarded
LENDING: Books and journals. Photocopies provided
COMPUTER DATA RETRIEVAL: Access to terminal.
HOLDINGS: 2,000 books; c4,000 bound journals, 60 current titles
SPECIAL COLLECTIONS: AL Woolf (neuropathology); Jack Small
 (neurosurgery and neurology); IA Guest Memorial collection
 (ca 200 vols in all)
CLASSIFICATION: Own
PUBLICATION: Library guide
NETWORK: West Midlands Regional Health Libraries

Warwick

638
SOUTH WARWICKSHIRE MEDICAL EDUCATION CENTRE LIBRARY
John Turner Building, S Warwickshire Hospital, Lakin Road,
Warwick CV34 5BW
Tel: 0926 495321 x4287
STAFF:Job share - Mrs H Hewison BA(Hons) ALA & Mrs VA Dalton
FOUNDED: 1986
TYPE: Medical, dental
HOURS: Mon-Fri 9-5.30
READERS: Medical staff (not nursing), GP's, Social Workers
STOCK POLICY: Books discarded after 5 years
LENDING: Books and journals. Photocopies provided
COMPUTER DATA RETRIEVAL: DATASTAR online - free
HOLDINGS: 2,000 books; 60 journals, 57 current titles;
                20 videotapes (VHS)
CLASSIFICATION: NLM
BRANCH: Psychiatric Library, Central Hospital, Warwick; Warneford
                Hospital, Leamington Spa
NETWORK: West Midlands Regional Health Libraries

Waterford

639
WATERFORD REGIONAL HOSPITAL
Ardkeen, Waterford, Republic of Ireland
Tel: 010 353 51 73321
STAFF: Miss A Tierney (Acting Librarian)
TYPE: Multidisciplinary
HOURS: Mon-Fri 9.20-1, 2-5.20

READERS: Staff and other users
LENDING: Books, videotapes only
HOLDINGS: 1,538 books, 75 bound journals; 20 current
 journals. 16 mm cine films, tape/slides, 35 mm slides,
 videotapes (VHS)
CLASSIFICATION: Title and author
NETWORK: SEHB

Watford

640
WATFORD POSTGRADUATE MEDICAL CENTRE
Watford General Hospital, Vicarage Road, Watford, Herts WD1 8HB
Tel: 0923 244366 x437
STAFF: Miss JE Reynolds BA MSc CertEd DipLib (part time)
TYPE: Medical
HOURS: Mon-Fri 9-5. Access available at other times.
                    Staffed Mon-Thu 9-4
READERS: Medical staff, other users for reference only
STOCK POLICY: Under review
LENDING: Books and journals. photocopies provided
COMPUTER DATA RETRIEVAL: DATASTAR online - charging policy under
                review. CD-ROM available
HOLDINGS: 1,100 books; 70 current journals; tape/slides,
                35mm slides, videotapes
CLASSIFICATION: Barnard (converting to NLM)
NETWORK: NW Thames Regional Library and Information Service

641
WEST HERTFORDSHIRE COLLEGE OF NURSING (SOUTH WEST DISTRICT)
Peace Prospect, Watford, herts, WD1 3HA
Tel: 0923 228343
STAFF: Miss MS Cowlard ALA, Miss SJ Kellett BA DipLib
FOUNDED: 1970
TYPE: Multidisciplinary
HOURS: Mon-Fri 8.30-4.30
READERS: Nursing staff
STOCK POLICY: Books discarded after 10 years, journals
 discarded after 5 years
LENDING: Books only. Photocopies provided
HOLDINGS: 6,000 books; 27 current journals
CLASSIFICATION: DDC
SPECIAL COLLECTIONS: Programmed texts; Students' projects
PUBLICATION: Additions list
BRANCHES: St Pauls, Hemel Hempstead; Leavesden Hospital, Abbots
                    Langley
NETWORK: NW Thames Regional Nursing Libraries; SW Herts Health
                    Authority Libraries

642
NORTH AND EAST HERTS SCHOOL OF NURSING (EAST SITE)
Queen Elizabeth II Hospital, Howlands, Welwyn Garden City,
  Hertfordshire AL7 4HQ
Tel: 0707 328111
STAFF: Mrs J Spruce ALA (part time)
FOUNDED: 1964
TYPE: NURSING
HOURS: 8.30-4.30 (First hour not staffed)
READERS: Staff, hospital and community nurses
STOCK POLICY: Books discarded after 5-10 years
LENDING: Books, AV material. Photocopies provided
COMPUTER DATA RETRIEVAL: Access to DATASTAR online. CD-ROM from 1983
HOLDINGS: 2,500 books; 30 current titles; 35mm slides, tape/slides,
             150 videotapes (VHS)
BRANCH: Hertford County Hospital
NETWORK: NW Thames; Hertfordshire County Library Service

643
QUEEN ELIZABETH II HOSPITAL
Howlands, Welwyn Garden City, Herts AL7 4HQ
Tel: 0707 328111 x4565
STAFF: Mrs JJ Roberts ALA
FOUNDED: 1963
TYPE: Multidisciplinary
HOURS: 9.30-5.15 daily
READERS: Staff, other users at discretion of Librarian
STOCK POLICY: Unbound journals discarded afer 5 years, bound
     journals discarded after 15 years. Books discarded after 10
LENDING: Books only. Photocopies provided
COMPUTER DATA RETRIEVAL: DATASTAR online - free. CD-ROM from 1989
HOLDINGS: 5,000 vols; 100 current journals
CLASSIFICATION: NLM
BRANCH: Hertford County Hospital
NETWORK: NW Thames Regional Library and Information Service

644
ROCHE PRODUCTS LIMITED
PO Box 8, 40 Broadwater Road, Welwyn Garden City, Herts, AL7 3AY
Tel: 0707 328128   Telex 262098 ROCHEW   Fax: 0707 338297
STAFF: NE Allen BSc ALA, 1 other (full-time), 1 (part-time) staff
TYPE: Medical, Pharmacology
HOURS: Mon-Fri 7.45-6
READERS: Staff only
STOCK POLICY: Books and journals discarded at varying intervals
LENDING: Books and journals. Photocopies provided
COMPUTER DATA RETRIEVAL: DATASTAR, BLAISE online. CD-ROM from 1988
HOLDINGS: 10,000 books; 15,000 journals, 850 current titles
CLASSIFICATION: UDC

645
SMITHKLINE BEECHAM PHARMACEUTICALS, RESEARCH AND DEVELOPMENT
The Frythe, Welwyn Garden City, Herts AL6 9AR
Tel: 0707 325111   Telex 261347   Fax: 0438 71 7612
Electronic mail: Telecom Gold 75: SNS001
STAFF: JR Sherwell MLib FLA MIInfSc, Mrs J Borutan BA ALA
FOUNDED: 1981
TYPE: Pharmaceutical
HOURS: Mon-Fri 9-4.45
READERS: Staff, other users by prior arrangement
STOCK POLICY: Out of date or duplicated stock discarded
LENDING: Books and journals. Photocopies provided
COMPUTER DATA RETRIEVAL: DATASTAR, DIALOG, STN, ORBIT online.
                        CD-ROM from 1988
HOLDINGS: 6,500 books; 400 journals, 325 current titles;
                       500 microfilms, 10 videotapes (VHS)
CLASSIFICATION: UDC (modified)
PUBLICATIONS: Accessions bulletin; Holdings list; Library guides
BRANCH: SKB Pharmaceuticals R & D, Tonbridge, Kent
NETWORK: HERTIS

West Bromwich

646
SANDWELL HEALTH AUTHORITY, MEDICAL DEPARTMENT LIBRARY
Kingston House, 438 High Street, West Bromwich, West
 Midlands B70 9LD
Tel: 021 553 6151 x262
STAFF: Dr M Harrison MB BS BA DPH FPCM (Honorary Librarian),
    Mrs CD Nash, Mrs J Bush
TYPE: Multidisciplinary
HOURS: Mon-Fri 9-5
READERS: Staff and other users
STOCK POLICY: Out of date books discarded
LENDING: Books and journals
COMPUTER DATA RETRIEVAL: Access to terminal.
HOLDINGS: 3,300 books; 35 current journals.
NETWORK: West Midlands Region Health Libraries

647
SANDWELL DISTRICT GENERAL HOSPITAL, MEDICAL LIBRARY
Lyndon, West Bromwich, West Midlands B71 4HJ
Tel: 021 553 1831 x3587   Electronic mail: DATAMAIL
STAFF: Mrs R Zalin BA(Econ) ALA (part-time), 1 other staff
FOUNDED: 1972
TYPE: Medical
HOURS: Mon-Fri 9-10. Staffed Mon-Fri 9.30-4.30
READERS: Staff only
STOCK POLICY: Books discarded after 10 years
LENDING: Books only. Photocopies provided
COMPUTER DATA RETRIEVAL: DATASTAR online - charged computer time
                    only
HOLDINGS: 1,500 books; 1,000 bound journals,100 current titles
CLASSIFICATION: NLM
NETWORK: West Midlands Region Health Libraries; BCLIP

648
SANDWELL SCHOOL OF NURSING LIBRARY
Sandwell District General Hospital, Lyndon, West Bromwich,
 West Midlands B71 4HJ
Tel: 021 553 1831 x3645
STAFF: Mrs G Grigson, Mrs J Turley
TYPE: Nursing
HOURS: Mon-Fri 8.30-4.30 (Tues to 6.30)
READERS: Nursing staff only
LENDING: Books only
COMPUTER DATA RETRIEVAL: In-house terminal.
HOLDINGS: 2,500 books; 30 current journals; Tape/slides,
                        videotapes (VHS)
CLASSIFICATION: Bliss
NETWORK: West Midlands Regional Health Libraries

Westcliff-on-Sea

649
SOUTHEND-ON-SEA POSTGRADUATE MEDICAL CENTRE/SE ESSEX SCHOOL OF
NURSING
Southend Hospital, Prittlewell Chase, Westcliff-on-Sea,
 Essex SS0 0RY
Tel: 0702 348911
STAFF: Miss NC Henwood BLS ALA, Mrs R Syers ALA (part-time)
TYPE: Multidisciplinary
HOURS: Nursing Library: 8.30-4.30. Medical Library: 33 hours pw)
READERS: Staff, other users on application to Librarian
STOCK POLICY: Books discarded when new edition published
LENDING: Books only. Photocopies provided
COMPUTER DATA RETRIEVAL: DATASTAR online - free to medical staff,
                other users charged
CLASSIFICATION: NLM
BRANCH: Rochford General Hospital, Rochford
NETWORKS: NE Thames; Essex County Libraries; Anglia Institute of
           Higher Education

Weston super Mare

650
WESTON SUPER MARE GENERAL HOSPITAL, EDUCATION CENTRE LIBRARY
Grange Rd, Uphill, Weston super Mare, Avon, BS23 4TQ
Tel: 0934 636363 x3806
STAFF: Mrs D Smithson ALA (part time)
TYPE: Multidisciplinary
HOURS: Open 24 hours (staffed part time)

READERS: Staff only
STOCK POLICY: Books discarded after 10 years
COMPUTER DATA RETRIEVAL: Access to DATASTAR online
HOLDINGS: 670 books; 46 journals; videotapes (66 Betamax, 11 VHS)
CLASSIFICATION: NLM
NETWORK: SWEHSLinC

Weybridge

651
MINISTRY OF AGRICULTURE, FISHERIES AND FOOD
Central Veterinary Laboratory, New Haw, Weybridge, Surrey
 KT15 3NB
Tel: 09323 4111   Telex 262318   Fax: 09323 47046
STAFF: Mrs EA Maclachlan MA DipLib ALA MIInfSc, Miss HE Johnson
 BA, Mrs J McCappin MSc ALA, Miss K Townsend MA,
 Miss L Hutchinson BSc DipLib
TYPE: Medical, pharmacy and veterinary
HOURS: Mon-Fri 8.30-6. Staffed Mon-Thurs 8.30-5, Fri 8.30-4.30
READERS: Staff. Other users for reference only, on application
STOCK POLICY: Out of date non-veterinary books and journals
                discarded
LENDING: Books and journals
COMPUTER DATA RETRIEVAL: In-house terminal. Free to MAFF staff,
                charged to non-MAFF staff
HOLDINGS: 21,650 books, 37,000 bound journals; 950 current
 journals. 16 mm cine films, tape/slides, 35 mm slides
CLASSIFICATION: Barnard (modified)
PUBLICATION: Current awareness list
NETWORK: Ministry of Agriculture, Fisheries and Food
BRANCH: Ministry of Agriculture, Fisheries and Food,
 Tolworth

Wickford

652
RUNWELL HOSPITAL, ASHLEY ROBIN LIBRARY
Wickford, Essex, SS11 7QE
Tel: 0268 735555 x420
STAFF: Miss NC Henwood BLS ALA (District Librarian),
             Mrs YP Abbott (part time)
FOUNDED: 1935
TYPE: Psychiatric
HOURS: Keyholders only
READERS: Staff only
STOCK POLICY: No stock discarded
LENDING: Books and journals. Photocopies provided
COMPUTER DATA RETRIEVAL: Access to terminal
HOLDINGS: 400 books; 60 current journals
CLASSIFICATION: Own
NETWORK: NE Thames

653
WIGAN AND LEIGH MEDICAL INSTITUTE
Thomas Linacre House, Wigan Infirmary, Wigan, Lancs WN1 2NN
Tel: 0942 822508
STAFF: Mrs MB Gerrard (part-time)
FOUNDED: 1974
TYPE: Multidisciplinary
HOURS: 24 hours to members. Staffed Mon-Fri 10-4
READERS: Staff only
STOCK POLICY: Journals discarded after 10 years, very few books
                        discarded
LENDING: Books only. Photocopies provided to other libraries
COMPUTER DATA RETRIEVAL: DATASTAR online - free
HOLDINGS: 1,800 books; 60 current journals.
CLASSIFICATION: LC
BRANCH: Leigh Postgraduate Centre

654
WIGAN AREA SCHOOL OF NURSING
Area Education Centre, The Elms, Wigan Lane, Wigan WN1 2NN
Tel: 0942 44000 x368
STAFF: Mrs R Melia BA ALA
TYPE: Multidisciplinary
HOURS: Mon-Fri 9-5
READERS: Nursing staff
STOCK POLICY: Books over 10 years old discarded
LENDING: Books only
HOLDINGS: 4,500 books; 35 current journals. 16mm cine
 films, tape/slides, 35mm slides, videotapes (Philips, VHS)
CLASSIFICATION: NLM
PUBLICATION: Library guide
NETWORK: NW Nursing Librarians Group

Winchester

655
WESSEX REGIONAL HEALTH AUTHORITY, HEADQUARTERS LIBRARY
Highcroft, Romsey Road, Winchester, Hants SO22 5DH
Tel: 0962 63511
STAFF: Mrs SF Pilsworth BA(Hons) ALA (part-time)
TYPE: Health administration
HOURS: STAFFED Mon-Fri 9-4
READERS: Staff only
STOCK POLICY: Varied, depends on subject matter
LENDING: Books and journals. Photocopies provided

COMPUTER DATA RETRIEVAL: DATASTAR online - free
HOLDINGS: c5,000 books; 166 journals, 100 current titles
CLASSIFICATION: NLM (amended)
NETWORK: HATRICS; WRLIS

656
WINCHESTER HEALTH AUTHORITY DISTRICT LIBRARY
Education Centre, Royal Hampshire County Hospital, Winchester,
Hants, SO22 5DG
Tel: 0962 824421   Fax: 0962 824659
STAFF: Ms C Dobson BA(Hons) CHSM ALA, Ms H Bingham BSc MSc,
      J Forni BA(Hons), Ms S Metcalfe BA(Hons)
TYPE: Multidisciplinary
READERS: Staff and other users
STOCK POLICY: Journals discarded after 30 years, books discarded
            after 10 years
LENDING: Books, journals, AV material. Photocopies provided
COMPUTER DATA RETRIEVAL: DATASTAR online . CD-ROM from 1989
HOLDINGS: books, journals, 35 mm slides, 86 tape/slides, 6 films,
            34 videotapes (VHS)
CLASSIFICATION: NLM (Wessex modification)
PUBLICATION: Guide to the District Library and Information Service
BRANCHES: at 9 hospitals/departments
NETWORK: WRLIS; HATRICS

Windlesham

657
LILLY RESEARCH CENTRE LIMITED
Erl Wood Manor, London Road, Windlesham, Surrey GU20 6PH
Tel: 0276 78344   Telex 858177   Fax: 0276 74390
STAFF: JA Wickenden ALA
FOUNDED: 1967
TYPE: Pharmacology
HOURS: Mon-Fri 8.30-4.30
READERS: Staff only
STOCK POLICY: Journals discarded
LENDING: Reference only. Photocopies provided
COMPUTER DATA RETRIEVAL: Online databases: DATASTAR, BLAISE,
        TELESYSTEMES, ORBIT, DIALOG, IRS, STN, PFDS.
            CD-ROM from 1978. PRESTEL available
HOLDINGS: 5,000 books; 450 journals, 370 current titles
CLASSIFICATION: UDC
NETWORK: HATRICS; SASLIC

Windsor

658
EAST BERKSHIRE DISTRICT LIBRARY AND INFORMATION SERVICE
John Lister Library, Postgraduate Medical Centre,
King Edward VII Hospital, Windsor, Berks SL4 3DR
Tel: 0753 860441 x6406/6407
STAFF: Ms S Pallot SRN ALA, Ms V Bonham ALA (part time)
TYPE: Multidisciplinary
HOURS: Open access at all times. Staffed Mon-Fri 9-5.30
READERS: Staff and other users
STOCK POLICY: Under revision
LENDING: Books and precurrent journals. Photocopies provided
COMPUTER DATA RETRIEVAL: DATASTAR, BLAISE online - charging policy
under review
HOLDINGS: 900 books; 90 current journals
CLASSIFICATION: NLM
BRANCHES: Heatherwood Hospital, Ascot; Churchill House, Bracknell;
Health Promotions Unit, Old Windsor
NETWORK: LASER; Oxford Region Library and Information Service; BLIP

Wolverhampton

659
COMBINED TRAINING CENTRE LIBRARY
New Cross Hospital, Wolverhampton Rd, Wolverhampton, WV10 0QP
Tel: 0902 732255 x2603
STAFF: Miss JH Paterson, Miss P Davis (Nursing Services),
Miss S Jukes
TYPE: Multidisciplinary
HOURS: Mon-Thu 9-5, Fri 9-4.30
READERS: All hospital staff
HOLDINGS: 10,000 books; 15 current journals
CLASSIFICATION: LC
NETWORK: West Midlands

660
ROYAL HOSPITAL, BELL LIBRARY
Royal Hospital, Cleveland Road, Wolverhampton WV2 1BT
Tel: 0902 351532 x4452
STAFF: Miss JH Paterson, Mrs ER Bayliss, Miss S Jukes
FOUNDED: 1879
TYPE: Multidisciplinary
HOURS: Mon-Thu 8.30-5, Fri 8.30-4.30
LENDING: Books only. Photocopies provided
COMPUTER DATA RETRIEVAL: Access to BLAISE
HOLDINGS: 1,329 books; 64 journals, 61 current titles
CLASSIFICATION: LC
NETWORK: West Midlands Region Health Libraries

661
SOUTH STAFFORDSHIRE POSTGRADUATE MEDICAL CENTRE
New Cross Hospital, Wednesfield, Wolverhampton WV10 0QP
Tel: 0902 732255 x2166
STAFF: Miss JH Paterson, Mrs EA Bayliss, Miss S Jukes
FOUNDED: 1970
TYPE: Multidisciplinary
HOURS: Mon-Thu 8.30-5, Fri 8.30-4.30
LENDING: Books only. Photocopies supplied
COMPUTER DATA RETRIEVAL: Access to BLAISE online
HOLDINGS: 2,184 books; 162 journals, 143 current titles
CLASSIFICATION: LC
NETWORK: West Midlands Region Health Libraries

662
WOLVERHAMPTON AND MIDLAND COUNTIES EYE INFIRMARY
Compton Road, Wolverhampton, WV3 9QR
Tel: 0902 26731 x428
STAFF: Miss JH Paterson
TYPE: Ophthalmology
HOURS: Staffed Wed 11.15-12.30
READERS: Staff only, other users for reference
COMPUTER DATA RETRIEVA: Access to terminal
HOLDINGS: 280 books; 7 current journals
NETWORK: West Midlands

Woodford Bridge

663
CLAYBURY HOSPITAL, DENIS MARTIN LIBRARY
Woodford Bridge, Essex IG8 8BY
Tel: 081 504 7171 x131
STAFF: Ms DM Hall BA ALA
FOUNDED: 1974
TYPE: Multidisciplinary
HOURS: Mon-Fri 9.30-5
READERS: Staff, other users for reference only
LENDING: Books only. Photocopies provided
COMPUTER DATA RETRIEVAL: Access to terminal.
HOLDINGS: 3,000 books; 50 journals, 40 current titles
CLASSIFICATION: DDC
NETWORK: NE Thames Regional Library and Information Service; PLCS

664
CHARLES HASTINGS POSTGRADUATE MEDICAL CENTRE LIBRARY
Worcester Royal Infirmary, Ronkswood Branch, Newtown Road,
 Worcester WR5 1HN
Tel: 0905 763333
STAFF: Dr I Davis (Honorary Librarian), Mrs C Spencer-Bamford
                                            (part-time)
TYPE: Multidisciplinary
HOURS: Mon-Fri 9-5. Staffed Mon, Fri 9-12, Wed, Thu 9-3
READERS: Consultants, doctors, GP's, and medical disciplines
STOCK POLICY: Books and journals discarded after 10 years
COMPUTER DATA RETRIEVAL: Access to terminal.
HOLDINGS: 800 books; 135 journals, 103 current titles
CLASSIFICATION: Own
BRANCH: Worcester Royal Infirmary (Castle St Branch)
NETWORK: West Midlands Regional Health Libraries

665
WORCESTER AND DISTRICT HEALTH AUTHORITY
Isaac Maddox House, Shrub Hill Road, Worcester, WR4 9RW
Tel: 0905 763333
STAFF: D Jones MA DipLib ALA (part time)
FOUNDED: 1986
TYPE: Health administration, medical
HOURS: Office hours (Staffed 2 mornings)
READERS: Staff only
STOCK POLICY: Books discarded
LENDING: Books and journals. Photocopies provided
COMPUTER DATA RETRIEVAL: DATASTAR online - charged
HOLDINGS: 3,000 books; 40 journals, 30 current titles
CLASSIFICATION: NLM (Wessex modification)
PUBLICATION: Guide; Bi-monthly bulletin
NETWORK: West Midlands

666
WORCESTER DISTRICT SCHOOL OF NURSING
Newtown Road, Worcester WR5 1HT
Tel: 0905 763333 x34309
STAFF: Mrs J Davis
TYPE: Nursing, Psychiatric
HOURS: Mon-Fri 8.15-4.15
READERS: Staff, other users for reference only
STOCK POLICY: Books over 10 years old discarded
LENDING: Books and AV material. Photocopies provided
HOLDINGS: c5,000 books; 50 journals, 35 current titles;
                tape/slides, 35mm slides, videotapes (U-matic, VHS)
CLASSIFICATION: DDC
NETWORK: West Midlands Region Health Libraries

667
WORCESTER ROYAL INFIRMARY, NEWTOWN BRANCH
Newtown Road, Worcester WR5 1JG
Tel: 0905 763333 x33161
STAFF: Mrs WP Schwab MA (part time)
FOUNDED: 1963. Moved to present site 1978
TYPE: Medical, psychiatric, psychology and addictions
HOURS: Mon-Thurs 8.30-12.30.
LENDING: Books and AV material only. Photocopies provided
COMPUTER DATA RETRIEVAL: Access to terminal.
HOLDINGS: 1,5 00 books; 48 journals, 30 current titles
CLASSIFICATION: Own
NETWORK: West Midlands Regional Health Libraries; Worcester
 and District Health Authority; PLCS

Wordsley

668
WORDSLEY HOSPITAL MEDICAL LIBRARY
Stream Road, Wordsley, West Midlands, DY8 5QX
Tel: 0384 288778
STAFF: Mrs BA Bolton ALA   (part time)
TYPE: Medica˙
HOURS: Open during day. Staffed Tue 12.30-1.30
READERS: Staff only
STOCK POLICY: Journals discarded after 12 years, books discarded
                after 10 years
LENDING: Books and journals
COMPUTER DATA RETRIEVAL: Access to DATASTAR - charged full cost
HOLDINGS: 600 books; 6 current journals
CLASSIFICATION: NLM
SPECIAL COLLECTION: Obstetric collection in Obstetric Unit
                Library (100 vols)
NETWORK: West Midlands

Worthing

669
SMITHKLINE BEECHAM PHARMACEUTICALS RESEARCH DIVISION
Clarendon Road, Worthing, Sussex BN14 8QH
Tel: 0903 39900 x423   Telex 87418
No furthur information available

670
WORTHING POSTGRADUATE CENTRE, DISTRICT HEALTH SCIENCES LIBRARY
Homefield Road, Worthing, West Sussex BN11 2HY
Tel: 0903 205111 x606
STAFF: Ms SJ Merriott ALA LCH (District Librarian), Mrs T Royce
       (part time), Mrs K Foxon (part time)
FOUNDED: c1975
TYPE: Multidisciplinary
HOURS: Mon-Fri 9-5
READERS: Staff, other users at discretion of Librarian
STOCK POLICY: Books discarded after 10 years
LENDING: Books and journals. Photocopies provided
COMPUTER DATA RETRIEVAL: DATASTAR, BLAISE online - free
HOLDINGS: 5,000 books; 220 journals, 156 current titles
CLASSIFICATION: NLM
NETWORK: SW Thames Regional Library and Information Service
BRANCH: Southlands Hospital, Shoreham-by-Sea

Wrexham

671
WREXHAM MEDICAL INSTITUTE, JOHN SPALDING LIBRARY
Technology Park Centre, Croesnewydd Rd, Wrexham, Clwyd LL13 7YP
Tel: 0978 291100
STAFF: Ms M McKeon BA DipLib ALA
TYPE: Medical
HOURS: Mon-Fri 9-5
READERS: Staff and other users
STOCK POLICY: Stock discarded
LENDING: Books and journals. Photocopies provided
COMPUTER DATA RETRIEVAL: DATASTAR, BLAISE online - free
        CD-ROM from 1990
HOLDINGS: 2,000 books; 150 journals
NETWORK: Clwyd Health Authority

Yeovil

672
SIR JOHN ENGLISH MEDICAL LIBRARY
Marsh-Jackson, Postgraduate Centre, Yeovil District Hospital,
  Higher Kingston, Yeovil, Somerset BA21 4AT
Tel: 0935 707495
STAFF: Mrs J Hill ALA (part time)
FOUNDED: 1974
TYPE: Multidisciplinary
HOURS: Always open. Staffed Mon-Fri 9-1.30

READERS: Staff, other users at discretion of librarian
STOCK POLICY: Books discarded after 10 years
LENDING: Books, journals, AV material. Photocopies provided
COMPUTER DATA RETRIEVAL: DATASTAR online - free
HOLDINGS: c1,500 books; 120 current journals; 35mm slides,
          tape/slides, videotapes (VHS)
CLASSIFICATION: NLM
NETWORK: SWEHSLinC

York

673
YORK AND SCARBOROUGH COLLEGE OF MIDWIFERY AND NURSING
Floor 3, Administration Block, York District Hospital,
 Wigginton Road, York YO3 7HE
Tel: 0904 631313 x4300/4301
STAFF: Mrs KM Smith C&G BEC DipLib
FOUNDED: 1975
TYPE: Multidisciplinary
HOURS: Mon-Thurs 9.15-4.30, Fri 9.15-3.
READERS: Staff , other users at Librarian's discretion
STOCK POLICY: Books discarded selectively after 10 years
LENDING: Books and non-current journals. Self service photocopying
COMPUTER DATA RETRIEVAL: DATASTAR online.
HOLDINGS: 10,000 books; 60 journals
CLASSIFICATION: Barnard
SPECIAL COLLECTION: Mental handicap (1,600 vols)
PUBLICATION: Acquisitions list
NETWORK: YRAHCLIS; Nursing Information Group (Yorkshire Region)

674
YORK DISTRICT HOSPITAL
 Wigginton Road, York YO3 7HE
Tel:0904 631313 x4300 & 4301
STAFF: Mrs MJ Rees MA DipLib ALA (part-time)
TYPE: Multidisciplinary
HOURS: Mon-Thu 9.15-4.30, Fri 9.15-1
READERS: Staff, other users for reference
STOCK POLICY: Books discarded after 7 years
LENDING: Books and journals
COMPUTER DATA RETRIEVAL: Access to DATASTAR. Free
HOLDINGS: 7,000 books; 160 journals, 130 current titles
CLASSIFICATION: Barnard
BRANCHES: Clifton Hospital, Bootham Hospital (both mental health)
NETWORK: YRAHCLIS

The following entry was received too late for inclusion at the correct place in the alphabet.

675
EAST RODING SCHOOL OF NURSING
Hedgecock Centre, Barking Hospital, Upney Lane, Barking, Essex, IG11 9LX
Tel: 081 594 5774
STAFF: SJ Johnson ALA
TYPE: Nursing, psychiatric
HOURS: Mon-Fri 8.30-4.30
READERS: Staff and students
STOCK POLICY: Books discarded at varying intervals
LENDING: Books only. photocopies provided
COMPUTER DATA RETRIEVAL: DATASTAR online. PRESTEL available
HOLDINGS: 7,000 books; 50 journals, 40 current titles; 30 tape/slides,
    100 35mm slides, 500 videotapes (VHS)
CLASSIFICATION: RCN
NETWORK: NE Thames

INDEXES

In all cases, reference is to entry number,
NOT to page number

Index of personal names

Boulton A, 82
Boulton C, 600, 602
Bradbury D, 69
Bradley A, 624
Bradley D, 544
Bradley E, 50
Brady D, 416
Brain S, 572
Brazier H, 173
Bremer R, 340
Brewer J, 371
Brewster PA, 313, 316
Brice LH, 453
Bridges H, 465
Brierley B, 504
Brooke ES, 359
Brophy P, 541
Brotherton SV, 41
Brown A, 381
Brown RC, 259
Brown RD, 219
Brown T, 128
Browne EF, 351
Bryson J, 129
Buchanan DS, 349
Bull E, 358
Bullimore A, 257
Bulman MJ, 143
Bunch AJ, 207
Burgess M, 138
Burgess VJ, 485
Burkinshaw K, 578
Burnett J, 28
Bush J, 646
Bush M, 78
Butler ME, 216
Bye V, 127

Campbell-Lendrum D, 228
Cann JC, 390
Cannell SE, 211
Cantwell IA, 355
Carley W, 66
Carlsen U-B, 302
Carmel MJ, 262
Carmichael A, 51
Carney BS, 338
Carney Sr de Lourdes, 172
Carr C, 583
Carter BA, 62, 266
Carter Mrs K, 163
Carter Ms K, 357
Carter MF, 508
Cartmell B, 65
Carver ME, 311, 315

Cawthorne MC, 107
Charlton A, 53
Chatarji DJ, 438
Checketts H, 388
Cheney C, 413
Chester S, 570
Chetwynd SM, 556
Christie M, 228
Clackson A, 250
Clapham A, 1
Claridge JM, 55
Clark K, 369
Clarke AG, 158
Clarke JM, 578
Clarke P, 372
Clarke Mrs P, 287
Clarke RE, 423
Clay D, 502
Clayton RM, 170
Clements B, 111
Clemo E, 608
Clennett MA, 334
Cobb A, 576
Coffey S, 459
Coggins AJ, 500
Colclough J, 430
Cole BJ, 496
Cole CA, 387
Coleman D, 365
Coleman M, 543
Colley AM, 253
Collings L, 606
Collins A, 496
Collins AMK, 313
Colman M, 549
Coltart IC, 203
Common DJ, 55
Compton P, 488
Connell D, 122
Connolly J, 74
Conway K, 165
Conyers T, 348
Cook S, 341
Cook SC, 353
Cooke R, 132
Cooney GdeL, 172
Cooper AB, 349
Cooper LD, 323
Corfe S, 325
Couch AS, 361
Couchman JD, 310
Coulshed J, 461
Court C, 155
Cover SE, 118
Cowan I, 184

Owen PD, 497

Pace C, 606
Packter E, 191
Padden SCR, 460
Padley C, 215
Padmore JH, 161
Pallot S, 658
Palmer ND, 418
Palmer RJ, 441
Pantry S, 575
Parker TA, 400
Parkin J, 350
Parkinson M, 145
Parr C, 606
Parr J, 66
Parr LJ, 389
Parry CD, 66
Paton E, 521
Paterson JH, 659, 660, 661
Patience EJ, 96
Patterson ME, 31
Paul AA, 109
Paull MA, 79
Paullada BL, 76
Payne JM, 204
Payne L, 379
Peacock GR, 435
Peacock S, 4
Pearson J, 16
Peeler L, 178
Pegg MA, 458
Pegler C, 83
Perkins VA, 443
Perrett AJ, 252
Perry HJ, 254
Perry M, 450
Phelps D, 542
Phillips CA, 599
Phillips J, 154
Picken FM, 386
Pilsworth SF, 655
Pirie W, 3
Pitman B, 537
Pitt R, 634
Plackett M, 407
Plaice C, 86
Playfair J, 199
Podmore W, 339
Polson J, 521
Poole G, 81
Poole VJ, 66
Porch L, 128
Porter C, 490

Powell A, 619
Poyner A, 281
Preston A, 552
Price RM, 441
Prior P, 624
Pritchard SJ, 123
Procter G, 454
Pullin C, 380
Pullum A, 62
Purry M, 136
Purry SJ, 123
Pye BC, 569

Radford E, 279
Raffan A, 389
Rampersad AM, 168
Randall J, 358
Rangeley PA, 458
Rawle P, 77
Ray A, 573
Reddy SN, 457
Reed E, 353
Rees JR, 617, 619
Rees MJ, 674
Reeves J, 535
Rehahn A, 372
Reid J, 223
Rendall JRS, 278
Renwick C, 370
Reynolds JE, 640
Reynolds WM, 105
Richards S, 625
Rigden P, 25
Riley CL, 63
Riley L, 528
Ritchie M, 305
Roach M, 296
Roberts FW, 115
Roberts J, 643
Roberts T, 465
Robertson B, 223
Robertson S, 351
Robertson WJ, 344
Robins ME, 243
Robinson BE, 288
Roddham M, 141
Roddis G, 576
Rodgers AM, 242
Rogers DJ, 140
Rossi PM, 278
Rothon L, 268
Rouse M, 75
Rowlands MJ, 66
Roy K, 300

Royce T, 670
Ruch A, 493
Rudd D, 66
Ruffle CC, 222
Rumsey DJ, 28
Rushford MA, 527
Russell CE, 352
Russell H, 348
Russell JA, 241
Russell-Edu W, 356
Ryan JH, 498
Ryan P, 378

Sadler L, 622
Saich BP, 553
St Aubyn PM, 206
Salehi-Jones M, 421, 424
Salter R, 353
Samuels M, 326
Sandeman N, 182
Sanderson M, 448
Sanson JM, 305
Saunders GO, 245
Saunders M, 632
Saunders MM, 31
Sawers C, 262
Scade L, 305
Schupbach WM, 441
Schwab WP, 667
Sclater C, 157, 185, 251
Scott J, 56
Scott Jane, 207
Sellers JM, 485
Semple P, 372
Sen A, 347
Senior KW, 66
Sewell RE, 109
Shapland-Howes P, 561
Sharma L, 570
Sharman J, 119
Shaw DF, 519
Shaw JG, 321
Shepherd A, 398
Shepherd L, 356
Sherwell J, 645
Sherwood FK, 402
Shewring L, 122
Shipton RC, 418
Sidoli E, 366
Simpson P, 298
Singleton VA, 85
Skene S, 496
Skinner AP, 491
Slade S, 570

Smalley P, 549
Smart H, 249
Smethurst J, 531
Smith A, 91
Smith C, 261
Smith CA, 160
Smith CM, 478, 479
Smith Mrs CM, 11
Smith D, 510
Smith EM, 555
Smith GHR, 219
Smith JE, 269
Smith JM, 206
Smith Km, 673
Smith Marianne 201
Smith Marie 306
Smith MC 184
Smith Mrs P, 552
Smith Mrs Paula 324
Smith PF, 438
Smith S, 570
Smith Mrs S, 340
Smith SE, 418
Smithson D, 650
Smurthwaite D, 624
Smyth S, 208
Smyth TM, 497
Snowball R, 511
Snowdon L, 489
Somers RL, 123
Soper R, 120, 123, 523
South E, 373
Sowerby Mrs , 65
Spencer B, 499
Spencer-Bamford C, 664
Springer JM, 597
Spruce J, 642
Spurrier HL, 620
Stallion S, 443
Stansbury T, 406
Stanton WJ, 500
Stephen D, 494
Stephen JM, 366
Stephens SE, 568
Stephenson GE, 288
Stephenson J, 598
Stevens D, 332
Stevens J, 123, 124
Stevenson AM, 201
Stevenson J, 319, 320
Stewart DC, 233
Stewart DWC, 411
Stockbridge-Bland C, 396
Stokes PC, 409

Stone JMC, 409
Storey C, 372
Storey S, 618
Strange A, 543, 544
Stratford D, 594
Stubbs I, 469
Summers P, 404
Summers R, 321
Sutton HB, 441
Swain SJ, 255
Swash GD, 451
Swerdlow S, 29
Syers R, 649
Symons HJM, 441
Szaygbuski W, 452

Tabor RB, 598
Tarbox S, 148
Taylor HE, 262
Taylor MR, 415
Taylor SL, 586
Teggart P, 447
Telford DR, 307
Thain A, 344
Tharratt PM, 432
Thevakarrunai N, 417
Thom M, 204
Thomas C, 633
Thomas H, 398
Thomas J, 14
Thomas JM, 374
Thomas M, 68
Thomas S, 121
Thompson Miss C, 268
Thompson Mrs C, 257
Thompson DI, 287
Thompson SM, 296
Thomson JLL, 375
Thorne CJR, 112
Thorpe J, 607
Thorpe JM, 276
Tierney A, 633
Tilley E, 584
Tillman S, 565
Titley GDC, 487
Todd I, 246
Todd M, 569
Todd Mrs M, 67
Todd-Jones MJ, 108
Tomkins B, 231
Townsend K, 651
Trigg AJ, 390
Trinder VM, 529
Trotter E, 80

Trounce L, 563
Tuite H, 301
Turner J, 272
Turtle K, 460
Tyrer JA, 324

Upson J, 223

Valentine P, 592
Vasarheiyl M, 159
Van Loo JR, 516
Vickers H, 555
Vose BM, 120, 523

Wade GR, 559
Wade J, 270
Waite M, 491
Wakeham M, 136
Walkden J, 125
Walker AR, 329
Walker D, 214
Walker ML, 426
Wall M, 92
Walley C, 312
Walton JG, 484
Want PC, 399
Ward C, 92
Ward MM, 632
Ward R, 365
Warden KA, 277
Warden L, 412
Warnock J, 579
Warren PJR, 519
Watson A, 398
Watson E, 100
Watt PNY, 31
Weaver E, 93
Weeks E, 79
Welch J, 596
Wells MR, 197
Wenham R, 377
Wensley M, 429
Wentz R, 344
Westmancoat HT, 390
Weston R, 283
Whalley Mrs, 65
Wharram P, 442
Wheeler M, 270
Whitaker J, 589
White Mrs Janice, 194
White Ms Joanne, 58
White JA, 468
Whitehouse BEH, 58
Whitlock DD, 384

Index of establishments

3M Health Care Limited, Loughborough , 448

Aberdeen School of Midwifery, 1
Abergele Hospital, 555
Addenbrooke's Hospital, Cambridge, 115
Administration Offices Library ESHA, Foxhall Rd,Ipswich, 294
Agricultural and Food Research Council, Institute of Animal Physiology and
          Genetics Research, Cambridge, 105
Agricultural and Food Research Council, Institute of Animal Physiology and
          Genetics Research, Roslin, 558
Agricultural Food Research Council, Institute of Food Research, Reading, 548
Ailsa Hospital, Ayr, 302
Airedale General Hospital Postgraduate Medical Centre, Keighley, 296
Aldeley House Work Library, Macclesfield, 451
Alexandra Hospital, Redditch, 551, 552
Alistair Mackenzie Library, Law Hospital, Carluke, 129
All Saints Hospital, Birmingham, 34
All Saints Hospital, Chatham, 233
Altnagelvin Hospital, Londonderry, 446
Amersham General Hospital, Staff Library, 7 , 283
Amersham General Hospital Medical/Nursing Library, 283, 284
Anglia Higher Education College, 136, 256
Animal Diseases Research Association, Edinburgh, 192
Arbroath Infirmary, 73
Argyll & Clyde College of Nursing, 258
Arnold Walker-Florence Mitchell Library, Royal College of Midwives, London,
          397
Arrowe Park Hospital, Upton, 629
Ashford Hospital, Middx, 9, 10
Ashford Postgraduate Medical Centre, Ashford, Middx, 9
Ashington Hospital, 11, 12
Ashley Robin Library, Runwell Hospital, Wickford, 652
Atkinson Morley's Hospital, Wimbledon , 417
Aubrey Keep Education Centre, Brentwood, 75
Avon College of Nursing & Midwifery, 79-83, 644
Ayr County Hospital, 302
Ayrshire & Arran Health Board, Area Medical library, 302
Ayrshire Central Hospital, Irvine, 302

BACUP, London, 33
Badsley Moor Lane Hospital, Rotherham, 559
Balfour Hospital, Orkney, 1
Ballochmyle Hospital, Mauchline, 302
Bangour General Hospital, Broxburn, 95, 96
Barking Hospital, 20, 291, 675
Barnes Library, University of Birmingham, 55

Barnet Community Health Services Library & Information Service, St Albans,
          561
Barnet Department of Nursing Studies, Barnet, 21
Barnet Department of Nursing Studies, Edgware 190
Barnet General Hospital, 21, 22
Barnet Postgraduate Medical Centre, 22
Barnsley Hall Hospital, Bromsgrove, 94
Barnsley Postgraduate Centre, 23
Basildon Hospital, 26
Basildon and Thurrock Health Authority, 26
Basingstoke District Hospital, 27
Bateman Centre for Postgraduate Medical Studies, Rochdale , 556
Bath District Medical Library, Bath, 28
Beaumont Hospital, Dublin, 173
Beccles Hospital, 257
Belfast City Hospital, 31
Belford Hospital, Fort William, 292
Bell Library, Royal Hospital, Wolverhampton , 660
Ben Wood Library, Birmingham Children's Hospital, 37
Birmingham Accident Hospital, 35, 53
Birmingham Accident Hospital and Rehabilitation Centre 35
Birmingham and Midland Eye Hospital, 36
Birmingham Children's Hospital, 37
Birmingham College of Nurse Education, Sutton Coldfield, 614
Bishop Auckland General Hospital, 61
Bishop Otter College, Chichester, 142
Blackburn Royal Infirmary, 63
Blood Products Laboratory, Elstree,215
Bloomsbury College of Nurse Education, London, 332
Boldero Library, University College and Middlesex School of Medicine,
          London, 434
Bolton General Hospital , 67
Bolton Institute of Higher Education, 66
Bolton & Salford College of Midwifery & Nursing, 67, 569
Booth Hall Children's Hospital, Manchester , 455
Bootham Hospital, York, 674
Boots Company Chemical Sciences Library , Nottingham, 497
Boots Company Consumer Products Development Library, Nottingham, 497
Boots Company Pharmaceutical Formulation, Nottingham, 497
Boots Company Toxicology/Pathology Library, Nottingham, 497
Boots Company plc, Research Library, Nottingham, 497

Gartnavel General Hospital, Glasgow, 241
George Eliot Centre Library, Nuneaton, 502
Gilbert Bain Hospital, Shetland, 1
Girdlestone Memorial Library, Oxford, 515
Glanadda School of Nursing, Gwynedd, 19
Glasgow Eastern College of Nursing and Midwifery, 235
Glasgow Northern College of Nursing, 236, 237
Glasgow Royal Infirmary, 237
Glasgow Southern College of Nursing and Midwifery, 238, 239
Glasgow Western College of Nursing and Midwifery, 240
Glasgow Western Infirmary, 241
Glenside Hospital, Bristol, 81
Gloucestershire Royal Hospital, 253, 254
Gloucestershire College of Nursing & Midwifery, Cheltenham, 138
Gloucestershire College of Nursing & Midwifery, Gloucester, 253
Good Hope General Hospital, Sutton Coldfield, 614, 615
Good Hope Hospital Postgraduate Medical Centre, Sutton Coldfield, 615
Goodmayes Hospital, Ilford, 290, 291
Grampian School of Occupational Therapy, 2
Grantham and Kesteven General Hospital Staff Library, 255
Graves Medical Audiovisual Library, Chelmsford, 135
Gravesend and North Kent Hospital, 160
Greater Glasgow Health Board, 237
Greaves Hospital, Southport, 328
Greenwich District Hospital, London, 352
Grimsby District General Hospital, 260
Guy's Hospital Medical School, London, 430
Guy's Hospital, London, 427, 433
Gwent Postgraduate Medical Centre, Newport, 487

Halifax General Hospital, 264
Halifax Postgraduate Medical Library, 264
Halley Stewart Library, St Christopher's Hospice, London, 416
Ham Green Hospital, Bristol, 88
Harefield, Hillingdon & Mount Vernon Education Division, Uxbridge, 630
Harefield and Northwood Postgraduate Medical Centre, Northwood, 495
Harold Wood Hospital, Romford, 267
Harperbury Hospital, Radlett, 546
Hartlepool General Hospital, 271
Hartwood Hospital, Shotts, 580
Hastings Postgraduate Medical Centre, 272
Health Buildings Library, DHSS, London, 349
Health Care Planning Library, Bexhill-on-Sea, 33
Health Education Authority, London, 353
Health Matters, Milton Keynes, 475

Institute of Food Research , Reading, 548
Institute of Laryngology and Otology, London , 436
Institute of Medical Laboratory Sciences, London , 361
Institute of Neurology, Rockefeller Medical Library, London, 362
Institute of Obstetrics and Gynaecology, London , 410
Institute of Occupational Medicine, Edinburgh , 193
Institute of Ophthalmology, London, 437
Institute of Orthopaedics, Francis Costello Library, Oswestry, 508
Institute of Orthopaedics, London, 438
Institute of Psychiatry Library, London , 363
Institute of Psycho-Analysis, London, 364
Institute of Urology, London, 439
Intake Trust Medical Library, Mansfield , 469
International Planned Parenthood Federation, London, 365
Inverclyde Royal Hospital, Greenock, 259
Ipswich Hospital, 294
Ipswich Medical Library , 294
Isle of Man Postgraduate Medical Centre, Douglas, 169
Islington District Library, London, 366

James Paget Hospital, Great Yarmouth, 257
Jersey General Hospital, St Helier, CI, 565
John Connolly Hospital, Birmingham, 43, 54
John Lister Library, King Edward VII Hospital, Windsor, 658
John Radcliffe Hospital, Cairns Library, Oxford, 510, 516
John Ross Postgraduate Medical Centre, Hereford , 278
John Rylands University Library of Manchester , 458
John Spalding Library, Wrexham Postgraduate Centre, 671
John Squire Medical Library, Clinical Research Centre, Harrow , 270
Joyce Green Hospital, Dartford, 160

Kennedy Institute of Rheumatology, London , 367
Kent and Canterbury Hospital, Canterbury, 118
Kent and Sussex Hospital, Tunbridge Wells , 628
Kent Postgraduate Medical Centre, Canterbury , 118
Keycol Hospital, Sittingbourne, 233
Kidderminster General Hospital, Nurse Education Centre, 298
Kidderminster General Hospital Postgraduate Medical Centre, 299
Killingbeck Hospital, Leeds, 312
King Edward VII Hospital, John Lister Library, Windsor, 658
King Edward VII Hospital Medical Library, Midhurst, 474
King George Hospital, Ilford, 291
King's College School of Medicine & Dentistry (Denmark Hill Campus),369
King's College School of Medicine & Dentistry (Strand Campus), 368
King's Fund Centre, London, 370

King's Lynn Health Science Library , 303
King's Mill Hospital, Sutton in Ashfield, 469
Kingston-upon-Thames Postgraduate Medical Centre, 304
Knowle Hospital, Fareham, 229

Ladybridge Hospital, Banff, 1
Lanarkshire College of Nursing and Midwifery, Carluke, 128
Lancashire Polytechnic Library, Preston, 541
Lancaster Postgraduate Medical Centre. 307
Law Hospital, Carluke , 128, 129
Laxton Library, Peterborough District Hospital, 527
Lea Castle Hospital, Kidderminster, 300
Leavesden Hospital, Abbots Langley, 641
Leeds College of Nursing, 310
Leeds University, Nuffield Centre for Health Services Studies, 310
Leicester General Hospital, 319
Leicester Royal Infirmary, Clinical Sciences Library, 321
Leigh Postgraduate Centre, Lancs, 653
Leighton Hospital, Crewe, 153
Les Cannon Memorial Library, Harefield and Northwood Postgraduate Medical
                Centre, Northwood , 495
Lewisham Hospital, London, 371
Lewisham and North Southwark Health Authority, Poisons Unit, 388
Lilly Research Centre Limited, Windlesham , 657
Linacre Library, Kent Postgraduate Medical Centre, Canterbury, 118
Lincoln Medical Library, 323
Lister Hospital, Stevenage, 606
Littlemore Hospital, Oxford, 514
Liverpool Medical Institution, 326
Liverpool School of Tropical Medicine, 327
Llandough Hospital, Medical Library, Penarth , 523
Llandough Hospital, Penarth , 123, 523
Llandudno School of Nursing, 19
Llanelli General Hospital, 330
Llanfairfechan School of Nursing, 19
Llanfrechfa Grange Hospital, Cwmbran, Gwent, 487
London College of Furniture, 372
London Foot Hospital and College of Podiatric Medicine, 373
London Hospital Medical College, 374
London Hospital, London, 389
London School of Hygiene and Tropical Medicine, 375
Long Grove Psychiatric Hospital, 220
Lord Mayor Treloar Hospital, Alton, 6
Lothian College of Nursing and Midwifery, 96, 194, 195
Lothian Health Board, Edinburgh, 196
Lovelock-Jones Nursing Education Centre, High Wycombe , 283
Loversall Hospital, Doncaster, 166
Lowestoft Hospital, 257

Lucy Wilmore Memorial Library, Stafford District General Hospital, 603
Luton and Dunstable Hospital Medical Centre , 449
Lynebank Hospital, Dunfermline, 185
Lynfield Mount Hospital, Bradford, 72

Macclesfield District General Hospital, 450
MacCurdy Psychopathology Library, Cambridge, 114
Macfarlan Smith Ltd, Edinburgh, 197
MacKenzie Medical Centre, Burnley, General Hospital, 98
Maidstone Hospital, 454
Malton Hospital, 573
Manchester Royal Infirmary, 457
Manor Hospital Postgraduate Medical Centre, Walsall, 633
Manor House Hospital, Aylesbury, 16
Mansfield and District General Hospital, Mansfield, 469
Mansfield and Worksop School of Nursing, Mansfield , 470
Mapperley Hospital Medical Library, Nottingham, 499
Mapperley Hospital, Nursing Branch Library, Nottingham, 500
Marsh-Jackson Postgraduate Medical centre, Yeovil, 672
Marylebone Library, London, 443
Mater Hospital Medical Library, Dublin, 172
Mayday Hospital, Thornton Heath, 156
Meanwood Park Hospital, Leeds, 312
Meanwood Park School of Nursing, Leeds, 310
Medical Research Council, Clinical Research Centre, Harrow, 270
Medical Research Council, Human Genetics Library, Edinburgh, 198
Medical Research Council, Dunn Nutritional Unit, Cambridge, 109
Medical Research Council, Laboratories, Carshalton , 131
Medical Research Council, Medical Research Unit, London, 376
Medical Research Council, National Institute for Medical Research,
                    Mill Hill, london, 377
Medical Research Council, Radiobiology Unit, Chilton, Oxon, 143
Medical Research Unit, MRC, London, 376
Medicines Library, DHSS, London, 349
Medway Hospital, Gillingham, 233
Mendip Nursing School, Wells, 622
Merck Sharp and Dohme Research Laboratories, Neuroscience Research Centre,
                    Harlow, 265
Merck Sharp and Dohme Limited, Hoddesdon , 285
Mid and West Essex Department of Nursing & Midwifery Education, 136, 217
Mid-Staffordshire Health Authority, Library & Information Unit, Stafford,
                    599
Mid-Staffordshire Health Authority, Training & Development Library,
                    Stafford, 600
Mid-Sussex Postgraduate Medical Centre, Haywards Heath, 276

PHLS Centre for Applied Microbiology and Research, Porton Down, 390
Papworth Hospital, Cambs, 522
Pembury Hospital, Nurse Education Centre, Tunbridge Wells, 627
Pembury Hospital, Tunbridge Wells, 626
Pen-y-fai Hospital, Bridgend, 77
Perth College of Nursing and Midwifery, 524
Perth Royal Infirmary, 525
Peter Gilroy Bevan Library, Dudley Rd Hospital, Birmingham, 38
Peter Thomas Nurse Education Centre, Birmingham, 45
Peterborough Department of Nurse Education, 526
Peterborough Postgraduate Medical Education Centre , 527
Pilgrim Hospital Staff Library, Boston, 68
Pinderfields General Hospital, Wakefield, 632
Plymouth School of Nursing, 530
Plymouth Health Authority District Library Service, 529, 530
Poisons Unit (Lewisham and North Southwark Healt Authority), 388
Pontefract General Infirmary, 531
Poole General Hospital, 533
Portsmouth School of Nursing, 534
Preston Hospital, North Shields, 489
Preston Postgraduate Medical Centre , 544
Preston School of Nursing, 542
Prestwich Hospital Professional Library , Manchester, 461
Prestwich Hospital School of Nursing, Manchester , 462
Prince Charles Hospital, Merthyr Tydfil , 472
Prince Philip Research Laboratories, London , 433
Prince William Postgraduate Medical Education Centre, Kettering, 297
Princess Alexandra Hospital, Harlow , 266
Princess Alexandra and Newham College of Nursing, London, 389
Princess Elizabeth Hospital, St Martin, CI, 567
Princess Margaret Hospital, Swindon, 620
Princess of Wales Hospital, Bridgend, 76
Public Health Laboratory Service, Central Public Health Laboratory,
          London, 390

Queen Alexandra Hospital, Cosham, 534
Queen Alexandra Hospital Postgraduate Medical Centre, Cosham, 535
Queen Charlotte's Hospital, London, 410
Queen Elizabeth Hospital for Children, London, 346, 392
Queen Elizabeth Hospital, Gateshead, 232
Queen Elizabeth Hospital, King's Lynn, 303
Queen Elizabeth II Hospital, Welwyn Garden City, 642, 643
Queen Elizabeth Military Hospital, London , 393
Queen Elizabeth School of Nursing, Birmingham 46
Queen Margaret College, Edinburgh, 199
Queen Mary's Hospital, Sidcup, 585
Queen Mary's University Hospital, London, 343, 394

Queen Victoria Hospital Medical Library, East Grinstead, 186
Queen's Medical Centre, University of Nottingham, 500
Queen's University Biomedical Library, Belfast, 31
Queen's University Medical Library, Belfast, 31

Radcliffe Infirmary, Cairns Library, Oxford, 511
Radcliffe Infirmary, Kilner Library of Plastic Surgery, Oxford, 513
Radiotherapy Library, Ivry Street, Ipswich, 294
Raigmore Hospital, Inverness, 292
Rainhill Hospital, Prescot, 539
Rauceby Hospital Staff Library, Sleaford, 68, 586
Reading Pathological Society, 549
Reckitt and Colman Pharmaceutical Division, Business & Commercial Library,
        Hull, 288
Redbridge District Library, Ilford, 291
Redhill Hospital, 553
Regional Radiotherapy Centre, Leeds, 310
Rhône-Poulenc Ltd, 158
Richmond House Library, DHSS, London, 349
Riverside College of Nursing, London, 345
Robert & Lilian Lindsay Library, British Dental Association, London, 334
Robert Jones and Agnes Hunt Orthopaedic Hospital, Oswestry, 508
Robert Lamb Medical library, Inverclyde Royal Hospital, Greenock, 259
Roche Products Limited, Welwyn Garden City , 644
Rochford General Hospital, 649
Rockefeller Medical Library, Institute of Neurology, London, 362
Romford College of Nursing and Midwifery, 268
Romford Medical Academic Centre, 557
Rorer Health Care Ltd, 188
Rotherham District General Hospital, 559
Rotherham Health Authority Staff Library and Information service, 559
Rotherham Memorial Library, Grimsby District General Hospital, 260
Royal (Dick) School of Veterinary Studies, University of Edinburgh, 212
Royal Air Force , Farnborough, 230
Royal Air Force Medical Library (MOD), Aylesbury 15
Royal Alexandra Hospital, Paisley, 521
Royal Army Medical College, London, 395
Royal Berkshire Hospital, Reading, 549, 550
Royal Berkshire Hospital, Postgraduate Medical Centre, Reading, 549
Royal College of General Practitioners, London, 396
Royal College of Midwives, London, 397
Royal College of Nursing, London, 393
Royal College of Obstetricians and Gynaecologists, London, 399
Royal College of Physicians and Surgeons of Glasgow, 242
Royal College of Physicians of Edinburgh, 200

Royal College of Physicians of London, 400
Royal College of Psychiatrists, London, 401
Royal College of Surgeons in Ireland, Dublin, 173
Royal College of Surgeons of Edinburgh, 201
Royal College of Surgeons of England, London, 402
Royal College of Veterinary Surgeons' Wellcome Library, London, 403
Royal Cornwall Hospital (Treliske), Truro , 625
Royal (Dick) School of Veterinary Studies, Edinburgh, 212
Royal Edinburgh Hospital, 210
Royal Free Hospital, School of Medicine, London , 404
Royal Free Hospital, School of Nursing, London , 405
Royal Halifax Infirmary, 264
Royal Hallamshire Hospital, Sheffield, 578
Royal Hampshire County Hospital, Winchester, 656
Royal Hospital, Wolverhampton, 660
Royal Hospital for Sick Children, Bristol, 87
Royal Infirmary, Blackburn, 63
Royal Infirmary, Huddersfield, 286
Royal Manchester Children's Hospital, 463
Royal National Hospital for Rheumatic Diseases, Bath, 28
Royal National Institute for the Blind, London, 406
Royal National Institute for the Blind, Peterborough, 528
Royal National Institute for the Deaf, London, 407
Royal National Orthopaedic Hospital, London , 438
Royal National Orthopaedic Hospital, Nurse Education Library, Stanmore, 605
Royal Northern Hospital, London, 366
Royal Oldham Hospital, Frank Lord Postgraduate Medical Centre, 503
Royal Orthopaedic Hospital, Birmingham , 53
Royal Pharmaceutical Society of Great Britain , London, 408
Royal Pharmaceutical Society of Great Britain (Scottish Branch), Edinburgh,
              202, 408
Royal Postgraduate Medical School, London , 409, 410
Royal Preston Hospital, 543
Royal Shrewsbury Hospital (Shelton), 582
Royal Shrewsbury Hospital (South), 583
Royal Shrewsbury Hospital School of Nursing, 584
Royal Society of Medicine, London, 411
Royal South Hants Hospital Staff Library, Southampton , 594
Royal Surrey County Hospital, Guildford, 261, 262
Royal United Hospital, Bath, 28
Royal Veterinary College (University of London) , 412
Royal Victoria Hospital, Bournemouth, 70
Runwell Hospital, Wickford, 652
Russell Square Library, DHSS, London, 349
Russells Hall Hospital, Dudley, 179
Ryder Postgraduate Medical Centre, Hexham, 282

Saint Albans City Hospital, 563
Saint Andrew's Hospital, London, 382, 389
Saint Andrew's Hospital, Northampton, 493
Saint Andrew's University Library, 564
Saint Ann's Hospital, Poole, 523
Saint Ann's Hospital, London, 415
Saint Augustine's Hospital, Canterbury , 119
Saint Bartholomew's Hospital Medical College, London, 413
Saint Bartholomew's School of Nursing, London , 414
Saint Cadoc's Hospital, Newport, Gwent, 487
Saint Charles Hospital, London, 415
Saint Christopher's Hospice, London, 416
Saint Clement's Hospital, London, 374
Saint Clement's Hospital, Psychiatric Library, Ipswich , 295
Saint Crispin Hospital, Mental Health Unit Library, Northampton, 494
Saint Francis Hospital (Psychiatric), Haywards Heath , 276
Saint George's Hospital, Morpeth, 479, 480
Saint George's Hospital Medical Library, Stafford , 601
Saint George's Hospital Medical School, London, 417
Saint Helens and Knowsley Postgraduate Centre, Prescot , 540
Saint Helier Hospital, Carshalton , 132
Saint James' University Hospital, Leeds, 310, 313, 316
Saint James' Hospital, Portsmouth, 536
Saint John's Hospital, Aylesbury , 16
Saint John's Hospital, Chelmsford, 134
Saint John's Hospital at Howden, Livingston, 329
Saint Joseph's Hospital, Clonmel, 144
Saint Lawrence's Hospital, Caterham, 156
Saint Leonard's Hospital, Ringwood, 523
Saint Loye's School of Occupational Therapy, 226
Saint Luke's Hospital, Bradford, 71, 72
Saint Margaret's Hospital, Epping, 217, 218
Saint Martin's Hospital, Bath, 28
Saint Mary's Hospital Medical Library, Manchester, 464
Saint Mary's Hospital Medical School, London, 418
Saint Mary's Hospital, Portsmouth, 537
Saint Mary's School of Nursing, London, 419
Saint Matthew's Hospital, Burntwood , 634
Saint Matthew's Hospital, Nurse Education Centre (Psychiatry), Burntwood,
          635
Saint Nicholas Psychiatric Hospital, Great Yarmouth , 258
Saint Paul's Hospital, Hemel Hempstead, 641
Saint Richard's Hospital, Chichester,141
Saint Thomas' Hospital Medical School, London, 430
Saint Thomas' Hospital, Nightingale School of Nursing, London, 421
Saint Thomas's Hospital, London, 430, 432
Saint Vincent's Hospital, Dublin, 174
Salford College of Technology, 570
Salford Royal Hospital, 571

Salisbury General Infirmary, 572
Salisbury Health Authority Library and Information Service, 572
Sally Howell Library, Epsom, 219
Sandhill Park Nursing School, Taunton, 622
Sandwell Area Health Authority, Community Medicine Library, West Bromwich,
          646
Sandwell District General Hospital, West Bromwich, 647
Sandwell School of Nursing, West Bromwich, 648
Scalebor Park Hospital (Psychiatric), Ilkley , 296
Scarborough Hospital, 573
Scarborough Health Authority District Library , 573
School of Midwifery, Aberdeen, 1
School of Nursing Library, St Luke's Hospital, Bradford, 72
School of Pharmacy, University of London, 422
Scottish Health Education Group, Edinburgh , 203
Scottish Health Service Centre, Edinburgh, 204
Scottish Health Service Common Services Agency, Edinburgh, 205
Scottish Office Library, Edinburgh, 206
Scottish Science Library, Edinburgh, 207
Seacroft Hospital, Leeds 312
Sefton School of Nursing, Liverpool, 328
Selly Oak Hospital, Birmingham, 49, 53
Selwyn Selwyn-Clarke Library, Queen Elizabeth Hospital for Children,
          London, 392
Severalls Hospital , Colchester, 146
Shelton Hospital, Shrewsbury, 582
Shetland Hospital, 1
Shotley Bridge General Hospital Postgraduate Medical Centre, Consett, 147
Shrewsbury Medical Institute, 583
Shropshire & Staffordshire College of Nursing & Midwifery, Shrewsbury, 602
Shropshire Health Authority, Shrewsbury, 581
Singleton Hospital, Swansea, 619
Sir John Black Library, Coventry, 152
Sir John English Medical Library, Yeovil, 672
Sir thomas Browne Library, Norfolk & Norwich Hospital, 496
Sister Dora School of Nursing, Birmingham, 50
Sister Dora School of Nursing, Walsall, 636
Skin Hospital, Birmingham, 51
Smithkline Beecham Pharmaceuticals Headquarters Medical Department,
          Reigate, 554
Smithkline Beecham Pharmaceuticals Headquarters Medical Library,
          Brentford,74
Smithkline Beecham Pharmaceuticals Research and Development, Welwyn, 645
Smithkline Beecham Pharmaceuticals Research and Development, Worthing, 669
Smithkline Beecham Pharmaceuticals Research Division, Betchworth, 32
Smithkline Beecham Research Division, Biosciences Research Centre, Epsom,
          221

Social Security Library, DHSS, London, 349
Solihull Health Authority Education Centre , 589
Somerset Postgraduate Centre, Nuffield Library, Taunton, 621
Somerset School of Nursing, Taunton, 622
South Bank Polytechnic, London, 423
South Birmingham Health Authority, 52
South Birmingham School of Nursing, 53
South Cheshire Postgraduate Medical Centre, Crewe, 153
South Cleveland Hospital, Middlesborough, 473
South Cumbria Health Authority, 25
South East Thames Regional Health Authority, Bexhill-on-Sea, 33
South Eastern Health Board, Kilkenny, 301
South Essex Department of Nursing and Midwifery Education, 256
South Lincolnshire Health District Library Service , 68
South Shields Postgraduate Medical Centre Library, 590
South Staffordshire Medical Centre Library, Wolverhampton, 661
South Tees Medical Library, Middlesbrough, 473
South Warwickshire Hospital, Warwick, 638
South West College of Health Studies, Plymouth, 530
South West Thames Regional Library Service , Guildford , 262
South Western Hospital Multidisciplinary Library, London, 424
South Western Regional Transfusion Centre, Bristol, 89
Southampton General Hospital, 595, 596, 598
Southend-on-Sea Postgraduate Medical Centre, 649
Southern General Hospital, Central Medical Library , Glasgow, 243
Southern General Hospital, Glasgow, 239, 243
Southmead Medical Information and Library Service, Bristol,88
Southmead Hospital College of Nursing, Bristol, 82
Spastics Society, London, 425
Springfield Hospital, Tooting, 417
Stafford District General Hospital, Postgraduate Medical Centre, 603
Staffordshire General Infirmary, Stafford, 600, 602, 603
Standish Hospital, Stonehouse, 254
State Hospital, Carstairs Junction,133
Stepping Hill Hospital Postgraduate Medical Library, Stockport, 607
Sterling Winthrop Group Limited, Guildford, 263
Stobhill General Hospital Medical Library, Glasgow, 244
Stoke Mandeville Hospital, Aylesbury, 14, 17
Stoke Park Hospital, Bristol, 83, 86
Stone House Hospital, Dartford, 160
Stracathro Hospital, Brechin, 73, 182
Stratheden Hospital, Cupar, 157
Sunnyside Hospital, Montrose, 182
Sussex Downs School of Nursing, Eastbourne , 189
Sussex Postgraduate Medical Centre, Brighton , 78

Tameside General Hospital, Ashton-under-Lyne, 13
Tavistock Joint Library, London, 426
Telford Hospital Education Centre, 623
Terence Mortimer Postgraduate Education Centre, Banbury , 18
Thane Medical Sciences Library, University College London, 440
Thanet district General Hospital, Margate, 471
Thomas Guy and Lewisham School of Nursing, London , 427
Tobacco Advisory Council, London, 428
Tone Vale Nursing School, Taunton , 622
Tooting Bec Hospital, London, 429
Torbay Hospital District Library, Torquay , 624
Towers Hospital, Leicester, 320
Trafford School of Nursing, Manchester, 466
Trent Regional Health Authority, Sheffield , 576

Uffculme and Charles Burns Clinics, Birmingham , 54
UK Transplant Service, SW Regional Transfusion Centre, Bristol, 89
United Medical and Dental School of Guy's & St Thomas's Hospital, London,
        430, 431, 432, 433
University College and Middlesex School of Medicine, London, 434, 435,
        436, 437, 438, 439, 440
University College Dublin, Medical Library , 175
University College Dublin, Veterinary Medicine Library, 176
University College Hospital, Galway, 231
University College London, Clinical Sciences Library , 435
University College London, Thane Medical Sciences Library, 440
University Hospital of Wales Combined Training Institute, Cardiff, 122
University Hospital of Wales, Cardiff, 123
University of Aberdeen, Medical School, 3
University of Birmingham, Barnes Library , 55
University of Birmingham, Clinical Teaching Block Library, 55, 56
University of Birmingham, Health Services Management Centre, 57
University of Bristol, Community Medicine Library, 90, 92
University of Bristol, Dental Library, 91, 92
University of Bristol, Medical Library, 89, 90, 91, 92
University of Bristol, Veterinary Library, 92, 93
University of Cambridge, Department of Biochemistry, Colman Library, 112
University of Cambridge, Department of Clinical Veterinary Medicine, 113
University of Cambridge, Department of Experimental Psychology, 114
University of Cambridge, Medical Library, 115
University of Cambridge, Physiological Laboratory , 116
University of Cambridge, Whipple Library, 117
University of Dundee, Ninewells Medical Library , 183
University of Edinburgh, Centre for Tropical Veterinary Medicine,
        Roslin, 208

Wigan and Leigh Medical Institute, 653
Wigan Infirmary, 653
Wigan Nurse Education Centre, 654
Wilfrid Stokes Medical library, Aylesbury, 17
William Harvey Hospital, Ashford, Kt, 8
Winchester Health Authority District Library, Winchester, 656
Wirral School of Nursing, Upton, 629
Winterton Hospital Teaching Centre Library, Stockton-on-Tees, 609
Wirral Postgraduate Medical Centre, Bebington, 29
Withington Hospital Medical Library, Manchester, 467
Withybush General Hospital, Haverfordwest , 275
Wolfson School of Nursing, London, 445
Wonford House Hospital, Exeter , 227
Woodilee Hospital, Glasgow, 236
Woodlands Orthopaedic Hospital, Bradford , 71, 72
Worcester and District Health Authority, Worcester, 665
Worcester District School of Nursing, Worcester, 660
Worcester Royal Infirmary, Newtown Branch, 667
Worcester Royal Infirmary, Ronkswood Branch, 664
Wordsley Hospital Medical Library, 668
Worthing Postgraduate Centre, District Health Sciences Library, 670
Wrexham Medical Institute, 671
Wycombe General Hospital, High Wycombe, 284
Wyeth Laboratories, Maidenhead, 452
Wynne Davies Postgraduate Medical Centre, Redditch, 552
Wythenshawe Hospital, Postgraduate Centre Medical Library, Manchester, 468

Yeovil Nursing School, 622
York and Scarborough College of Nursing & Midwifery, York, 673
York District Hospital, 674
Ysbyty Glan Clwyd, Rhyl, 555
Ysbyty Gwynedd District General Hospital, Bangor, 19

Index to counties

Avon: 79-93, 650

Bedfordshire: 449
Berkshire: 154, 452, 481, 548-550, 587, 588, 658
Buckinghamshire: 7, 14, 15, 16, 17, 283, 284, 475, 476, 477

Cambridgeshire: 105-117, 522, 526, 527, 528
Cheshire: 139, 153, 450, 451, 607
Cleveland: 271, 473, 608, 609
Cornwall: 625
Cumbria: 25, 126, 127

Derbyshire: 140, 161, 162, 163, 164
Devon: 24, 224-227, 529, 530, 624
Dorset: 168, 533
Durham: 61, 147, 159

East Sussex: 33, 78, 134, 135, 136, 187, 188, 189, 272
Essex: 20, 26, 75, 145, 146, 158, 217, 218, 256, 265-268, 290, 291, 557,
    649, 652, 663, 675

Gloucestershire: 137, 138, 252, 253, 254
Greater Manchester: 13, 66, 67, 101, 102, 455-468, 504, 556, 568-571,
    653-654

Hampshire: 6, 27, 70, 229, 230, 535-538, 593-598, 655, 656
Hereford & Worcester: 94, 278-281, 551, 552, 664-667
Hertfordshire: 21, 22, 62, 215, 277, 285, 546, 547, 561, 562, 563, 640-645
Humberside: 260, 287, 288, 289

Isle of Man: 169

Kent: 8, 30, 118, 119, 160, 233, 453, 454, 506, 507, 585, 626, 627, 628

Lancashire: 63, 64, 65, 97, 98, 307, 463, 541-545
Leicestershire: 318, 319, 320, 321, 447, 448
Lincolnshire: 68, 255, 323, 586
London: 331-445

Merseyside: 29, 324-328, 539, 540, 629
Middlesex: 9, 10, 74, 190, 191, 216, 269, 270, 495, 591, 592, 605,
    630, 631

Norfolk: 257, 496
North Yorkshire: 447, 573, 673, 674

Northamptonshire: 297, 303, 478, 479, 480, 491, 492, 493, 494
Northumberland: 11, 12, 282
Nottinghamshire: 469, 470, 497, 498, 499, 500

Oxfordshire: 18, 143, 510-520

Shropshire: 508, 581, 582, 583, 584, 623
Somerset: 28, 621, 622, 672
South Yorkshire: 23, 166, 167, 559, 575, 576, 577, 578, 579
Staffordshire: 99, 100, 317, 599-603, 610, 611
Suffolk: 103, 293, 294, 295
Surrey: 32, 104, 131, 132, 148, 155, 156, 219-223, 261-263, 304, 553, 554, 651, 657

Tyne & Wear: 232, 482-486, 489, 590

Warwickshire: 273, 274, 308, 501, 502, 560, 638
West Midlands: 34-60, 150, 151, 152, 177, 178, 179, 589, 612-616, 633-637, 646, 647, 648, 659, 660, 661, 662, 668
West Sussex: 141, 142, 186, 276, 474, 669, 670
West Yorkshire: 69, 71, 72, 165, 264, 286, 296, 309-313, 509, 531, 632
Wiltshire: 572, 620

SCOTLAND
Borders: 574
Central: 228
Dumfries & Galloway: 180, 181
Fife: 157, 184, 185, 251, 305, 306, 564
Grampian: 1, 2, 3
Highlands: 292
Lothian: 95, 96, 192-214, 329, 558
Strathclyde: 5, 128, 129, 138, 234-250, 258, 259, 302, 521
Tayside: 73, 182, 183, 524, 525

WALES
Clwyd: 555, 671
Dyfed: 4, 130, 275, 330
Gwent: 487
Gwynedd: 19
Mid-Glamorgan: 76, 77, 472, 532
South Glamorgan: 120-125, 523
West Glamorgan: 617, 618, 619

NORTHERN IRELAND   31, 446, 488

CHANNEL ISLANDS   565, 566, 567

IRISH REPUBLIC
Dublin: 171-176, 301
Galway: 231
Limerick: 322
Tipperary: 144
Waterford: 639

Index to named collections

Ballantyne, JW, 200
Barber-Lomax historical collection, 169
Bedford, Evan, 400
Bevan, Frank, 18
Brighton and Sussex Medico-Chirurgical Society, 78
Bruner, Julian 402

Campbell, Menzies 402
Carswell, Sir Robert 435
Chick, Dame Harriet, 109
Comfort collection, 411

Dorchester, Marquis of, 400

Elias Jones collection, 237
Exeter Cathedral library, 224

Fairbairn collection, 210
Ferguson collection, 245
Freud, Sigmund, 41
Friel, Sheldon, 171

Gray, Henry 403
Guest, IA 637

Harvey, William: historical collection, 8
Hastings collection, 338
Hunter, John 402
Hunter-Baillie collection, 402
Hunterian collection, 245

Keith, Arthur 402

Leicestershire Medical Society, 321
Lister, Joseph 402

MacCurdy library, 114
Macewen, 242
Mackenzie, 242
Manchester medical collection 458
Meiklejohn, Andrew 611

Newcastle collection 483
Nottingham Medico-Chirurgical Society 500

Oppenheimer medical biographies, 348
Owen, Richard 402

Parry , Caleb Hillier, 92
Pybus collection, 486

Selected subject index

N.B. This index only includes major collections

Prosthetics 249

Psychiatry 44, 54, 114, 115, 133, 183, 187, 210, 220, 294, 295, 321, 363,
    401, 417, 426, 480, 504, 514, 560, 582, 586, 592, 634

Psychiatric nursing 10, 58, 83, 150, 166, 217, 235, 268, 494, 542, 635, 553,
    602, 614, 666

Psychology 114, 318, 364

Public health, 90

Radiology 335, 456

Radiotherapy 310, 421

Rheumatology 367

Science 202, 348, 548

Sociology 429

Speech therapy 381

Sports medicine 442

Statistics 387

Surgery 173, 201, 242, 402

Tropical medicine, 327, 375

Urology 439

Veterinary medicine 93, 105, 176, 192, 208, 212, 213, 248, 285, 403, 412,
    481, 558, 651

Welfare 66, 365, 372, 406, 407, 423, 425, 475, 488, 528, 569